Medical Education in the United States and Canada

PUBLIC HEALTH ECONOMICS

UNIVERSITY OF MICHIGAN

MEDICAL EDUCATION
IN THE
UNITED STATES AND CANADA

A REPORT TO
THE CARNEGIE FOUNDATION
FOR THE ADVANCEMENT OF TEACHING

BY
ABRAHAM FLEXNER

WITH AN INTRODUCTION BY
HENRY S. PRITCHETT
PRESIDENT OF THE FOUNDATION

BULLETIN NUMBER FOUR

576 FIFTH AVENUE
NEW YORK CITY

D. B. UPDIKE, THE MERRYMOUNT PRESS, BOSTON

TABLE OF CONTENTS

CONTENTS

CONTENTS

APPENDIX

INTRODUCTION

THE present report on medical education forms the first of a series of papers on professional schools to be issued by the Carnegie Foundation. The preparation of these papers has grown naturally out of the situation with which the trustees of the Foundation were confronted when they took up the trust committed to them.

When the work of the Foundation began five years ago the trustees found themselves intrusted with an endowment to be expended for the benefit of teachers in the colleges and universities of the United States, Canada, and Newfoundland. It required but the briefest examination to show that amongst the thousand institutions in English-speaking North America which bore the name college or university there was little unity of purpose or of standards. A large majority of all the institutions in the United States bearing the name college were really concerned with secondary education.

Under these conditions the trustees felt themselves compelled to begin a critical study of the work of the college and of the university in different parts of this wide area, and to commend to colleges and universities the adoption of such standards as would intelligently relate the college to the secondary school and to the university. While the Foundation has carefully refrained from attempting to become a standardizing agency, its influence has been thrown in the direction of a differentiation between the secondary school and the college, and between the college and the university. It is indeed only one of a number of agencies, including the stronger colleges and universities, seeking to bring about in American education some fair conception of unity and the attainment ultimately of a system of schools intelligently related to each other and to the ambitions and needs of a democracy.

At the beginning, the Foundation naturally turned its study to the college, as that part of our educational system most directly to be benefited by its endowment. Inevitably, however, the scrutiny of the college led to the consideration of the relations between the college or university and the professional schools which had gathered about it or were included in it. The confusion found here was quite as great as that which exists between the field of the college and that of the secondary school. Colleges and universities were discovered to have all sorts of relations to their professional schools of law, of medicine, and of theology. In some cases these relations were of the frailest texture, constituting practically only a license from the college by which a proprietary medical school or law school was enabled to live under its name. In other cases the medical school was incorporated into the college or university, but remained an *imperium in imperio*, the college assuming no responsibility for its standards or its support. In yet other cases the college or university assumed partial obligation of support, but no responsibility for the standards of the professional school, while in only a relatively small number of cases was the school of law or of medicine an integral part of the university, receiving from it university standards and adequate maintenance. For the past two decades there has been a marked tendency to set up some connection between universities and detached medical schools, but under the very loose construction just referred to.

Meanwhile the requirements of medical education have enormously increased. The fundamental sciences upon which medicine depends have been greatly extended. The laboratory has come to furnish alike to the physician and to the surgeon a new means for diagnosing and combating disease. The education of the medical practitioner under these changed conditions makes entirely different demands in respect to both preliminary and professional training.

Under these conditions and in the face of the advancing standards of the best medical schools it was clear that the time had come when the relation of professional education in medicine to the general system of education should be clearly defined. The first step towards such a clear understanding was to ascertain the facts concerning medical education and the medical schools themselves at the present time. In accordance, therefore, with the recommendation of the president and the executive committee, the trustees of the Carnegie Foundation at their meeting in November, 1908, authorized a study and report upon the schools of medicine and law in the United States and appropriated the money necessary for this undertaking. The present report upon medical education, prepared, under the direction of the Foundation, by Mr. Abraham Flexner, is the first result of that action.

No effort has been spared to procure accurate and detailed information as to the facilities, resources, and methods of instruction of the medical schools. They have not only been separately visited, but every statement made in regard to each detail has been carefully checked with the data in possession of the American Medical Association, likewise obtained by personal inspection, and with the records of the Association of American Medical Colleges, so far as its membership extends. The details as stated go forth with the sanction of at least two, and frequently more, independent observers.

In making this study the schools of all medical sects have been included. It is clear that so long as a man is to practise medicine, the public is equally concerned in his right preparation for that profession, whatever he call himself,—allopath, homeopath, eclectic, osteopath, or whatnot. It is equally clear that he should be grounded in the fundamental sciences upon which medicine rests, whether he practises under one name or under another.

It will be readily understood that the labor involved in visiting 150 such schools is great, and that in the immense number of details dealt with it is altogether impossible to be sure that every minute fact concerning these institutions has been ascertained and set down. While the Foundation cannot hope to obtain in so great an undertaking absolute completeness in every particular, such care has been exercised, and the work has been so thoroughly reviewed by independent authorities, that the statements which are given here may be confidently accepted as setting forth the essential facts respecting medical education and respecting the institutions which deal with it.

In this connection it is perhaps desirable to add one further word. Educational institutions, particularly those which are connected with a college or a university, are peculiarly sensitive to outside criticism, and particularly to any statement of the circumstances of their own conduct or equipment which seems to them unfavorable in comparison with that of other institutions. As a rule, the only knowledge which the public has concerning an institution of learning is derived from the statements given out by the institution itself, information which, even under the best circumstances, is colored by local hopes, ambitions, and points of view. A considerable number of colleges and universities take the unfortunate position that they are private institutions and that the public is entitled to only such knowledge of their operations as they choose to communicate. In the case of many medical schools the aversion to publicity is quite as marked as it is reputed to be in the case of certain large industrial trusts. A few institutions questioned the right of any outside agency to collect and publish the facts concerning their medical schools. The Foundation was called upon to answer the question: Shall such an agency as the Foundation, dedicated to the betterment of American education, make public the facts concerning the medical schools of the United States and Canada?

The attitude of the Foundation is that all colleges and universities, whether supported by taxation or by private endowment, are in truth public service corporations, and that the public is entitled to know the facts concerning their administration and development, whether those facts pertain to the financial or to the educational side. We believe, therefore, that in seeking to present an accurate and fair statement of the work and the facilities of the medical schools of this country, we are serving the best possible purpose which such an agency as the Foundation can serve; and, furthermore, that only by such publicity can the true interests of education and of the universities themselves be subserved. In such a reasonable publicity lies the hope for progress in medical education.

I wish to add with pleasure that notwithstanding reluctance in some quarters to furnish information, the medical schools of the colleges and universities, as well as proprietary and independent medical schools, have generally accepted the view just stated and have seconded the work of the Foundation by offering to those who were engaged in this study every facility to learn their opportunities and resources; and I beg to express the thanks of the trustees of the Foundation to each of these institutions for the coöperation which it has given to a study which, in the very nature of the case, was to bear sharply in the way of criticism upon many of those called on for coöperation.

The report which follows is divided into two parts. In the first half the history of medical education in this country and its present status are set forth. The story is there told of the gradual development of the commercial medical school, distinctly an American product, of the modern movement for the transfer of medical education to university surroundings, and of the effort to procure stricter scrutiny of those seeking to enter the profession. The present status of medical education is then fully described and a forecast of possible progress in the future is attempted. The second part of the report gives in detail a description of the schools in existence in each state of the Union and in each province of Canada.

It is,the purpose of the Foundation to proceed at once with a similar study of medical education in Great Britain, Germany, and France, in order that those charged with the reconstruction of medical education in America may profit by the experience of other countries.

The striking and significant facts which are here brought out are of enormous consequence not only to the medical practitioner, but to every citizen of the United States and Canada; for it is a singular fact that the organization of medical education in this country has hitherto been such as not only to commercialize the process of education itself, but also to obscure in the minds of the public any discrimination between the well trained physician and the physician who has had no adequate training whatsoever. As a rule, Americans, when they avail themselves of the services of a physician, make only the slightest inquiry as to what his previous training and preparation have been. One of the problems of the future is to educate the public itself to appreciate the fact that very seldom, under existing conditions, does a patient receive the best aid which it is possible to give him in the present state of medicine, and that this is due mainly to the fact that a vast army of men is admitted to the practice of medicine who are untrained in sciences fundamental to the profession and quite without a sufficient experience with disease. A right education of public opinion is one of the problems of future medical education.

The significant facts revealed by this study are these:

(1) For twenty-five years past there has been an enormous over-production of uneducated and ill trained medical practitioners. This has been in absolute disregard of the public welfare and without any serious thought of the interests of the public. Taking the United States as a whole, physicians are four or five times as numerous in proportion to population as in older countries like Germany.

(2) Over-production of ill trained men is due in the main to the existence of a very large number of commercial schools, sustained in many cases by advertising methods through which a mass of unprepared youth is drawn out of industrial occupations into the study of medicine.

(3) Until recently the conduct of a medical school was a profitable business, for the methods of instruction were mainly didactic. As the need for laboratories has become more keenly felt, the expenses of an efficient medical school have been greatly increased. The inadequacy of many of these schools may be judged from the fact that nearly half of all our medical schools have incomes below $10,000, and these incomes determine the quality of instruction that they can and do offer.

Colleges and universities have in large measure failed in the past twenty-five years to appreciate the great advance in medical education and the increased cost of teaching it along modern lines. Many universities desirous of apparent educational completeness have annexed medical schools without making themselves responsible either for the standards of the professional schools or for their support.

(4) The existence of many of these unnecessary and inadequate medical schools has been defended by the argument that a poor medical school is justified in the interest of the poor boy. It is clear that the poor boy has no right to go into any profession for which he is not willing to obtain adequate preparation; but the facts set forth in this report make it evident that this argument is insincere, and that the excuse which has hitherto been put forward in the name of the poor boy is in reality an argument in behalf of the poor medical school.

(5) A hospital under complete educational control is as necessary to a medical school as is a laboratory of chemistry or pathology. High grade teaching within a hospital introduces a most wholesome and beneficial influence into its routine. Trustees of hospitals, public and private, should therefore go to the limit of their authority in opening hospital wards to teaching, provided only that the universities secure sufficient funds on their side to employ as teachers men who are devoted to clinical science.

In view of these facts, progress for the future would seem to require a very much smaller number of medical schools, better equipped and better conducted than our schools now as a rule are; and the needs of the public would equally require that we have fewer physicians graduated each year, but that these should be better educated and better trained. With this idea accepted, it necessarily follows that the medical school will, if rightly conducted, articulate not only with the university, but with the general system of education. Just what form that articulation must take will vary in the immediate future in different parts of the country. Throughout the eastern and central states the movement under which the medical school articulates with the second year of the college has already gained such impetus that it can be regarded as practically accepted. In the southern states for the present it would seem that articulation with the four-year high school would be a reasonable starting-point for the future. In time the development of secondary education in the south and the growth of the colleges will make it possible for southern medical schools to accept the two-year college basis of preparation. With reasonable prophecy the time is not far distant when, with fair respect for the interests of the public and the need for physicians, the articulation of the medical school with the university may be the same throughout the entire country. For in the future the college or the university which accepts a medical school must make itself responsible for university standards in the medical school and for adequate support for medical education. The day has gone by when any university can retain the respect of educated men, or when it can fulfil its duty to education, by retaining a low grade professional school for the sake of its own institutional completeness.

If these fundamental principles can be made clear to the people of the United States and of Canada, and to those who govern the colleges and the universities, we may confidently expect that the next ten years will see a very much smaller number of medical schools in this country, but a greatly increased efficiency in medical education, and that during the same period medical education will become rightly articulated with, and rightly related to, the general educational system of the whole country.

In the suggestions which are made in this report looking toward the future development of medicine, it ought to be pointed out that no visionary or impossible achievement is contemplated. It is not expected that a Johns Hopkins Medical School can be erected immediately in cities where public support of education has hitherto been meager. Nevertheless, it is quite true that there is a certain minimum of equipment and a minimum of educational requirement without which no attempt ought to be made to teach medicine. Hitherto not only proprietary medical schools, but colleges and universities, have paid scant attention to this fact. They have been ready to assume the responsibility of turning loose upon a helpless community men licensed to the practice of medicine without any serious thought as to whether they had received a fair training or not. To-day, under the methods pursued in modern medicine, we know with certainty that a medical school cannot be conducted without a certain minimum of expense and without a certain minimum of facilities. The institution which attempts to conduct a school below this plane is clearly injuring, not helping, civilization. In the suggestions which are made in this report as to what constitutes a reasonable minimum no visionary ideal has been pursued, but only such things have been insisted upon as in the present light of our American civilization every community has a right to demand of its medical school, if medicine is to be taught at all.

It seems desirable also in connection with both the medical school and the university or college to add one word further concerning the relation of financial support to efficiency and sincerity. Where any criticism is attempted of inadequate methods or inadequate facilities, no reply is more common than this: "Our institution cannot be judged from its financial support. It depends upon the enthusiasm and the devotion of its teachers and its supporters, and such devotion cannot be measured by financial standards."

Such an answer contains so fine a sentiment and so pregnant a truth that it oftentimes serves to turn aside the most just criticism. It is true that every college must ultimately depend upon the spirit and devotion of those who work in it, but behind this noble statement hides most of the insincerity, sham, and pretense not only of the American medical school, but of the American college. The answer quoted is commonly made by the so-called university that, with an income insufficient to support a decent college, is trying to cover the whole field of university education. It is the same answer that one receives from the medical school which, with wholly inadequate facilities, is turning out upon an innocent and long-suffering community men who must get their medical education after they get out of the institution. In many of these ill manned and poorly equipped institutions there is to be found a large measure of devotion, but the fact remains that such devotion is usually ill placed, and the individual who gives it loses sight of the interests of education and of the general public in his desire to keep alive an institution without reason or right to exist.

It will, however, be urged by weak schools that the fact that an institution is ill manned and poorly equipped is inconclusive; that in the time devoted to the examination of a single school it is impossible to do it justice. Objection of this kind is apt to come from schools of two types,—ineffective institutions in large cities, and schools attached to colleges in small towns in which clinical material is scarce. In my opinion the objection is without force. A trained observer of wide experience can go directly to the heart of a problem of this character. The spirit, ideals, and facilities of a professional or technical school can be quickly grasped. In every instance in which further inquiry has been made, the conclusions reached by the author of the report have been sustained.

The development which is here suggested for medical education is conditioned largely upon three factors: first, upon the creation of a public opinion which shall discriminate between the ill trained and the rightly trained physician, and which will also insist upon the enactment of such laws as will require all practitioners of medicine, whether they belong to one sect or another, to ground themselves in the fundamentals upon which medical science rests; secondly, upon the universities and their attitude towards medical standards and medical support; finally, upon the attitude of the members of the medical profession towards the standards of their own practice and upon their sense of honor with respect to their own profession.

These last two factors are moral rather than educational. They call for an educational patriotism on the part of the institutions of learning and a medical patriotism on the part of the physician.

By educational patriotism I mean this: a university has a mission greater than the formation of a large student body or the attainment of institutional completeness, namely, the duty of loyalty to the standards of common honesty, of intellectual sincerity, of scientific accuracy. A university with educational patriotism will not take up the work of medical education unless it can discharge its duty by it; or if, in the days of ignorance once winked at, a university became entangled in a medical school alliance, it will frankly and courageously deal with a situation which is no longer tenable. It will either demand of its medical school university ideals and give it university support, or else it will drop the effort to do what it can only do badly.

By professional patriotism amongst medical men I mean that sort of regard for the honor of the profession and that sense of responsibility for its efficiency which will enable a member of that profession to rise above the consideration of personal or of professional gain. As Bacon truly wrote, "Every man owes a duty to his profession," and in no profession is this obligation more clear than in that of the modern physician. Perhaps in no other of the great professions does one find greater discrepancies between the ideals of those who represent it. No members of the social order are more self-sacrificing than the true physicians and surgeons, and of this fine group none deserve so much of society as those who have taken upon their shoulders the burden of medical education. On the other hand, the profession has been diluted by the presence of a great number of men who have come from weak schools with low ideals both of education and of professional honor. If the medical education of our country is in the immediate future to go upon a plane of efficiency and of credit, those who represent the higher ideals of the medical profession must make a stand for that form of medical education which is calculated to advance the true interests of the whole people and to better the ideals of medicine itself.

There is raised in the discussion of this question a far-reaching economic problem to which society has as yet given little attention; that is to say, What safeguards may society and the law throw about admission to a profession like that of law or of medicine in order that a sufficient number of men may be induced to enter it and yet the unfit and the undesirable may be excluded?

It is evident that in a society constituted as are our modern states, the interests of the social order will be served best when the number of men entering a given profession reaches and does not exceed a certain ratio. For example, in law and medicine one sees best in a small village the situation created by the over-production of inadequately trained men. In a town of two thousand people one will find in most of our states from five to eight physicians where two well trained men could do the work efficiently and make a competent livelihood. When, however, six or eight ill trained physicians undertake to gain a living in a town which can support only two, the whole plane of professional conduct is lowered in the struggle which ensues, each man becomes intent upon his own practice, public health and sanitation are neglected, and the ideals and standards of the profession tend to demoralization.

A similar state of affairs comes from the presence of too large a number of ill trained lawyers in a community. When six or eight men seek to gain their living from the practice of the law in a community in which, at the most, two good lawyers could do all the work, the demoralization to society becomes acute. Not only is the process of the law unduly lengthened, but the temptation is great to create business. No small proportion of the American lack of respect for the law grows out of the presence of this large number of ill trained men seeking to gain a livelihood from the business which ought in the nature of the case to support only a much smaller number. It seems clear that as nations advance in civilization, they will be driven to throw around the admission to these great professions such safeguards as will limit the number of those who enter them to some reasonable estimate of the number who are actually needed. It goes without saying that no system of standards of admission to a profession can exclude all the unfit or furnish a perfect body of practitioners, but a reasonable enforcement of such standards will at least relieve the body politic of a large part of the difficulty which comes from over-production, and will safeguard the right of society to the service of trained men in the great callings which touch so closely our physical and political life.

The object of the Foundation in undertaking studies of this character is to serve a constructive purpose, not a critical one. Unless the information here brought together leads to constructive work, it will fail of its purpose. The very disappearance of many existing schools is part of the reconstructive process. Indeed, in the course of preparing the report a number of results have already come about which are of the highest interest from the constructive point of view. Several colleges, finding themselves unable to carry on a medical school upon right lines, have, frankly facing the situation, discontinued their medical departments, the result being a real gain to medical education. Elsewhere, competing medical schools which were dividing the students and the hospital facilities have united into a single school. In still other instances large sums of money have been raised to place medical education on a firmer basis.

In the preparation of this report the Foundation has kept steadily in view the interests of two classes, which in the over-multiplication of medical schools have usually been forgotten,— first, the youths who are to study medicine and to become the future practitioners, and, secondly, the general public, which is to live and die under their ministrations.

No one can become familiar with this situation without acquiring a hearty sympathy for the American youth who, too often the prey of commercial advertising methods, is steered into the practice of medicine with almost no opportunity to learn the difference between an efficient medical school and a hopelessly inadequate one. A clerk who is receiving $50 a month in the country store gets an alluring brochure which paints the life of the physician as an easy road to wealth. He has no realization of the difference between medicine as a profession and medicine as a business, nor as a rule has he any adviser at hand to show him that the first requisite for the modern practitioner of medicine is a good general education. Such a boy falls an easy victim to the commercial medical school, whether operating under the name of a university or college, or alone.

The interests of the general public have been so generally lost sight of in this matter that the public has in large measure forgot that it has any interests to protect. And yet in no other way does education more closely touch the individual than in the quality of medical training which the institutions of the country provide. Not only the personal well-being of each citizen, but national, state, and municipal sanitation rests upon the quality of the training which the medical graduate has received. The interest of the public is to have well trained practitioners in sufficient number for the needs of society. The source whence these practitioners are to come is of far less consequence.

In view of this fact, the argument advanced for the retention of medical schools in places where good clinical instruction is impossible is directly against the public interest. If the argument were valid, it would mean that the sick man is better off in the hands of an incompetent home-grown practitioner than in those of one well trained in an outside school. Such an argument ought no longer to blind the eyes of intelligent men to the actual situation. Any state of the Union or any province of Canada is better off without a medical school than with one conducted in a commercial spirit and below a reasonable plane of efficiency. No state and no section of a state capable of supporting a good practitioner will suffer by following this policy. The state of Washington, which has no medical school within its borders, is doubtless supplied with as capable and well trained a body of medical practitioners as is Missouri with its eleven medical schools or Illinois with its fourteen.

The point of view which keeps in mind the needs and qualifications of the medical student and the interests of the great public is quite a different one from that which the institution which conducts a medical department ordinarily occupies. The questions which look largest to the institutions are: Can we add a medical school to our other departments? and if so, where can we find the students? The questions which the other point of view suggest are: Is a medical school needed? Cannot those qualified to study medicine find opportunities in existing schools? If not, are the means and the facilities at hand for teaching medicine on a right basis?

While the aim of the Foundation has throughout been constructive, its attitude towards the difficulties and problems of the situation is distinctly sympathetic. The report indeed turns the light upon conditions which, instead of being fruitful and inspiring, are in many instances commonplace, in other places bad, and in still others, scandalous. It is nevertheless true that no one set of men or no one school of medicine is responsible for what still remains in the form of commercial medical education. Our hope is that this report will make plain once for all that the day of the commercial medical school has passed. It will be observed that, except for a brief historical introduction, intended to show how present conditions have come about, no account is given of the past of any institution. The situation is described as it exists today in the hope that out of it, quite regardless of the past, a new order may be speedily developed. There is no need now of recriminations over what has been, or of apologies by way of defending a régime practically obsolete. Let us address ourselves resolutely to the task of reconstructing the American medical school on the lines of the highest modern ideals of efficiency and in accordance with the finest conceptions of public service.

It is hoped that both the purpose of the Foundation and its point of view as thus stated may be remembered in any consideration of the report which follows, and that this publication may serve as a starting-point both for the intelligent citizen and for the medical practitioner in a new national effort to strengthen the medical profession and rightly to relate medical education to the general system of schools of our nation.

The Foundation is under the greatest obligation in the preparation of this report to leading representatives of medicine and surgery in this country for their coöperation and advice. The officers of the various medical associations and of the Association of American Medical Colleges have furnished information which was invaluable and have given aid in the most cordial way. We are particularly indebted for constant and generous assistance to Dr. William H. Welch of Johns Hopkins University, Dr. Simon Flexner of the Rockefeller Institute, and Dr. Arthur D. Bevan, chairman of the Council on Education of the American Medical Association. In addition, our acknowledgments are due to Dr. N. P. Colwell, secretary of the Council on Education of the American Medical Association, and to Dr. F. C. Zapffe, secretary of the Association of American Medical Colleges, for most helpful coöperation. I wish to acknowledge also our indebtedness to a number of eminent men connected with various schools of medicine who have been kind enough to read the proof of this report and to give us the benefit of their comment and criticism.

HENRY S. PRITCHETT.

April 16, 1910.

PART I
MEDICAL EDUCATION
IN THE UNITED STATES AND CANADA

CHAPTER I

HISTORICAL AND GENERAL

THE American medical school is now well along in the second century of its history.[1] It began, and for many years continued to exist, as a supplement to the apprenticeship system still in vogue during the seventeenth and eighteenth centuries. The likely youth of that period, destined to a medical career, was at an early age indentured to some reputable practitioner, to whom his service was successively menial, pharmaceutical, and professional: he ran his master's errands, washed the bottles, mixed the drugs, spread the plasters, and finally, as the stipulated term drew towards its close, actually took part in the daily practice of his preceptor,—bleeding his patients, pulling their teeth, and obeying a hurried summons in the night. The quality of the training varied within large limits with the capacity and conscientiousness of the master. Ambitious spirits sought, therefore, a more assured and inspiring discipline. Beginning early in the eighteenth century, having served their time at home, they resorted in rapidly increasing numbers to the hospitals and lecture-halls of Leyden, Paris, London, and Edinburgh. The difficulty of the undertaking proved admirably selective; for the students who crossed the Atlantic gave a good account of themselves. Returning to their native land, they sought opportunities to share with their less fortunate or less adventurous fellows the rich experience gained as they "walked the hospitals" of the old world in the footsteps of Cullen, Munro, and the Hunters. The voices of the great masters of that day thus reëchoed in the recent western wilderness. High scientific and professional ideals impelled the youthful enthusiasts, who bore their lighted torches safely back across the waters.

Out of these early essays in medical teaching, the American medical school developed. As far back as 1750 informal classes and demonstrations, mainly in anatomy, are matters of record. Philadelphia was then the chief center of medical interest. There, in 1762, William Shippen the younger, after a sojourn of five years abroad, began in the very year of his return home, a course of lectures on midwifery. In the following autumn he announced a séries of anatomical lectures "for the advantage of the young gentlemen now engaged in the study of physic in this and the neighboring provinces, whose circumstances and connections will not admit of their going abroad for improvement to the anatomical schools in Europe; and also for the entertainment of any gentlemen who may have the curiosity to understand the anatomy of the Human Frame." From these detached courses the step to an organized medical school was taken at the instigation of Shippen's friend and fellow student abroad,

[1] This statement has reference only to the United States and Canada, with which the present account alone deals. As a matter of fact, a chair of medicine was established at the University of Mexico towards the close of the sixteenth century. A complete medical school was there developed. James J. Walsh: "First American Medical School," in *New York Medical Journal*, Oct. 10, 1908 (based on *Historia de la medicina en Mexico des de la epoca de los Indios, hasta la presente.* Por Francisco Flores. Mexico, 1886).

John Morgan, who in 1765 proposed to the trustees of the College of Philadelphia the creation of a professorship in the theory and practice of medicine. At the ensuing Commencement, Morgan delivered a noble and prophetic discourse, still pertinent, upon the institution of medical schools in America. The trustees were favorable to the suggestion; the chair was established, and Morgan himself was its first occupant. Soon afterwards Shippen became professor of anatomy and surgery. Thirteen years previously the Pennsylvania Hospital, conceived by Thomas Bond, had been established through the joint efforts of Bond himself and Benjamin Franklin. Realizing that the student "must Join Examples with Study, before he can be sufficiently qualified to prescribe for the sick, for Language and Books alone can never give him Adequate Ideas of Diseases and the best methods of Treating them," Bond now argued successfully in behalf of bedside training for the medical students. "There the Clinical professor comes in to the Aid of Speculation and demonstrates the Truth of Theory by Facts," he declared in words that a century and a half later still warrant repetition; "he meets his pupils at stated times in the Hospital, and when a case presents adapted to his purpose, he asks all those Questions which lead to a certain knowledge of the Disease and parts Affected; and if the Disease baffles the power of Art and the Patient falls a Sacrifice to it, he then brings his Knowledge to the Test, and fixes Honour or discredit on his Reputation by exposing all the Morbid parts to View, and Demonstrates by what means it produced Death, and if perchance he finds something unexpected, which Betrays an Error in Judgement, he like a great and good man immediately acknowledges the mistake, and, for the benefit of survivors, points out other methods by which it might have been more happily treated."[1] The writer of these sensible words fitly became our first professor of clinical medicine,[2] with unobstructed access to the one hundred and thirty patients then in the hospital wards. Subsequently the faculty of the new school was increased and greatly strengthened when Adam Kuhn, trained by Linnaeus, was made professor of materia medica, and Benjamin Rush, already at twenty-four on the threshold of his brilliant career, became professor of chemistry.

Our first medical school was thus soundly conceived as organically part of an institution of learning and intimately connected with a large public hospital. The instruction aimed, as already pointed out, not to supplant, but to supplement apprenticeship. A year's additional training, carrying the bachelor's degree, was offered to students who, having demonstrated a competent knowledge of Latin, mathematics, natural and experimental philosophy, and having served a sufficient apprenticeship to some reputable practitioner in physic, now completed a prescribed lecture curriculum, with attendance upon the practice of the Pennsylvania Hospital for one

[1] An essay on *The Utility of Clinical Lectures*, by Thomas Bond, 1766.

[2] There is no record of Dr. Bond's appointment, but in the minutes of the Hospital trustees he "is requested by the Trustees and Professors to continue his Clinical Lectures at the Hospital as a Branch of Medical Education." Quoted by Packard: *History of Medicine in the United States*, p. 201.

year. This course was well calculated to round off the young doctor's preparation, reviewing and systematizing his theoretical acquisitions, while considerably extending his practical experience.

Before the outbreak of the Revolution, the young medical school was prosperously started on its career. The war of course brought interruption and confusion. More unfortunate still, for the time being, was the local rivalry—ominous as the first of its kind—of the newly established medical department of the University of Pennsylvania; but wise counsels averted disaster, and in 1791 the two institutions joined to form a single faculty, bearing, as it still bears, the name of the university,—the earliest of a long and yet incomplete series of medical school mergers. Before the close of the century three more "medical institutes," similar in style, had been started: one in 1768 in New York, as the medical department of King's College, which, however, temporarily collapsed on the British occupation and was only indirectly restored to vigor by union in 1814 with the College of Physicians and Surgeons, begun by the Regents in 1807; another, the medical department of Harvard College, opened in Cambridge in 1783, and twenty-seven years later removed to Boston so as to gain access to the hospitals there;[1] last of the group, the medical department of Dartmouth College, started in 1798 by a Harvard graduate, Dr. Nathan Smith, who was himself for twelve years practically its entire faculty—and a very able faculty at that.

The sound start of these early schools was not long maintained. Their scholarly ideals were soon compromised and then forgotten. True enough, from time to time seats of learning continued to create medical departments,—Yale in 1810, Transylvania in 1817, among others. But with the foundation early in the nineteenth century at Baltimore of a proprietary school, the so-called medical department of the so-called University of Maryland,[2] a harmful precedent was established.[3] Before that a college of medicine had been a branch growing out of the living university trunk.

[1] The removal took place in 1810. But definite arrangements for clinical teaching long remained vague. Dr. R. C. Cabot quotes the *Harvard Catalogue* of 1833 as follows: "The lectures for medical students are delivered in Boston. . . . During lectures the students may find in the city various opportunities for practical instruction." A hospital is first mentioned in 1835, "when it is stated that students may attend the medical visits at the Massachusetts General Hospital." R. C. Cabot: "Sketch of the Development of the Department of Clinical Medicine," in *Harvard Medical Alumni Quarterly*, Jan., 1904, p. 666.

[2] In recent years an effort has been made to fill out the non-existent university by an affiliation with St. John's College (Annapolis), whereby it becomes nominally the department of arts of the University of Maryland. This is, of course, a makeshift. A university begins with a school of arts and sciences; it cannot be formed of loosely associated schools of dentistry, pharmacy, and even law, whether with or without still looser connection with a remote college of arts. Analogous in type are the so-called medical departments of the Universities of Buffalo, Toledo, and Memphis, which at this writing still lack academic affiliation. Their titles cannot disguise the fact that they are in essence independent medical schools, nor does a university charter make a university.

[3] This was in imitation of London, as against the Edinburgh or the Leyden example, followed by the four earlier schools. But the London schools never conferred the degree or gave the right to practise: for the bestowal of degrees is the function of a university, the qualification for practice is determined by the state. The American departure in both these respects developed evils from which England has never suffered.

This organic connection guaranteed certain standards and ideals, modest enough at that time, but destined to a development which medical education could, as experience proved, ill afford to forego. Even had the university relation been preserved, the precise requirements of the Philadelphia College would not indeed have been permanently tenable. The rapid expansion of the country, with the inevitable decay of the apprentice system in consequence, must necessarily have lowered the terms of entrance upon the study. But for a time only: the requirements of medical education would then have slowly risen with the general increase in our educational resources. Medical education would have been part of the entire movement instead of an exception to it. The number of schools would have been well within the number of actual universities, in whose development as respects endowments, laboratories, and libraries they would have partaken; and the country would have been spared the demoralizing experience in medical education from which it is but now painfully awakening.

Quite aside from the history, achievements, or present merits of any particular independent medical school, the creation of the type was the fertile source of unforeseen harm to medical education and to medical practice. Since that day medical colleges have multiplied without restraint, now by fission, now by sheer spontaneous generation. Between 1810 and 1840, twenty-six new medical schools sprang up; between 1840 and 1876, forty-seven more;[1] and the number actually surviving in 1876 has been since then much more than doubled. First and last, the United States and Canada have in little more than a century produced four hundred and fifty-seven medical schools, many, of course, short-lived, and perhaps fifty still-born.[2] One hundred and fifty-five survive to-day.[3] Of these, Illinois, prolific mother of thirty-nine medical colleges, still harbors in the city of Chicago fourteen; forty-two sprang from the fertile soil of Missouri, twelve of them still "going" concerns; the Empire State produced forty-three, with eleven survivors;[4] Indiana, twenty-seven, with two survivors; Pennsylvania, twenty, with eight survivors; Tennessee, eighteen, with nine survivors. The city of Cincinnati brought forth about twenty, the city of Louisville eleven. These enterprises — for the most part they can be called schools or institutions only by courtesy — were frequently set up regardless of opportunity or need: in small towns as readily as in large, and at times almost in the heart of the wilderness. No field, however limited, was ever effectually preëmpted. Wherever and whenever the roster of untitled practitioners rose above half a dozen, a medical school was likely at any moment to be precipitated. Nothing was really essential but

[1] *Contrib. to History of Med. Educat.*, N. S. Davis (Washington, 1877, p. 41).

[2] These were usually frauds, suppressed by police or by post-office departments. Postgraduate and osteopathic schools are not included in these figures.

[3] Including osteopathic schools, of which there are eight, but not including postgraduate schools, of which there are thirteen, one of them in Kansas City without students at present. The last-named institution retains its organization in order to obtain staff recognition at the Kansas City Hospital.

[4] Not including four postgraduate schools.

professors. The laboratory movement is comparatively recent; and Thomas Bond's wise words about clinical teaching were long since out of print. Little or no investment was therefore involved. A hall could be cheaply rented and rude benches were inexpensive. Janitor service was unknown and is even now relatively rare. Occasional dissections in time supplied a skeleton—in whole or in part—and a box of odd bones. Other equipment there was practically none. The teaching was, except for a little anatomy, wholly didactic. The schools were essentially private ventures, money-making in spirit and object. A school that began in October would graduate a class the next spring; it mattered not that the course of study was two or three years; immigration recruited a senior class at the start.[1] Income was simply divided among the lecturers, who reaped a rich harvest, besides, through the consultations which the loyalty of their former students threw into their hands. "Chairs" were therefore valuable pieces of property, their prices varying with what was termed their "reflex" value: only recently a professor in a now defunct Louisville school, who had agreed to pay $3000 for the combined chair of physiology and gynecology, objected strenuously to a division of the professorship assigning him physiology, on the ground of "failure of consideration;" for the "reflex" which constituted the inducement to purchase went obviously with the other subject.[2] No applicant for instruction who could pay his fees or sign his note was turned down. State boards were not as yet in existence. The school diploma was itself a license to practise. The examinations, brief, oral, and secret, plucked almost none at all; even at Harvard, a student for whom a majority of nine professors "voted" was passed.[3] The man who had settled his tuition bill was thus practically assured of his degree, whether he had regularly attended lectures or not. Accordingly, the business throve. Rivalry between different so-called medical centers was ludicrously bitter. Still more acrid were—and occasionally are—the local animosities bound to arise in dividing or endeavoring to monopolize the spoils. Sudden and violent feuds thus frequently disrupted the faculties. But a split was rarely fatal: it was more likely to result in one more school. Occasionally, a single too masterful individual became the strategic object of a hostile faculty combination. Daniel Drake, indomitable pioneer in medical education up and down the Ohio Valley, thus tasted the ingratitude of his colleagues. As presiding officer of the faculty of the Medical College of Ohio, at Cincinnati, cornered by a cabal of men, only a year since indebted to him for their professorial titles and profits, he was compelled to put a motion for his own expulsion and to announce to his enemies a large major-

---

[1] This is recent as well as ancient history, e.g.:

Tufts College Medical School	opened 1893	first class graduated	1894
Illinois Medical College	" 1894	" " "	1895
Birmingham Medical College	" 1894	" " "	1895
College of Physicians and Surgeons, Little Rock	" 1906	" " "	1907
College of Physicians and Surgeons, Memphis	" 1906	" " "	1907

[2] The sale of chairs is not even now wholly unknown. At the North Carolina Medical College (Charlotte, N. C.) the faculty owns the stock, and the sale of one's stock carries with it one's chair.

[3] There were at Harvard at one time only seven professors and an examination was conducted even if only a majority was present.

ity in its favor. It is pleasant to record that the indefatigable man was not daunted.
He continued from time to time to found schools and to fill professorships—at Lexington, at Philadelphia, at Oxford in Ohio, at Louisville, and finally again in that
beloved Cincinnati, where he had been so hardly served. In the course of a busy
and fruitful career, he had occupied eleven different chairs in six different schools,
several of which he had himself founded; and he had besides traversed the whole
country, as it then was, from Canada and the Great Lakes to the Gulf, and as far
westward as Iowa, collecting material for his great work, historically a classic, *The
Diseases of the Interior Valley of North America.*

In the wave of commercial exploitation which swept the entire profession so far
as medical education is concerned, the original university departments were practically torn from their moorings. The medical schools of Harvard, Yale, Pennsylvania,
became, as they expanded, virtually independent of the institutions with which they
were legally united, and have had in our own day to be painfully won back to their
former status.[1] For years they managed their own affairs, disposing of professorships by common agreement, segregating and dividing fees, along proprietary lines.
In general, these indiscriminate and irresponsible conditions continued at their
worst until well into the eighties. To this day it is as easy to establish a medical
school as a business college,[2] though the inducement and tendency to do so have
greatly weakened. Meanwhile, the entire situation had fundamentally altered. The
preceptorial system, soon moribund, had become nominal. The student registered in
the office of a physician whom he never saw again. He no longer read his master's
books, submitted to his quizzing, or rode with him the countryside in the enjoy-
ment of valuable bedside opportunities. All the training that a young doctor got
before beginning his practice had now to be procured within the medical school. The
school was no longer a supplement; it was everything. Meanwhile, the practice of
medicine was itself becoming quite another thing. Progress in chemical, biological,
and physical science was increasing the physician's resources, both diagnostic and
remedial. Medicine, hitherto empirical, was beginning to develop a scientific basis
and method. The medical schools had thus a different function to perform: it took
them upwards of half a century to wake up to the fact. The stethoscope had been
in use for over thirty years before, as Dr. Cabot notes,[3] its first mention in the catalogue of the Harvard Medical School in 1868–9; the microscope is first mentioned

[1] The first step towards depriving the medical school of virtual autonomy was taken when the university undertook to collect the fees and thenceforward to administer the finances of the department by
means of an annual budget. This took place at Harvard in 1871, at Yale in 1880, at the University
of Pennsylvania in 1896. The scope of the medical faculty has gradually shrunk since. Columbia,
which gave up its medical department to the College of Physicians and Surgeons in 1814, contracted
a nominal relation with that school in 1860; in 1891 the connection became organic.

[2] In New York, however, the chartering of educational institutions is in the hands of the Regents,
who have large powers. Nevertheless, they have recently given a limited charter to the Brooklyn
Postgraduate School, a corporation practically without resources and relying on hospital and student
fee income (the latter thus far small) to carry it through.

[3] Cabot, *loc. cit.*, p. 673.

the following year. The schools had not noticed at all when the vital features of the apprentice system dropped out. They continued along the old channel, their ancient methods aggravated by rapid growth in the number of students and by the lowering in the general level of their education and intelligence. Didactic lectures were given in huge, badly lighted amphitheaters, and in these discourses the instruction almost wholly consisted. Personal contact between teacher and student, between student and patient, was lost. No consistent effort was made to adapt medical training to changed circumstances. Many of the schools had no clinical facilities whatsoever, and the absence of adequate clinical facilities is to this day not prohibitive. The school session had indeed been lengthened to two sessions; but they were of only sixteen to twenty weeks each. Moreover, the course was not graded and the two classes were not separated. The student had two chances to hear one set of lectures—and for the privilege paid two sets of fees. To this traffic many of the ablest practitioners in the country were parties, and with little or no realization of its enormity at that! "It is safe to say," said Henry J. Bigelow, professor of surgery at Harvard in 1871, "that no successful school has thought proper to risk large existing classes and large receipts in attempting a more thorough education."[1] A minority successfully wrung a measure of good from the vicious system which they were powerless to destroy. They contrived to reach and to inspire the most capable of their hearers. The best products of the system are thus hard to reconcile with the system itself. Competent and humane physicians the country came to have,—at whose and at what cost, one shudders to reflect; for the early patients of the rapidly made doctors must have played an unduly large part in their practical training. An annual and increasing exodus to Europe also did much to repair the deficiencies of students who would not have neglected better opportunities at home. The Edinburgh and London tradition, maintained by John Bell, Abernethy, and Sir Astley Cooper, persisted well into the century. In the thirties, Paris became the medical student's Mecca, and the statistical and analytical study of disease, which is the discriminating mark of modern scientific medicine, was thence introduced into America by the pupils of Louis,[2]—the younger Jackson, "dead ere his prime," Gerhard, and their successors. With the generation succeeding the civil war, the tide turned decisively towards Germany, and thither continues to set. These men subsequently became teachers in the colleges at Philadelphia, New York, Boston, Charleston, and elsewhere; and from them the really capable and energetic students got much. One of the latter, who in recent years has wielded perhaps the greatest single influence in the country towards the reconstruction of medical education, says of his own school, the College of Physicians and Surgeons of New York, in the early seventies: "One can decry the system of those days, the inadequate preliminary requirements, the short courses, the dominance of the didactic lecture, the meager appliances for

[1] *Medical Education in America*, by Henry J. Bigelow, Cambridge, the University Press, 1871, p. 79.
[2] Osler: "Influence of Louis on Modern Medicine," *Bulletin Johns Hopkins Hospital*, vol. iii., nos. 77, 78.

demonstrative and practical instruction, but the results were better than the system. Our teachers were men of fine character, devoted to the duties of their chairs; they inspired us with enthusiasm, interest in our studies and hard work, and they imparted to us sound traditions of our profession; nor did they send us forth so utterly ignorant and unfitted for professional work as those born of the present greatly improved methods of training and opportunities for practical studies are sometimes wont to suppose. Clinical and demonstrative teaching for undergraduates already existed. Of laboratory training there was none."[1] As much could perhaps be said of a half-dozen other institutions. The century was therefore never without brilliant names in anatomy, medicine, and surgery; but they can hardly be cited in extenuation of conditions over which unusual gifts and perseverance alone could triumph. Those conditions made uniform and thorough teaching impossible; and they utterly forbade the conscientious elimination of the incompetent and the unfit.

From time to time, of course, the voice of protest was heard, but it was for years a voice crying in the wilderness. Delegates from medical schools and societies met at Northampton, Massachusetts, in 1827, and agreed upon certain recommendations lengthening the term of medical study and establishing a knowledge of Latin and natural philosophy as preliminary thereto. The Yale Medical School actually went so far as to procure legislation to this end. But it subsequently beat a retreat when it found itself isolated in its advanced position, its quondam allies having failed to march.[2] As far back as 1835, the Medical College of Georgia had vainly suggested concerted action looking to more decent methods; but no step was taken until, eleven years later, an agitation set up by Nathan Smith Davis resulted in the formation of the American Medical Association, committed to two propositions, viz., that it is desirable "that young men received as students of medicine should have acquired a suitable preliminary education," and "that a uniform elevated standard of requirements for the degree of M.D. should be adopted by all the medical schools in the United States." This was in 1846; much water has flowed under the bridge since then; and though neither of these propositions has even yet been realized, there is no denying that, especially in the last fifteen years, substantial progress has been made.

In the first place, the course has now at length been generally graded[3] and ex-

[1] Wm. H. Welch: "Development of American Medicine," *Columbia University Quarterly Supplement*, Dec., 1907.

[2] Wm. H. Welch: "The Relation of Yale to Medicine" (reprinted from *Yale Medical Journal* for Nov., 1901), p. 20, and note 28, pp. 30, 31.

[3] A certain amount of ungraded teaching is still to be found, especially in the south and west. For example, at Chattanooga, no examinations are held at the close of the first year; the examinations at the close of the second year are supposed to cover two years' work, the practical outcome of which is obvious. More frequently, clinical lectures are delivered to the juniors and seniors together,—at least, as far as a single amphitheater is capable of containing the combined classes. This is the case at the University of Louisville. At certain other schools, the work is only partially graded, *e.g.*, the Memphis Hospital Medical College, Tennessee Medical College, University of Arkansas, Birmingham Medical College, Ensworth Medical College (St. Joseph, Mo.), Hahnemann, San Francisco, Kansas Medical (Topeka), Woman's Medical (Baltimore), Maryland Medical, Mississippi Medical, American

tended to four years, still varying, however, from six [1] to nine months each in duration. Didactic teaching has been much mitigated. Almost without exception the schools furnish some clinical teaching; many of them provide a fair amount, though it is still only rarely used to the best teaching advantage; a few are quite adequately equipped in this respect. Relatively quicker and greater progress has been made on the laboratory side since, in 1878,[2] Dr. Francis Delafield established the laboratory of the Alumni Association of the College of Physicians and Surgeons of New York;[3] in the same autumn Dr. William H. Welch opened the pathological laboratory of the Bellevue Hospital Medical College, from which, six years later, he was called to organize the Johns Hopkins Medical School in Baltimore. It is at length everywhere conceded that the prospective student of medicine should prove his fitness for the undertaking. Not a few schools rest on a substantial admission basis; the others have not yet abandoned the impossible endeavor at one and the same time to pay their own way and to live up to standards whose reasonableness they cannot deny. Finally, the creation of state boards has compelled a greater degree of conscientiousness in teaching, though in many places, unfortunately, far too largely the conscientiousness of the drillmaster.

In consequence of the various changes thus briefly recounted, the number of medical schools has latterly declined. Within a twelvemonth a dozen have closed their doors. Many more are obviously gasping for breath. Practically without exception, the independent schools are scanning the horizon in search of an unoccupied university harbor. It has, in fact, become virtually impossible for a medical school to comply even in a perfunctory manner with statutory, not to say scientific, requirements and show a profit. The medical school that distributes a dividend to its professors or pays for buildings out of fees must cut far below the standards which its own catalogue probably alleges. Nothing has perhaps done more to complete the discredit of commercialism than the fact that it has ceased to pay. It is but a short step from an annual deficit to the conclusion that the whole thing is wrong anyway.

In the first place, however, the motive power towards better conditions came from genuine professional and scientific conviction. The credit for the actual initiative belongs fairly to the institutions that had the courage and the virtue to make the start. The first of these was the Chicago school, which is now the medical de-

Medical (St. Louis), St. Louis College of Physicians and Surgeons, Barnes Medical, Western Eclectic (Kansas City), Éclectic Medical (New York), Eclectic Institute (Cincinnati).

[1] The low-grade southern schools have a nominal seven months' course; but as they allow students to enter without penalty several weeks later and have liberal Christmas holidays besides, the course is actually less than six months.

[2] Prior to this date Drs. Francis Delafield, E. G. Janeway, and others had given courses at Bellevue Hospital and elsewhere in histology, pathology, etc. See George C. Freeborn: *History of the Association of the Alumni of the College of Physicians and Surgeons*, New York, p. 10, etc. Instruction in pathological anatomy in the Harvard Medical School had begun in 1870 with the appointment of Dr. R. H. Fitz to an instructorship in that subject.

[3] This laboratory was at first independent of the faculty of the College of Physicians and Surgeons.

partment of Northwestern University, and which in 1859 initiated a three-year graded course. Early in the seventies the new president of Harvard College startled the bewildered faculty of its medical school into the first of a series of reforms that began with the grading of the existing course and ended in 1901 with the requirement of an academic degree for admission.[1] In the process, the university obtained the same sort of control over its medical department that it exercises elsewhere.[2] Towards this consummation President Eliot had aimed from the start; but he was destined to be anticipated by the establishment in 1893 of the Johns Hopkins Medical School on the basis of a bachelor's degree, from which, with quite unprecedented academic virtue, no single exception has ever been made.[3] This was the first medical school in America of genuine university type, with something approaching adequate endowment, well equipped laboratories conducted by modern teachers, devoting themselves unreservedly to medical investigation and instruction, and with its own hospital, in which the training of physicians and the healing of the sick harmoniously combine to the infinite advantage of both. The influence of this new foundation can hardly be overstated. It has finally cleared up the problem of standards and ideals; and its graduates have gone forth in small bands to found new establishments or to reconstruct old ones. In the sixteen years that have since elapsed, fourteen more institutions have actually advanced to the basis of two or more years of college work; others have undertaken shortly to do so. Besides these, there are perhaps a dozen other more or less efficient schools whose entrance requirements hover hazily about high school graduation. In point of organization, the thirty-odd schools now supplying the distinctly better quality of medical training are not as yet all of university type. Thither they are unquestionably tending; for the moment, however, the very best and some of the very worst[4] are alike known as university departments. Not a few so-called university medical departments are such in name only. They are practically independent enterprises, to which some university has good-naturedly lent its prestige. The College of Physicians and Surgeons of Chicago is the medical department of the University of Illinois, but the relation between them is purely contractual; the state university contributes nothing to its support. The Southwestern University of Texas possesses a medical department at Dallas, but the university is legally protected against all responsibility for its debts.[5] These fictitious alignments retard

[1] See page 28.

[2] A vein of unmistakable uneasiness runs through Bigelow's address on *Medical Education in America*, previously referred to: "Most American medical colleges are virtually close corporations, ... administered by their professors, who receive the students' fees, and upon whose tact and ability the success of these institutions depends. A university possesses over all its departments a legal jurisdiction; but it may be a question of expediency how far this shall be enforced" (p. 59).

[3] See, however, p. 28.

[4] *e.g.*, University of Arkansas, Willamette University, Cotner University (Lincoln, Nebraska), Western University (London, Ontario), Epworth University, Fort Worth University, etc.

[5] Other university departments of this nominal character are: medical department of the University of Arkansas (Little Rock); College of Physicians and Surgeons (Los Angeles), which is nominally the medical department of the University of Southern California; Denver and Gross College of

the readjustment of medical education through further reduction in the number of schools, because the institutions involved are enabled to live on hope for perhaps another decade or more. It is important that our universities realize that medical education is a serious and costly venture; and that they should reject or terminate all connection with a medical school unless prepared to foot its bills and to pitch its instruction on a university plane. In Canada conditions have never become so badly demoralized as in the United States. There the best features of English clinical teaching had never been wholly forgotten. Convalescence from a relatively mild over-indulgence in commercial medical schools set in earlier and is more nearly completed.

With the creation of the heterogeneous situation thus bequeathed to us, it is clear that consideration for the public good has had on the whole little to do; nor is it to be expected that this situation will very readily readjust itself in response to public need. A powerful and profitable vested interest tenaciously resists criticism from that point of view; not, of course, openly. It is too obvious that if the sick are to reap the full benefit of recent progress in medicine, a more uniformly arduous and expensive medical education is demanded. But it is speciously argued that improvements thus accomplished will do more harm than good: for whatever makes medical education more difficult and more costly will deplete the profession and thus deprive large numbers of all medical attention whatsoever, in order that a fortunate minority may get the best possible care. It is important to forestall the issue thus raised; otherwise it will crop out at every turn of the following discussion, in the effort to justify the existing situation and to break the force of constructive suggestion. It seems, therefore, necessary to refer briefly at this point to the statistical aspects of medical education in America, so far as they are immediately pertinent to the question of improvement and reform.

The problem is of course practical and not academic. Pending the homogeneous filling up of the whole country, inequalities must be tolerated. Man has been not inaptly differentiated as the animal with "the desire to take medicine."[1] When sick, he craves the comfort of the doctor,—any doctor rather than none at all, and in this he will not be denied. The question is, then, not merely to define the ideal training of the physician; it is just as much, at this particular juncture, to strike the solution that, economic and social factors being what they are, will distribute as widely as possible the best type of physician so distributable. Doubtless the chaos above characterized is in part accounted for by crude conditions that laughed at regular methods of procedure. But this stage of our national existence has gone by. What with widely ramifying railroad and trolley service, improving roads, automobiles, and

Medicine, which is nominally the medical department of the University of Denver; School of Medicine of the University of Georgia; Albany (New York) Medical College, which is nominally the medical department of Union University; medical department of Western University (London, Ont.), etc. For none of these alliances is there a valid reason; on the contrary, there is in every instance a good reason why the university concerned should break off the connection.

[1] Osler: *Aequanimitas*, p. 131.

rural telephones, we have measurably attained some of the practical consequences of homogeneity. The experience of older countries is therefore suggestive, even if not altogether conclusive.

Professor Paulsen, describing in his book on the *German Universities* the increased importance of the medical profession, reports with some astonishment that "the number of physicians has increased with great rapidity so that now there is, in Germany, one doctor for every 2000 souls, and in the large cities one for every 1000."[1] What would the amazed philosopher have said had he known that in the entire United States there is already on the average one doctor for every 568 persons, that in our large cities there is frequently one doctor for every 400[2] or less, that many small towns with less than 200 inhabitants each have two or three physicians apiece![3]

Over-production is stamped on the face of these facts; and if, in its despite, there are localities without a physician, it is clear that even long-continued over-production of cheaply made doctors cannot force distribution beyond a well marked point. In our towns health is as good and physicians probably as alert as in Prussia; there is, then, no reason to fear an unheeded call or a too tardy response, if urban communities support one doctor for every 2000 inhabitants. On that showing, the towns have now four or more doctors for every one that they actually require,—something worse than waste, for the superfluous doctor is usually a poor doctor. So enormous an overcrowding with low-grade material both relatively and absolutely decreases the number of well trained men who can count on the profession for a livelihood. According to Gresham's law, which, as has been shrewdly remarked, is as valid in education as in finance, the inferior medium tends to displace the superior. If then, by having in cities one doctor for every 2000 persons, we got four times as good a doctor as now when we provide one doctor for every 500 or less, the apothecaries would find time hanging somewhat more heavily on their hands. Clearly, low standards and poor training are not now needed in order to supply physicians to the towns.

[1] Thilly's translation, p. 400.

[2] New York, 1 : 460; Chicago, 1 : 580; Washington, 1 : 270; San Francisco, 1 : 370. These ratios are calculated on the basis of figures obtained from Polk's *Medical Register*, the *American Medical Directory*, and estimates prepared by the U. S. Census Bureau. The force of the figures as to the number of physicians cannot be broken by urging that many physicians no longer practise. Such have been carefully excluded by the compilers of the *American Medical Directory*. Figures used throughout this report were obtained from these sources.

[3] Examples may be cited at random from every section of the country in proof of the fact that overcrowding is general, not merely local or exceptional, *e.g.*:

Ohio:	Killbrook, population	307,	has three doctors		
	Houston	"	227	" " "	
Texas:	Wellington	"	87	" five	"
	Whitt	"	378	" four	"
	Whitney	"	766	" six	"
Massachusetts:	Colerain	"	80	" two	"
	Harding	"	100	" "	"
Nebraska:	Eustin	"	232	" "	"
	Crofton	"	46	" "	"
Oregon:	Fossil	"	370	" "	"
	Gaston	"	182	" "	"

(From the *American Medical Directory*. 1909.)

In the country the situation follows one of two types. Assuming that a thousand people in an accessible area will support a competent physician, one of two things will happen if the district contains many less. In a growing country, like Canada or our own middle west, the young graduate will not hesitate to pitch his tent in a sparsely settled neighborhood, if it promises a future. A high-grade and comparatively expensive education will not alter his inclination to do this. The more exacting Canadian laws rouse no objection on this score. The graduates of McGill and Toronto have passed through a scientific and clinical discipline of high quality; but one finds them every year draining off into the freshly opened Northwest Territory. In truth, it is an old story. McDowell left the Kentucky backwoods to spend two years under Bell in Edinburgh; and when they were over, returned contentedly to the wilderness, where he originated the operation for ovarian tumor in the course of a surgical practice that carried him back and forth through Kentucky, Ohio, and Tennessee. Benjamin Dudley, son of a poor Baptist preacher, dissatisfied with the results first of his apprenticeship, then of his Philadelphia training, hoarded his first fees, and with them subsequently embarked temporarily in trade; he loaded a flat-boat with sundries, which he disposed of to good advantage at New Orleans, there investing in a cargo of flour, which he sold to the hungry soldiers of Wellington in the Spanish peninsula. The profits kept Dudley in the hospitals of Paris for four years, after which he came back to Lexington, and for a generation was the great surgeon and teacher of surgery in the rough country across the Alleghanies. The pioneer is not yet dead within us. The self-supporting students of Ann Arbor and Toronto prove this. For a region which holds out hope, there is no need to make poor doctors, — still less to make too many of them.

In the case of stranded small groups in an unpromising environment the thing works out differently. A century of reckless over-production of cheap doctors has resulted in general overcrowding; but it has not forced doctors into these hopeless spots. It has simply huddled them thickly at points on the extreme margin. Certain rural communities of New England may, for example, have no physician in their midst, though they are in most instances not inaccessible to one. But let never so many low-grade doctors be turned out, whether in Boston or in smaller places like Burlington or Brunswick, that are supposed not to spoil the young man for a country practice, these unpromising places, destined perhaps to disappear from the map, will not attract them. They prefer competition in some already over-occupied field. Thus, in Vermont, Burlington, the seat of the medical department of the University of Vermont, with a population of less than 21,000, has 60 physicians, one for every 333 inhabitants;[1] nor can these figures be explained away on the ground that the largest city in the state is a vortex which absorbs more than its proper share; for the state abounds in small towns in which several doctors compete in the service of less than a thousand persons: Post Mills, with 105 inhabitants, has two doctors;

[1] *American Medical Directory;* Polk (1908) gives 75 active physicians, a ratio of 1 : 280.

Jeffersonville, with 400, has two; Plainfield, with 341, has three. Other New England states are in the same case. It would appear, then, that over-production on a low basis does not effectually overcome the social or economic obstacles to spontaneous dispersion. Perhaps the salvation of these districts might, under existing circumstances, be better worked out by a different method. A large area would support one good man, where its separate fragments are each unable to support even one poor man. A physician's range, actual and virtual, increases with his competency. A well qualified doctor may perhaps at a central point set up a small hospital, where the seriously ill of the entire district may receive good care. The region is thus better served by one well trained man than it could possibly be even if over-production on a low basis ultimately succeeded in forcing an incompetent into every hamlet of five and twenty souls. This it cannot compel. It cannot keep even the cheap man in a place without a "chance;" it can only demoralize the smaller places which are capable of supporting a better trained man whose energies may also reach out into the more thinly settled surrounding country. As a last resort, it might conceivedly become the duty of the several states to salary district physicians in thinly settled or remote regions, — surely a sounder policy than the demoralization of the entire profession for the purpose of enticing ill trained men where they will not go.[1] We may safely conclude that our methods of carrying on medical education have resulted in enormous over-production at a low level, and that, whatever the justification in the past, the present situation in town and country alike can be more effectively met by a reduced output of well trained men than by further inflation with an inferior product.

The improvement of medical education cannot therefore be resisted on the ground that it will destroy schools and restrict output: that is precisely what is needed. The illustrations already given in support of this position may be reinforced by further examples from every section of the Union, — from Pennsylvania with one doctor for every 636 inhabitants, Maryland with one for every 658, Nebraska with one for every 602, Colorado with one for every 328, Oregon with one for every 646. It is frequently urged that, however applicable to other sections, this argument does not for the present touch the south, where continued tolerance of commercial methods is required by local conditions. Let us briefly consider the point. The section as a whole contains one doctor for every 760 persons. In the year 1908, twelve states[2] showed a gain in population of 358,837. If now we allow in cities one additional physician for every increase of 2000, and outside cities an additional one for every increase of 1000 in population, — an ample allowance in any event, — we may in general figure on one more physician for every gain of 1500 in total population. We are not now arguing that a ratio of 1 : 1500 is correct; we are under no necessity of proving that. Our conten-

---

[1] These officials would combine the duties of county health officer with those now assigned in large towns to the city physician.

[2] This includes Kentucky, Virginia, Tennessee, North Carolina, South Carolina, Georgia, Florida, Alabama, Mississippi, Louisiana, Texas, Arkansas.

tion is simply that, starting with our present overcrowded condition, production henceforth at the ratio of one physician to every *increase* of 1500 in population will prevent a shortage, for the next generation at least. In 1908 the south, then, needed 240 more doctors to take care of its increase in population. In the course of the same year, it is estimated that 500 vacancies in the profession were due to death.[1] If every vacancy thus arising must be filled, conditions will never improve. Let us agree to work towards a more normal adjustment by filling two vacancies due to death with one new physician,—once more, a decidedly liberal provision. This will prove sufficiently deliberate; it would have called for 250 more doctors by the close of the year. In all, 490 new men would have amply cared for the increase in population and the vacancies due to death. As a matter of fact, the southern medical schools turned out in that year 1144 doctors; 78 more southerners were graduated from the schools of Baltimore and Philadelphia. The grand total would probably reach 1300,—1300 southern doctors to compete in a field in which one-third of the number would find the making of a decent living already difficult. Clearly, the south has no cause to be apprehensive in consequence of a reduced output of higher quality.[2] Its requirements in the matter of a fresh supply are not such as to make it necessary to pitch their training excessively low.

The rest of the country may be rapidly surveyed from the same point of view. The total gain in population, outside the southern states already considered, was 975,008,—requiring on the basis of one more doctor for every 1500 more people, 650 doctors. By death, in the course of the year there were in the same area 1730 vacancies. Replacing two vacancies by one doctor, 865 men would have been required; in most sections public interest would be better cared for if they all remained unfilled for a decade to come. On the most liberal calculation, 1500 graduates would be called for, and 1000 would be better still. There were actually produced in that year, outside the south, 3497, *i.e.*, between two and three times as many as the country could possibly assimilate; and this goes on, and has been going on, every year.

It appears, then, that the country needs fewer and better doctors; and that the way to get them better is to produce fewer. To support all or most present schools at the higher level would be wasteful, even if it were not impracticable; for they can-

[1] Based on figures collected by the American Medical Association.

[2] As Kentucky is one of the largest producers of low-grade doctors in the entire Union, it is interesting to observe conditions there. The following is the result of a careful study of Henderson County made for me by one thoroughly acquainted with it.
Total population, 35,000 ; number of doctors, 56; ratio, 1 : 624.

DISTRIBUTION

Place	Population	No. Drs.	Ratio	Place	Population	No. Drs.	Ratio
City of Henderson	17,500	27	1 : 644	Zion	250	3	1 : 84
Anthaston	24	1	1 : 24	Robards	500	3	1 : 167
Baskett	200	2	1 : 100	Niagara	100	3	1 : 34
Cairo	200	1	1 : 200	McDonald's Landing	25		
Corydon	1,000	4	1 : 250	Alzey	25	1	1 : 25
Dixie	300	1	1 : 300	Smith Mills	200	3	1 : 67
Geneva	100	2	1 : 50	Spottsville	700	3	1 : 234
Hebardsville	400	2	1 : 200				

Throughout the county there are doctors within five miles everywhere.

not be manned. Some day, doubtless, posterity may reëstablish a school in some place where a struggling enterprise ought now to be discontinued. Towards that remote contingency nothing will, however, be gained by prolonging the life of the existent institution.

The statistics just given have never been compiled or studied by the average medical educator. His stout asseveration that "the country needs more doctors" is based on "the letters on file in the dean's office," or on some hazy notion respecting conditions in neighboring states. As to the begging letters: selecting a thinly settled region, I obtained from the dean of the medical department of the University of Minnesota a list of the localities whence requests for a physician have recently come. With few exceptions, they represent five states:[1] fifty-nine towns in Minnesota want a doctor; but investigation shows that these fifty-nine towns have already one hundred and forty-nine doctors between them![2] Forty-one places in North Dakota apply; they have already one hundred and twenty-one doctors. Twenty-one applications come from South Dakota, from towns having already forty-nine doctors; seven from Wisconsin, from places that had twenty-one physicians before their prayer for more was made; six from Iowa, from towns that had seventeen doctors at the time. It is clear that the files of the deans will not invalidate the conclusion which a study of the figures suggests. They are more apt to sustain it: for the requests in question are less likely to mean "no doctor" than poor doctors,[3]—a distemper which continued over-production on the same basis can only aggravate, and which a change to another of the same type will not cure. As to general conditions, no case has been found in which a single medical educator contended that his own vicinity or state is in need of more doctors: it is always the "next neighbor." Thus the District of Columbia, with one doctor for every two hundred and sixty-two souls, maintains two low-grade medical schools. "Do you need more doctors in the District?" was asked of one of the deans. "Oh, no, we are making doctors for Maryland, Virginia, and Pennsylvania,"—for Maryland, with seven medical schools of its own and one doctor for every six hundred and fifty-eight inhabitants; for Virginia, with three medical schools of its own and one doctor for every nine hundred and eighteen; for Pennsylvania, with its eight schools and one doctor for every six hundred and thirty-six persons.

With the over-production thus demonstrated, the commercial treatment of medical education is intimately connected. Low standards give the medical schools access to a large clientele open to successful exploitation by commercial methods. The

[1] The general distribution in these states shows that over-production prevails in new states as in old ones: Minnesota 1:981; South Dakota 1:821; Iowa 1:605; North Dakota 1:971; Wisconsin 1:936.

[2] Ten of the fifty-nine were without registered physicians; but of these ten, two are not to be found on the map, two more are not in the *Postal Guide;* of the other six, four are in easy reach of doctors; two, with a combined population of one hundred and fifty, are out of reach.

[3] Occasionally these applications, which create the impression of a dearth, come from apothecaries who have a rear office to rent, a physician with a practice to sell, etc.

crude boy or the jaded clerk who goes into medicine at this level has not been moved by a significant prompting from within; nor has he as a rule shown any forethought in the matter of making himself ready. He is more likely to have been caught drifting at a vacant moment by an alluring advertisement or announcement, quite commonly an exaggeration, not infrequently an outright misrepresentation. Indeed, the advertising methods of the commercially successful schools are amazing.[1] Not infrequently advertising costs more than laboratories. The school catalogues abound in exaggeration, misstatement, and half-truths.[2] The deans of these institutions occasionally know more about modern advertising than about modern medical teaching. They may be uncertain about the relation of the clinical laboratory to bedside instruction; but they have calculated to a nicety which "medium" brings the largest "return." Their dispensary records may be in hopeless disorder; but the card system by which they keep track of possible students is admirable. Such exploitation of medical education, confined to schools that admit students below the level of actual high school graduation, is strangely inconsistent with the social aspects of medical practice. The overwhelming importance of preventive medicine, sanitation, and public health indicates that in modern life the medical profession is an organ differentiated by society for its own highest purposes, not a business to be exploited by individuals according to their own fancy. There would be no vigorous campaigns led by enlightened practitioners against tuberculosis, malaria, and diphtheria, if the commercial point of view were tolerable in practice. And if not in practice, then not in education. The theory of state regulation covers that point. In the act of granting the right to confer degrees, the state vouches for them; through protective boards it still further seeks to safeguard the people. The public interest is then paramount, and when public interest, professional ideals, and sound educational procedure concur in the recommendation of the same policy, the time is surely ripe for decisive action.

[1] One school offers any graduate who shall have been in attendance three years a European trip.

[2] See chapter viii., "Financial Aspects of Medical Education," especially p. 135.

[3] A few instances may be cited at random:

Medical Department, University of Buffalo: "The dispensary is conducted in a manner unlike that usually seen. . . . Each one will secure unusually thorough training in taking and recording of histories" (p. 25). There are no dispensary records worthy the name.

Halifax Medical College: "First-class laboratory accommodation is provided for histology, bacteriology and practical pathology" (p. 9). One utterly wretched room is provided for all three.

Medical Department, University of Illinois: "The University Hospital . . . contains one hundred beds, and its clinical advantages are used exclusively for the students of this college" (p. 56). Over half of these beds are private, and the rest are of but limited use.

Western University (London, Ontario): Clinical instruction. "The Victoria Hospital . . . now contains two hundred and fifty beds, and is the official hospital of the City of London," etc. (p. 14). On the average, less than thirty of these beds are available for teaching.

The Medical Department of the University of Chattanooga: "The latest advances" are taught "in the most entertaining and instructive manner;" professors are "chosen for their proficiency;" "speculative research pertains" to the department of physiology; the department of pathology is "provided with a costly collection of specimens and generous supply of the best microscopes" (one, as a matter of fact); "the hospitals afford numerous cases of labor"!

CHAPTER II

THE PROPER BASIS OF MEDICAL EDUCATION

WE have in the preceding chapter briefly indicated three stages in the development of medical education in America,—the preceptorship, the didactic school, the scientific discipline. We have seen how an empirical training of varying excellence, secured through attendance on a preceptor, gave way to the didactic method, which simply communicated a set body of doctrines of very uneven value; how in our own day this didactic school has capitulated to a procedure that seeks, as far as may be, to escape empiricism in order to base the practice of medicine on observed facts of the same order and cogency as pass muster in other fields of pure and applied science. The apprentice saw disease; the didactic pupil heard and read about it; now once more the medical student returns to the patient, whom in the main he left when he parted with his preceptor. But he returns, relying no longer altogether on the senses with which nature endowed him, but with those senses made infinitely more acute, more accurate, and more helpful by the processes and the instruments which the last half-century's progress has placed at his disposal. This is the meaning of the altered aspect of medical training: the old preceptor, be he never so able, could at best feel, see, smell, listen, with his unaided senses. His achievements are not indeed to be lightly dismissed; for his sole reliance upon his senses greatly augmented their power. Succeed as he might, however, his possibilities in the way of reducing, differentiating, and interpreting phenomena, or significant aspects of phenomena, were abruptly limited by his natural powers. These powers are nowadays easily enough transcended. The self-registering thermometer, the stethoscope, the microscope, the correlation of observed symptoms with the outgivings of chemical analysis and biological experimentation, enormously extend the physician's range. He perceives more speedily and more accurately what he is actually dealing with; he knows with far greater assurance the merits or the limitations of the agents which he is in position to invoke. Though the field of knowledge and certainty is even yet far from coextensive with the field of disease and injury, it is, as far as it goes, open to quick, intelligent, and effective action.

Provided, of course, the physician is himself competent to use the instrumentalities that have been developed! There is just now the rub. Society reaps at this moment but a small fraction of the advantage which current knowledge has the power to confer. That sick man is relatively rare for whom actually all is done that is at this day humanly feasible,—as feasible in the small hamlet as in the large city, in the public hospital as in the private sanatorium. We have indeed in America medical practitioners not inferior to the best elsewhere; but there is probably no other country in the world in which there is so great a distance and so fatal a difference between the best, the average, and the worst.

The attempt will be made in this chapter and the next to account for these discrepancies in so far as they are traceable to circumstances that antedate the formal beginning of medical education itself. The mastery of the resources of the profession in the modern sense is conditioned upon certain definite assumptions, touching the medical student's education and intelligence. Under the apprentice system, it was not necessary to establish any such general or uniform basis. The single student was in personal contact with his preceptor. If he were young or immature, the preceptor could wait upon his development, initiating him in simple matters as they arose, postponing more difficult ones to a more propitious season; meanwhile, there were always the horses to be curried and the saddle-bags to be replenished. In the end, if the boy proved incorrigibly dull, the perceptor might ignore him till a convenient excuse discontinued the relation. During the ascendancy of the didactic school, it was indeed essential to good results that lecturers and quizmasters should be able to gauge the general level of their huge classes; but this level might well be low, and in the common absence of conscientiousness usually fell far below the allowable minimum. In any event, the student's part was, parrot-like, to absorb. His medical education consisted largely in getting by heart a prearranged system of correspondences,—an array of symptoms so set off against a parallel array of doses that, if he noticed the one, he had only to write down the other: a coated tongue—a course of calomel; a shivery back—a round of quinine. What the student did not readily apprehend could be drilled[1] into him — towards examination time — by those who had themselves recently passed through the ordeal which he was now approaching; and an efficient apparatus that spared his senses and his intellect as entirely as the drillmaster spared his industry was readily accessible at temptingly low prices in the shape of "essentials" and "quiz-compends." Thus he got, and in places still gets, his materia medica, anatomy, obstetrics, and surgery. The medical schools accepted the situation with so little reluctance that these compends were—and occasionally still are—written by the professors[2] and sold on the pre-

---

[1] "A reiteration of undisputed facts in their simplest expression," is Bigelow's way of putting it. *Loc. cit.*, p. 11.

[2] From the last catalogues of certain medical publishers:

"Quiz-compends:"
Physiology, by A. P. Brubaker, Professor of Physiology, Jefferson Medical College, Philadelphia.
Gynecology, by Wm. H. Wells, Demonstrator of Clinical Obstetrics, Jefferson Medical College, Philadelphia.
Surgery, by Orville Horwitz, Prof. of Genito-Urinary Surgery, Jefferson Medical College, Philadelphia.
Diseases of Children, by Marcus P. Hatfield, Professor of Diseases of Children, Chicago Medical College.
Special Pathology, by A. E. Thayer, Professor of Pathology, University of Texas.
"Essentials:"
Surgery, by Edward Martin, Professor of Clinical Surgery, University of Pennsylvania.
Anatomy, by C. B. Nancrede, Professor of Surgery, University of Michigan.
Obstetrics, by W. E. Ashton, Professor of Gynecology, Medico-Chirurgical College, Philadelphia.
Gynecology, by E. B. Cragin, Professor of Obstetrics, Columbia University.
Histology, by Louis Leroy, Professor of Medicine, College of Physicians and Surgeons, Memphis.
Diseases of the Skin, by H. W. Stelwagon, Prof. of Dermatology, Jefferson Medical College, Phila.
Diseases of the Eye, by Edward Jackson, Professor of Ophthalmology, University of Colorado.

mises.[1] Under such a régime anybody could, as President Eliot remarked, "walk into a medical school from the street," and small wonder that of those who did walk in, many "could barely read and write."[2] But with the advent of the laboratory, in which every student possesses a locker where his individual microscope, reagents, and other paraphernalia are stored for his personal use; with the advent of the small group bedside clinic, in which every student is responsible for a patient's history and for a trial diagnosis, suggested, confirmed, or modified by his own microscopical and chemical examination of blood, urine, sputum, and other tissues, the privileges of the medical school can no longer be open to casual strollers from the highway. It is necessary to install a doorkeeper who will, by critical scrutiny, ascertain the fitness of the applicant: a necessity suggested in the first place by consideration for the candidate, whose time and talents will serve him better in some other vocation, if he be unfit for this; and in the second, by consideration for a public entitled to protection from those whom the very boldness of modern medical strategy equips with instruments that, tremendously effective for good when rightly used, are all the more terrible for harm if ignorantly or incompetently employed.

A distinct issue is here presented. A medical school may, the law permitting, eschew clinics and laboratories, cling to the didactic type of instruction, and arrange its dates so as not to conflict with seedtime and harvest; or it may equip laboratories, develop a dispensary, and annex a hospital, pitching its entrance requirements on a basis in keeping with its opportunities and pretensions. But it cannot consistently open the latter type of school to the former type of student. It cannot provide laboratory and bedside instruction on the one hand, and admit crude, untrained boys on the other. The combination is at once illogical and futile. The funds of the school may indeed procure facilities; but the intelligence of the students can alone ensure their proper use. Nor can the dilemma be evaded by alleging that a small amount of laboratory instruction administered to an unprepared medical student makes a "practitioner," while the more thorough training of a competent man makes a "scientist."[3] At the level at which under the most favorable circumstances the medical student gets his education, it is absurd to speak of an inherent conflict between science and practice. We shall have occasion later to touch on the relation of teaching and

[1] For example, in the Atlanta College of Physicians and Surgeons; Medical Department, University of Nashville; North Carolina Medical College (Charlotte); Medical Department, University of Pittsburgh; John A. Creighton Medical College (Omaha, Nebraska); Starling-Ohio Medical College (Columbus); George Washington University (D. C.).

[2] The *American Medical Association Bulletin*, vol. iii., no. 5, p. 262.

[3] At a medical convention recently held, a professor in an institution on the basis of a "high school education or its equivalent," made this point in a speech, as against the medical department of a university, which requires for entrance college work: The lower-grade institution made "doctors," it was averred; the higher made only "scientists." Now it chances that for the last two years both sets of students have submitted to a practical examination in subjects like urinalysis, which assuredly it behooves the "doctor" as well as the "scientist" to master. At these examinations the "doctors" show an average of 59 per cent; the "scientists," 77 per cent. On the combined written and practical examinations this year, the "doctors" in question averaged 65.2 per cent, the "scientists" averaged 83.1 per cent.

research,[1] between which it is necessary to establish a *modus vivendi*. But that problem has nothing to do with the point now under discussion,—*viz.*, as to how much education or intelligence it requires to establish a reasonable presumption of fitness to undertake the study of medicine under present conditions.

Taking, then, modern medicine as an attempt to fight the battle against disease most advantageously to the patient, what shall we require of those who propose to enlist in the service? To get a somewhat surer perspective in dealing with a question around which huge clouds of dust have been beaten up, let us for a moment look elsewhere. A college education is not in these days a very severe or serious discipline. It is compounded in varying proportions of work and play; it scatters whatever effort it requires, so that at no point need the student stand the strain of prolonged intensive exertion. Further, the relation of college education to specific professional or vocational competency is still under dispute. It is clear, then, that a college education is less difficult, less trying, less responsible, than a professional education in medicine. It is therefore worth remarking that the lowest terms upon which a college education is now regularly accessible are an actual four-year high school training, scholastically determined, whether by examination of the candidate or by appraisement of the school.

Technical schools of engineering and the mechanic arts afford perhaps an even more illuminating comparison. These institutions began, like the college, at a low level; but they did not long rest there. Their instruction was too heavily handicapped by ignorance and immaturity. To their graduates, tasks involving human life and welfare were committed: the building of bridges, the installation of power plants, the construction of sewage systems. The technical school was thus driven to seek students of greater maturity, of more thorough preliminary schooling, and strictly to confine its opportunities to them. Now it is noteworthy that, though in point of intensive strain the discipline of the modern engineer equals the discipline of the modern physician, in one important respect, at least, it is less complex and exacting. The engineer deals mainly with measurable factors. His factor of uncertainty is within fairly narrow limits. The reasoning of the medical student is much more complicated. He handles at one and the same time elements belonging to vastly different categories: physical, biological, psychological elements are involved in each other. Moreover, the recent graduate in engineering is not at once exposed to a decisive responsibility; to that he rises slowly through a lengthy series of subordinate positions that search out and complete his education.[2] Between the young graduate in medicine and his ultimate responsibility—human life—nothing interposes. He cannot nowadays begin with easy tasks under the surveillance of a superior; the issues of life

[1] See page 55.

[2] It is interesting to observe the tendency towards conferring only a bachelor's degree in engineering at graduation instead of the degree of C.E., etc. The bachelor in engineering usually goes to work at laborer's wages; he is years reaching the degree of responsibility with which the graduate in medicine usually begins.

and death are all in the day's work for him from the very first. The training of the doctor is therefore more complex and more directly momentous than that of the technician. Be it noted, then, that the minimum basis upon which a good school of engineering to-day accepts students is, once more, an actual high school education, and that the movement towards elongating the technical course to five years confesses the urgent need of something more.

There is another aspect of the problem equally significant. The curriculum of the up-to-date technical school is heavily weighted, to be sure; but except for mathematics, the essential subjects with which it starts are separate sciences that presuppose no prior mastery of contributory sciences. Take at random the College of Engineering of the University of Wisconsin. In the first year the science work is chemistry, and though the course is difficult, it demands no preceding acquaintance with chemistry itself or with any other science; second-year physics is in the same case, and the mechanics of the second semester looks back no further than to the physics of the first.

Very different is the plight of the medical school. There the earliest topics of the curriculum proper—anatomy, physiology, physiological chemistry—already hark back to a previous scientific discipline. Every one of them involves already acquired knowledge and manipulative skill. They are laboratory sciences at the second, not the primary, stage. Consider, for example, anatomy, the simplest and most fundamental of them all. It used to begin and end with the dissection of the adult cadaver. It can neither begin nor end there to-day; for it must provide the basis upon which experimental physiology, pathology, and bacteriology may intelligently be built up. Mere dissection does not accomplish this; in addition to gross anatomy, the student must make out under the microscope the normal cellular structure of organ, muscle, nerve, and blood-vessel; he must grasp the whole process of structural development. Histology and embryology are thus essential aspects of anatomical study. No treatment of the subject including these is possible within the time-limits of the modern medical curriculum unless previous training in general biology has equipped the student with the necessary fundamental conceptions, knowledge, and technical dexterity. It has just been stated that physiology presupposes anatomy on lines involving antecedent training in biology; it leans just as hard on chemistry and physics. The functional activities of the body propound questions in applied chemistry and applied physics. Nutrition and waste—what are these but chemical problems within the realm of biology? The mechanism of circulation, of seeing, or hearing—what are these but physical problems under the same qualifications? The normal rhythm of physiological function must then remain a riddle to students who cannot think and speak in biological, chemical, and physical language.

All this is, however, only preliminary. The physician's concern with normal process is not disinterested curiosity; it is the starting-point of his effort to comprehend and to master the abnormal. Pathology and bacteriology are the sciences concerned with abnormalities of structure and function and their causation. Now the agents and forces which invade the body to its disadvantage play their game, too, according to law. And to learn that law one goes once more to the same fundamental sciences upon which the anatomist and the physiologist have already freely drawn,—*viz.*, biology, physics, and chemistry.

Nor do these apparently recondite matters concern only the experimenting investigator, eager to convert patiently acquired knowledge of bacterial and other foes into a rational system of defense against them. For the practical outcome of such investigation is not communicable by rote; it cannot be reduced to prescriptions for mechanical use by the unenlightened practitioner. Modern medicine cannot be formulated in quiz-compends; those who would employ it must trouble to understand it. Moreover, medicine is developing with beneficent rapidity along these same biological and chemical lines. Is our fresh young graduate of five and twenty to keep abreast of its progress? If so, he must, once more, understand; not otherwise can he adopt the new agents and new methods issuing at intervals from each of a dozen fertile laboratories; for rote has no future: it stops where it is. "There can be no doubt," said Huxley, "that the future of pathology and of therapeutics, and *therefore of practical medicine*, depends upon the extent to which those who occupy themselves with these subjects are trained in the methods and impregnated with the fundamental truths of biology."[1] Now the medical sciences proper—anatomy, physiology, pathology, pharmacology—already crowd the two years of the curriculum that can be assigned to them; and in so doing, take for granted the more fundamental sciences—biology, physics, and chemistry—for which there is thus no adequate opportunity within the medical school proper. Only at the sacrifice of some essential part of the medical curriculum—and for every such sacrifice the future patients pay—can this curriculum be made to include the preliminary subjects upon which it presumes.

From the foregoing discussion, these conclusions emerge: By the very nature of the case, admission to a really modern medical school must at the very least depend on a competent knowledge of chemistry, biology,[2] and physics. Every departure from this basis is at the expense of medical training itself. From the exclusive standpoint of the medical school it is immaterial where the student gets the instruction. But it is clear that if it is to become the common minimum basis of medical education, some recognized and organized manner of obtaining it must be devised: it cannot be left to the initiative of the individual without greatly impairing its quality. Regular provision must therefore be made at a definite moment of normal educational progress. Now the requirement above agreed on is too extensive and too difficult to be incorporated in its entirety within the high school or to be substituted for a considerable

---

[1] Quoted by F. T. Lewis in "The Preparation for the Study of Medicine," *Popular Science Monthly*, vol. lxxv., no. 1, p. 66.

[2] Including botany.

portion of the usual high school course; besides, it demands greater maturity than the secondary school student can be credited with except towards the close of his high school career. The possibility of mastering the three sciences outside of school may be dismissed without argument. In the college or technical school alone can the work be regularly, efficiently, and surely arranged for. The requirement is therefore necessarily a college requirement, covering two years, because three laboratory courses cannot be carried through in a briefer period,—a fortunate circumstance, since it favors the student's simultaneous development along other and more general lines. It appears, then, that a policy that at the outset was considered from the narrow standpoint of the medical school alone shortly involves the abandonment of this point of view in favor of something more comprehensive. The preliminary requirement for entrance upon medical education must therefore be formulated in terms that establish a distinct relation, pedagogical and chronological, between the medical school and other educational agencies. Nothing will do more to steady and to improve the college itself than its assumption of such definite functions in respect to professional and other forms of special training.

So far we have spoken explicitly of the fundamental sciences only. They furnish, indeed, the essential instrumental basis of medical education. But the instrumental minimum can hardly serve as the permanent professional minimum. It is even instrumentally inadequate. The practitioner deals with facts of two categories. Chemistry, physics, biology enable him to apprehend one set; he needs a different apperceptive and appreciative apparatus to deal with other, more subtle elements. Specific preparation is in this direction much more difficult; one must rely for the requisite insight and sympathy on a varied and enlarging cultural experience. Such enlargement of the physician's horizon is otherwise important, for scientific progress has greatly modified his ethical responsibility. His relation was formerly to his patient—at most to his patient's family; and it was almost altogether remedial. The patient had something the matter with him; the doctor was called in to cure it. Payment of a fee ended the transaction. But the physician's function is fast becoming social and preventive, rather than individual and curative. Upon him society relies to ascertain, and through measures essentially educational to enforce, the conditions that prevent disease and make positively for physical and moral well-being. It goes without saying that this type of doctor is first of all an educated man.

How nearly our present resources—educational and economic—permit us to approach the standards above defined is at bottom a question of fact to be investigated presently. We have concluded that a two-year college training, in which the sciences are "featured," is the minimum basis upon which modern medicine can be successfully taught. If the requisite number of physicians cannot at one point or another be procured at that level, a temporary readjustment may be required; but such an expedient is to be regarded as a makeshift that asks of the sick a sacrifice that must not be required of them a moment longer than is necessary. Before accepting such a measure, however, it is exceedingly important not to confuse the basis on which society can actually get the number of doctors that it needs with the basis on which our present number of medical schools can keep going. Much depends upon which end we start from.

CHAPTER III

THE ACTUAL BASIS OF MEDICAL EDUCATION

TAKING a two-year college course, largely constituted of the sciences, as the normal point of departure, let us now survey the existing status. The one hundred and fifty-five medical schools of the United States and Canada fall readily into three divisions: the first includes those that require two or more years of college work for entrance; the second, those that demand actual graduation from a four-year high school or oscillate about its supposed "equivalent;" the third, those that ask little or nothing more than the rudiments or the recollection of a common school education.

To the first division sixteen institutions already belong;[1] six more, now demanding one year of college work, will fully enter the division in the fall of 1910 by requiring a second;[2] and several more, at this date still in the second division, will shortly take the step from the high school to the two-year college requirement.[3] The Johns Hopkins requires for entrance a college degree which, whatever else it represents, must include the three fundamental sciences, French, and German. No exception has ever been made to this degree requirement; but recently admission to the second-year class has been granted to students holding an A.B. degree earned by four years' study, the last of them devoted to medical subjects in institutions where those subjects were excellently taught.[4] At Harvard the degree requirement has been somewhat unsettled by a recent decision to admit students without degree, provided they have had two years of college science; they are to be grouped as "spe-

[1] Johns Hopkins, Harvard, Western Reserve, Rush (University of Chicago), Cornell, Stanford, Wake Forest (N. C.), Yale, and the state universities of California, Minnesota, North Dakota, Wisconsin, Michigan (exclusive of the homeopathic department), Kansas, Nebraska, South Dakota.

[2] Universities of Indiana, Iowa (exclusive of the homeopathic department), Missouri, Pennsylvania, Utah, Syracuse. Several institutions ask one year of college work, without as yet definite announcement as to requirement of the second, *e.g.*, Virginia, Fordham, Northwestern, North Carolina. In general, the one-year college requirement is hard to distinguish from the high school requirement, for if conditions are allowed, — and they always are, — it adds but little to the better type of high school education. Northwestern has had two years' experience under the one-year college requirement, but has not yet really enforced it. The University of North Carolina was to require a year of college work, 1909-10, but students were admitted on the strength of their unsupported statements "as having had a college year. . . . Practically, this means that the entrance requirements were not enforced."

[3] Columbia, Dartmouth, Colorado.

[4] Practically, this amounts to a recognition of the A.B. degree won after three years of study,—a movement deserving encouragement rather than criticism, as matters now stand. In fact, the Johns Hopkins degree was originally conferred at the close of three years of study, but the academic matriculation requirement was considerably higher than in institutions granting the A.B. degree after four years of study. Recently the academic matriculation has been lowered and the A.B. course lengthened to four years. In consequence, the action of the medical department above described involves unwittingly a curious discrimination against the Johns Hopkins A.B. degree, for this degree now requires four years and may not include medical subjects. To get the Johns Hopkins M.D., a student has two roads open to him: he may work four years for the Johns Hopkins A.B. and four more for its M.D.,—eight in all; or, starting at exactly the same point, he may get his A.B. in four years at an institution that includes in its A.B. the first year in medicine, then enter the Johns Hopkins medical school and get its M.D. in three years,—that is, seven years in all. A B.S. degree earned in three years, followed by the M.D. earned in four, gives the same result,—a preference, once more, that operates against the Johns Hopkins A.B.

cial" students, and are required to maintain higher standing in order to qualify for the M.D. degree. But as these students enter on a general rule and as a matter of course, and are, under a slight handicap, eligible to the M.D. degree, they are not accurately described as special. A special student is properly one whom no rule fits, one whose admission presents certain individual features requiring consideration on their merits. Such is not the case with the students under discussion: they enter just as regularly as the degree men, and without that limitation as to number which makes of the "special student" device something of a privilege. Harvard can thus, admit any student who is eligible to the schools with the two-year college requirement.[1] The other institutions under discussion telescope the college and medical courses: the preliminary medical sciences constitute the bulk of two college years;[2] the next two years are reckoned twice. They count simultaneously as third and fourth years of the college and as first and second years of the medical course. At their close the student gets the A.B. degree, but his medical education is already half over. Without exception, the schools belonging to this group are high-grade institutions. They differ considerably, however, in the degree of rigor with which their elevated entrance requirements have been enforced from the start. At the University of Pennsylvania, for example, in a class of 114, admitted this year (1909–10) on a one-year college basis, 75 (66 per cent) are conditioned; at Ann Arbor, of 36 entering on the two-year college basis, only 8 are conditioned at all, and those mainly in organic chemistry; at Yale, which advanced in 1909–10 from the high school to the two-year college basis, in a class of 23, there was only one partial condition in biology, and, best of all, failed members of last year's class on the old basis were refused re-admission. Experience elsewhere indicates that the percentage of conditions declines rapidly as students learn by forethought to adjust their work to their ultimate purpose, and as the colleges facilitate adjustment by providing the requisite opportunities: both of which processes will be accelerated, if the medical schools have the courage—and the financial strength—to close their doors to students who labor under anything more than a slight handicap. Here as elsewhere development follows hard upon actual responsibility.

Our second division constitutes the real problem; out of it additional high-grade medical schools to the number actually required must be developed. About fifty institutions, whose entrance standard approximates high school graduation, belong here. Great diversity exists in the quality of the student body of these institutions: the regents' certificates in New York, state board supervision in Michigan, the control of admission to their medical departments by the academic authorities of McGill

[1] The rule just described went into effect 1909–10; two students took advantage of it in a class of 62. In 1908 there were 254 students with degrees, 23 without.

[2] Cornell, Western Reserve, and Stanford combine academic and college courses to the extent of one year only. The pedagogical aspect of the combined course is discussed pp. 73, 74.

and Toronto, insure as capable and homogeneous an enrolment as is obtainable at
or about the high school level. A few others, not so well protected, are within measurable distance of the same category,—the medical department of Tulane University and Jefferson Medical College (Philadelphia), for example. In general, however,
the schools of this division are difficult to classify;[1] for they freely admit students
on bases that are not only hopelessly unequal to each other, but are even incapable
of reduction to a common denominator. On their actual standards the catalogue
statements throw little light: there the requirements are cast in the form of a de-
scending scale, running from the top, down. Equally acceptable in their sight are a
bachelor's degree from a college or a university, a diploma from an "accredited"
high school, an examination in a few specified and several of a wide range of optional studies, and a certificate from the principal of a high school, normal school,
or academy, from a "reputable instructor," from a state or city superintendent of
education, or from a state board of medical examiners, that stamps the applicant
as possessing the "equivalent" of a high school education. Now it is clear that the
alternatives at the top are mainly decorative. The real standard is perilously close
to the "equivalent" that creeps in modestly at the bottom. There is, of course,
no active prejudice anywhere against Ph.D.'s and A.M.'s and A.B.'s and B.Sc.'s;
they are apt to be rather conspicuously exploited, when they drift in. But they do
not set the pace; they do not determine or even vitally affect the character of the
school. In these instances the medical curriculum either contains the pre-medical
subjects in an elementary form, or, what may be worse, tries to go ahead entirely
without them. The real standard is not influenced by the presence of degree men,
and the wonder is that any of them sacrifice the advantage of a superior education by
resorting to these institutions. The minimum is, then, the real standard; all else is
permissive; for to the needs of those admitted at the bottom the quantity and quality
of the instruction must in fairness conform.

   To get at the real admission standard, then, of these medical schools, one must
make straight for the "equivalent." On the methods of ascertaining and enforcing
that, the issue hangs. Now the "equivalent" may be defined as a device that concedes the necessity of a standard which it forthwith proceeds to evade. The professed high school basis is variously sacrificed to this so-called "equivalent." The
medical schools under discussion agree to accept at face value only graduation diplomas[2] from "approved" or "accredited" high schools. These terms have a definite
meaning: they indicate schools which, upon proper investigation, have been recognized by the state universities of their respective states, or by some other competent
educational organization,—in New England, by the College Entrance Certificate
Board; in the middle west, by the North Central Association. High schools and acad-
emies not acceptable at full value to state universities or to the bodies just named

[1] In Part II each school is separately characterized.
[2] As a matter of fact, nongraduates are also admitted on certificates—a violation of standard, of course.

do not belong to the "approved" or "accredited" class: their diplomas and certificates are not, therefore, entitled to be received in satisfaction of the announced standard. They are nevertheless freely accepted. At Tufts, for example, the first year class (1909–10) numbers 151, of whom only little more than half submit credentials that actually comply with the standard; of the others, 80 are accepted from non-accredited schools on the strength of diplomas and certificates entitled to no weight on the professed standard of the Tufts Medical School.[1] This is a common occurrence. It is defended on the ground that "we know the schools." That is, however, quite impossible. The wisdom of Solomon would not suffice to determine the actual value of credentials so heterogeneous in origin and content. Universities dealing with far less various material organize registration and inspection bureaus for their protection and enlightenment. But not infrequently the medical departments of these very institutions, pretending to stand on the same basis as the academic department, refrain from seeking the aid of the university registration office. The medical department of Bowdoin is on the college campus, yet its authorities accept certificates that the college would refuse; the medical departments of Vanderbilt, Tufts, George Washington University, Creighton (Omaha), Northwestern, the Universities of Vermont and Pennsylvania,[2] are in easy reach of intelligent advice which they do not systematically utilize. In striking contrast, the medical department of the University of Texas at Galveston refers all credentials to the registration office of the university at Austin, the action of which is final.

If the standard were enforced, the candidates in question, not offering a graduation diploma from an accredited high school, would be compelled to enter by written examination. But the examination is, as things stand, only another method of evasion. Neither in extent nor in difficulty do the written examinations, in the relatively rare cases in which they are given, even approximate the high school standard. Nor are they meant to do so. Colleges with medical departments of the kind under discussion do not expect academic and medical students to pass the same or the same kind of examination: a special set of questions is prepared for the medical candidates, including perhaps half the subjects, and each of these traversing about half the ground covered by the academic papers. At Tufts, the medical matriculate attempts six papers, representing, all told, less than two years of high school work; and he is accepted on condition if he passes three.[3] Papers of similar quality are put forward at Boston University; those at Bowdoin are more extensive and more difficult, though still below the supposedly equal academic standard. The written examinations held under the authority of the state boards in Kentucky, Pennsylvania, Missouri,[4] are of

[1] Those still remaining are commented on below.
[2] The academic authorities here pass on the college year.
[3] Of the class above mentioned 38 were admitted by examination.
[4] A St. Louis cramming establishment, conducted by the wife of a teacher in a local medical school, offers to prepare in a single year, according to the Missouri standard, a boy who has never had any

the same insufficient character. In Michigan they fairly well approximate high school value,—in consequence of which they are decidedly unpopular.[1] In Illinois the written examination has been transformed into an informal after-dinner conversation between candidate and examiner, as we shall presently discover.

There remains still a third method of cutting below an actual high school standard,—the method indeed that provides much the most capacious loophole for the admission of unqualified students under the cloak of nominal compliance with the high school standard. The agent in the transactions about to be described is the medical examiner, appointed in some places by voluntary agreement between the schools, elsewhere delegated by the state board,[2] or by the superintendent of public instruction acting in its behalf, for the purpose of dealing with students who present written evidence other than the diploma of an accredited high school. It is intended and expected that this official shall enforce a high school standard. In few states is this standard achieved. The education department in New York, the state boards in Minnesota and Michigan, maintain what may be fairly called a scholastically honest high school requirement; for they require a diploma representing an organically complete secondary school education, properly guaranteed, or, in default thereof, a written examination covering about the same ground: there is no other recourse.

Elsewhere the state board is legally powerless, as in Maryland, or unwilling to antagonize the schools, as in Illinois and Kentucky. The outside examiners, agreed on by the schools in the former case, designated by law in the latter, fall far short of enforcing a high school standard. The examiner, even where distinctly well intentioned, as in Kentucky, never gets sufficient control. The schools do not want the rule enforced, and the boards are either not strong enough or not conscientious enough to withstand them. Besides, the examiners lack time, machinery, and encouragement for the proper performance of their ostensible office. They are busy men: here, a county official; there, a school principal; elsewhere, a high school professor.[3] A single individual, after his regular day's work is over, without assistance of any kind, is thus expected to perform a task much more complicated than that for which Harvard, Columbia, and the University of Michigan maintain costly establishments. There is

high school training at all. It is pointed out that by matriculating at once the student may escape any subsequent advance in entrance requirements.

[1] In Ohio the examinations are fairly representative of high school values, as far as they go. But up to this time they have not covered a complete high school course and they have little influence on enrolment, as tutor-certificates are freely accepted in their stead.

[2] In these cases, the requirement is really a practice, not an educational regulation. But the effect is the same.

[3] Occasionally the school has an "arrangement" by which defective candidates are referred to a "coach," who is simultaneously "examiner;" he thus approves his own work. This is the practice of the George Washington University medical department. Again, the school refers defective candidates to the preparatory department of its own university, and shortly after admits them on an assurance of the "equivalent" from that source. This is the Creighton school (Omaha) plan; out of 56 members of its first-year class (1908-9), 23 were admitted on certificates (not diplomas) of this kind.

no set time when candidates must appear. They drop in as they please, separately: now, before the medical school opens, again, long after; sometimes with their credentials, sometimes without them. There is no definite procedure. At times, the examiner concludes from the face of the papers; at times from the face of the candidate. The whole business is transacted in a free and easy way. In Illinois, for example, the law speaks of "preliminary" educational requirements; the state board graciously permits them to become subsequents. Students enter the medical schools, embark on the study of medicine, and at their convenience "square up"[1] with one of the examiners. An evening call is arranged; there is an informal talk, aiming to elicit what "subjects" the candidate "has had." He may, after an interview lasting from thirty minutes to two hours, and rarely including any writing, be "passed" with or without "conditions;" if with conditions, the rule requires him to reappear for a second "examination" before the beginning of the sophomore year; but nothing happens if he postpones his reappearance until a short time before graduation.[2] Besides, a condition in one subject may be removed by "passing" in another! "No technical questions are asked; the presumption is that the applicant won't remember details." Formerly, written examinations were used in part; but they were given up "because almost everybody failed." And it may at any moment happen that an applicant actually turned down by one examiner will be passed by another. The most flagrantly commercial of the Chicago schools[3] operate "pre-medical" classes, where a hasty cram, usually at night, suffices to meet the academic requirements of the Illinois state board: "the examiner's no prude, he'll give a man a chance," said the dean of one of them.

In Pennsylvania there was until quite lately no high school requirement by law; but recent legislation fixes the high school or its equivalent, on which the better schools had previously agreed, as the legal minimum. Its value has hitherto varied. In the first place, the examiners have accepted three-year high school graduates: "They come every day and are not turned down." In the second place, the alternatives in the matter of studies are so many that he must indeed have had narrow op-

---

[1] Quotation marks indicate throughout words taken down on the spot in the course of interviews with officials.

[2] New York, while dealing strictly with applicants for practice who have been educated in New York state, deals somewhat more leniently with the outsider. The New York law provides that to be "registered as maintaining a proper medical standard," a school must, among other things, "require that *before* beginning the course for the degree, all matriculates afford evidence of a general preliminary education equivalent to at least a four-year high school course," etc. (*Handbook* 9, April, 1908, p. 45.) As a matter of fact, a student who received his degree from a school on the accredited or registered list (*ibid.*, pp. 48–70) may, on applying for registration in New York, find his preliminary education to have been below the New York standard. In certain circumstances, he may be allowed to make good his defects, provided they are of limited scope. He is thus bringing his "*preliminary*" education up to standard, *after* he has received his M.D. degree. This is a concession that the New York Education Department makes to the loose educational administration of other states. It is to be hoped that after due notice given it may be discontinued. The offending schools may very properly be excluded from the list.

[3] Bennett Medical College, Illinois Medical College, Jenner Medical College, Chicago Night University, Reliance Medical College.

portunities who cannot piece together scraps enough to gain conditional admission. "The more subjects, the more points," one dean is quoted as saying. Partial certificates—a year's work taken here, a subject or part of a subject taken there—may be added up until the sum equals arithmetically the "units" of a high school course. Moreover, the same subject can be counted twice: English grammar and rhetoric are two subjects, not one; so are English literature and English classics; so biology and zoölogy. Now, aside from these duplications, it is absurd to sum up fragmentary or isolated "credits" of this kind as "equivalent" to a high school course, even if the details were each adequately tested, as they are not. For a school curriculum is an organic thing in whose continuity and interrelations its educational virtue resides. One subject bears upon another; one year reinforces another. A curriculum has, as such, unity, purpose, method. It is not merely a question of time, still less of detached specified amounts without reference to time.[1]

Things are not essentially different in Baltimore, where the entire matter is regulated by voluntary action on the part of the three schools belonging to the division under consideration. The "examination" is of the usual kind: "on a strict accounting they would all fail." In Louisville, students are admitted into the local school, the medical department of the University of· Louisville, by either examination or certificate. The examination covers less than a four-year high school course; certificates are accepted from two-year high schools as full satisfaction of the requirements. Worse still, the school also admits students without either, in flat disregard of its professed standard and of the state board. St. Louis, Denver, Nashville, Pittsburgh, furnish further illustration. In none of these does the examiner exact, whether through examination or in evaluation of certificates, the preliminary standard which he is ostensibly appointed to enforce. In most cases the very word "preliminary" is a misnomer, just as we have found it to be in Illinois. For example, the Ohio requirement is not really preliminary to medical education. The schools on the so-called high school or equivalent basis admit students who have not completely satisfied the examiner. Strictly speaking, these students should not be allowed to proceed to the sophomore class; for their medical school credits beyond the first year cannot count until after the admission requirements have been satisfied. Meanwhile they may have reached the senior class. And the moment they satisfy the examiner in respect to "preliminaries," now "subsequents" to the extent of two or three years, that moment their previous work in the medical school automatically becomes "good." At Vanderbilt the first-year class had been studying two months,—yet not a single "preliminary" credential had been even submitted to the examiner; at Louisville

[1] It is useless to review all the states separately, for the differences are not very significant. Ohio, however, may be instanced as a state in transit towards the Michigan standard. At present, the examiner accepts as equivalent to graduation from an approved high school several alternatives, none of which is really equivalent: (1) whole years taken in different institutions, provided they sum up four; (2) certificates from "known instructors," testifying that candidates have "made up" conditions,—no fixed periods of study being required in such cases; (3) examinations, covering hitherto less than the high school course.

work begins November 15, but students have until January 8 before even calling on that functionary. Even Michigan wavers here: for March 1, 1910, had come around before all the first-year students of the Detroit School of Medicine had satisfied the state board. In such cases the requirement may be preliminary to graduation, or to practice, or to what-not; it is absurd to regard it as preliminary to medical education. For the whole purpose of a preliminary is to guarantee a certain degree of training, maturity, and knowledge before the student crosses the threshold of the medical school, on the ground that he is not fit to cross the threshold without it; and this purpose is abandoned if he is allowed to enter without it and subsequently, by hook or crook, in hastily snatched moments, to go through the form of a perfunctory compliance that becomes complete some time before he comes up for his M.D. degree. There is no retroactive virtue in such a feat. Educational futility can go no farther. A high school "preliminary requirement," scrappily accumulated as a side issue incidental to attendance in the medical school, is worse than nothing to the extent that it has interfered with undivided attention to medical study.[1]

To all the disorder that prevails in schools of this grade in the United States, the Canadian schools at the same level present, with two exceptions,[2] a forcible contrast. There, too, "equivalents" are accepted; but they are equivalents in fact as in name, for they are probed by a series of written examinations, each three hours in length, held at a stated time and place, only and actually in advance of the opening of the medical school, entrance to which is absolutely dependent on their outcome.

The quality of the student body thus accumulated in the schools under discussion bears out the above description. "The facilities are better than the students;" "the boys are imbued with the idea of being doctors; they want to cut and prescribe; all else is theoretical;" students accepted in chemistry or physics "don't know a barometer when they see it;" "it is difficult to get a student to *want* to repeat an experiment (in physiology). They have neither curiosity nor capacity." "The machinery does n't stop the unfit." "Men get in, not because the country needs the doctors, but because the schools need the money." "What is your honest opinion of your own enrolment?" a professor in a Philadelphia school was asked. "Well, the most I would claim," he answered, "is that nobody who is absolutely worthless gets in"!

[1] Some state boards are already in possession of the legal right to enforce a preliminary requirement. The Illinois law, for example, says: "The State Board of Health shall be empowered to establish a standard of *preliminary education* deemed requisite to *admission* to a medical college in good standing" (par. 6 b, ch. 91, Hurd's *Revised Statutes*, 1908). The board is apparently free to refuse examination to any applicant whose completed entrance certificate does not bear date four years prior to his M.D. diploma. The present policy of the Illinois board thus squarely contravenes the obvious intention of the statute. Contrast with this lax procedure the Scotch requirement: "The student must within fifteen days of the commencement of study, obtain registration." (*Regulations for the Triple Qualification*, ch. i. § 2.)

[2] Laval University, Montreal, which admits students below grade; but they must come to the United States to practise, for they have no standing in Canada; and Western University, London, Ont., which leaves the entire question to the discretion of the student, who, it is supposed, will conform to the local requirement of the place in which he expects to settle.

We have still to deal with schools of our third division. They are most numerous in the south, but they exist in almost all medical "centers,"—San Francisco, Chicago, —there plainly on the sufferance of the state board, for the law, if enforced, would stamp them out,—St. Louis and Baltimore. Outside the south they usually make some pretense of requiring the "equivalent" of a high school education; but no examiner of any kind is employed, and the deans are extremely reluctant to be pinned down. Southern schools of this division, after specifying an impressive series of acceptable credentials ranging once more from university degrees downward, announce their satisfaction with a "grammar school followed by two years of a high school," or in default thereof a general assurance of adequate "scholastic attainments" by a state, city, or county superintendent, or some other person connected with education or purporting to be such; but the lack of such credentials is not very serious, for the student is admitted without them, with leave to procure them later. Many of the schools accept students from the grammar schools. Credentials, if presented, are casually regarded and then usually returned; a few may be found, rolled up in a rubber band, in a dusty pigeonhole. There is no protection against fraud or forgery. At the College of Medicine and Surgery, Chicago, a thorough search for credentials or some record of them was made by the secretary and several members of the faculty, through desk drawers, safe, etc., but without avail. The school is nevertheless in "good standing" with the Illinois state board, and is "accredited" by the New York Education Department to the extent of three years' work. At the medical department of the University of Georgia I was told: "We go a long way on faith." In visits to medical colleges certificates were found from non-existent schools as well as from non-existent places.[1] Of course a few fairly competent students may be found sprinkled in these institutions. But for the most part, the student body gets in on the "equivalent." At the Atlanta School of Medicine, 73 per cent of last year's first-year class entered thus; at the Mississippi Medical College (Meridian, Mississippi), 80 per cent; at Birmingham Medical College, 62 per cent. In point of quality, the classes are not competent to use such opportunities as are provided. In Atlanta the Grady Hospital is open for bedside clinics to groups of six students; on the average, two come. In Chattanooga it is "rare to get a medical student who knows even a little algebra; it is impossible to use with medical students the text-books in science used in freshman academic classes." At Charlotte I was told that "it is idle to talk of real laboratory work for

---

[1] Accepted certificates are in this form:

To.............................., Dean:
Sir: I have examined Mr. ...., of ...., and find his scholastic attainments equal to those requisite for a first-grade teacher's certificate in our public schools, with the equivalent of two years of high school study.
                    Yours very truly,
                         (Sign here) ...., Superintendent of Public Instruction.

These are furnished to the student by the medical college; he needs only to have them signed. The college does not investigate the signature: no official mark or seal is asked. Even the medical department of Vanderbilt accepts preliminary certificates in this form.

students so ignorant and clumsy. Many of them, gotten through advertising, would make better farmers. There's no use in having apparatus for experimental physiology—the men could n't use it; they're all thumbs."

Statistical proof of inadequacy of preparation is furnished by what one may fairly call the abnormal mortality within schools operating on the basis of "equivalents." The standards of promotion in these schools watch narrowly the action of the state boards, which are usually lenient. The schools are too weak financially to do otherwise; doubtful points are resolved in the boy's favor.[1] Hence the school examinations play less havoc than would follow tests strictly constructed in the public interest. Yet the mortality from one cause or another by the close of the first year runs from 20 to 50 per cent. At the Medico-Chirurgical College of Philadelphia an initial first-year enrolment of 152 in October fell to 100[2] by the following January first; of these, 60 passed without conditions, much less than one-half the original class enrolment; at Tufts the entering class 1908-9 shows in the catalogue an enrolment of 141; 75 were promoted, with or without conditions, into the sophomore class;[3] at Cornell, on its former high school basis, the failures at the close of the first year in a period of ten years averaged 28 per cent; at Buffalo, the failed and conditioned of three successive first-year classes amounted to 40 per cent of the total enrolment; at Vanderbilt, out of a class of 70, the dropped, conditioned, and failed amounted to 44 per cent; at the College of Physicians and Surgeons, Atlanta, 70 per cent, out of a class of 99. In schools on the higher basis, i.e., two years of college work or better, the instruction is more elaborate, the work more difficult, and the examinations harder; for scientific ideals rather than chances with the state board dominate. Yet the mortality drops decisively. At the Johns Hopkins, the mortality during three successive years averages less than 5 per cent, only half of which is due to failure; at Ann Arbor, on the one-year college basis, the mortality is below 10 per cent. The exhibit made by institutions that have tried both standards is especially instructive. At the University of Missouri, during the last three years of the high school or equivalent basis, there was a mortality due to actual failure of 35 per cent; during the following three years, when one year of college work was required, the mortality fell to 12½ per cent. At the medical department of the University of Minnesota, during the last three years of the high school requirement, the mortality was

---

[1] The dean of one school admitted that he carried "men easily from class to class, but plucked them in the last year,"—an excellent thing for the school: it collects three years' fees and still avoids a low record in the state board examinations.

[2] Some dropped out because unable to qualify, a few for lack of funds, others because of inability to do the work; but the enormous number that drop or fail throws a strong light on the miscellaneous character of the enrolment obtained on the "equivalent" basis.

[3] It is relatively immaterial to our argument what became of the other 66; they represent fatalities for most of which low standards are to blame. As a matter of fact they are thus accounted for: 14 were dropped students (not catalogued with their class on account of conditions); 20 failed of promotion; 17 took all or a portion of first-year examinations 1908-9, but did not return 1909-10; 15 left before the final examinations.

18 per cent;[1] in the three years following, on the basis of one year of college work, the mortality was about 10 per cent. At the University of Virginia, in the last two years on the old basis, 38 per cent of the students failed in one or more subjects; an increase in entrance requirements by one college year reduces the fatalities to 14 per cent, despite the augmented difficulty of the work. The medical department of the University of Texas has gradually advanced from a two-year high school basis to a four-year high school basis; on the lower standard there were 34 per cent of hopeless failures in 1903, as against 13 per cent of hopeless failures in 1908, on the higher. The requirement of a college year assists doubly,—first, in eliminating the sham equivalents; next, in strengthening the equipment of those who actually persist. Canada accomplishes the former by means of the examinations already noticed, with the result that the mortality there is distinctly less than ours, at something like the same ostensible level.[2]

The breaches made by the fatalities above described are repaired by immigration, which on investigation proves to be in most instances only another way of evading standards,—entrance and other. To some extent, good students who find themselves in a poor school endeavor to retrieve their error by transferring themselves to a better; again, there is a certain amount of enforced emigration annually from schools that, like the University of Wisconsin, offer medical instruction in the first two years only. In the main, however, the "lame ducks" move, and, strangely enough, into schools that are at the moment engaged in rejecting a number equally lame. The interchange is veiled by pretended examinations; but the character of the examination can be guessed from the quality of the students that pass it. Two standards are thus often broken at once: An ill equipped student registers in a low-grade Chicago school. At the close of a year or two, he transfers to the College of Physicians and Surgeons, which might have declined him originally. He has thus circumvented its admission requirements. If, now, he has previously failed in the medical courses so far pursued, and succeeds "on examination" in passing, he has simultaneously circumvented the professional requirements as well. Instances of both kinds abound in schools at and below the high school basis. In 1908–9 the Medico-Chirurgical College of Philadelphia accepted failures from the Jefferson Medical College and

---

[1] This relatively low mortality is to be ascribed to the fact that the student body, though on the high school basis, contained no "equivalents."

[2] A tabular statement will perhaps help to bring these facts home. Three institutions on the high basis (Johns Hopkins, Harvard, University of Minnesota) show:

Total enrolment	Dropped before examinations	Failed and conditioned	Passed without conditions
757	2 per cent	17 per cent	81 per cent

Seven of the strongest schools in the United States on the high school or equivalent basis (Jefferson Medical, New York University, University of Maryland, Medico-Chirurgical, Tufts, Yale, and University of Pennsylvania (the last two before elevating their standard) show:

2280	11 per cent	38 per cent	51 per cent

McGill and Toronto show:

945	5 per cent	28 per cent	67 per cent

the University of Pennsylvania and advanced them to the classes to which they had been denied promotion by the teachers who knew them best; at the same time the Jefferson Medical College[1] itself accepted and in the same way advanced failures from New York University and the University of Pennsylvania; Tufts admits as "specials" students failed at Dartmouth, Queen's (Kingston, Ontario), and the Medico-Chirurgical of Philadelphia; the medical department of the University of Illinois (College of Physicians and Surgeons, Chicago) fairly abounds in rejected students from other schools, and in emigrated students from the low-grade institutions of Chicago and elsewhere; of the same character is a large part of the enrolment of the medical department of Valparaiso University. Failures from Ann Arbor are regarded as worthy of advancement by Northwestern (Chicago). The Physicians and Surgeons of Baltimore gives time and subject credit — after "examination," of course — to failures turned out of the University of Buffalo, New York University, the University of Pennsylvania, the Jefferson Medical College, and Yale; the University of Maryland is equally indiscriminate, advancing to the classes which they had failed to reach students from most of the same institutions and some from the local College of Physicians and Surgeons and the Baltimore Medical College, besides. Other Jefferson Medical failures, not to be found in the two Baltimore schools just named, should be looked for in the Baltimore Medical College, together with failures from Tufts, Long Island Hospital Medical College, etc. The upper classes of two Baltimore schools — the Maryland Medical College and the Atlantic Medical College — are largely recruited by emigration from other schools;[2] the latter of these had (1908–9) a senior class of 31, a freshman class of 1, — and every member of the senior class had been admitted to advanced standing from some other school.[3]

Is this the best that can be done? Will the actual enforcement of a real and adequate standard starve any section of the country in the matter of physicians?

The question can be answered without guesswork or speculation. The south requires something like 400 doctors annually.[4] How high a standard can it enforce, and still get them? In the year 1908–9 there were 15,791 male students in four-year high schools in six southern states,[5] — Alabama, Georgia, Louisiana, South Carolina, Vir-

---

[1] This institution, like others, admits to advanced standing a considerable number of students from schools whose entrance requirements are much below its own; *e.g.*, in the session above referred to, there were several students from the medical department of Fort Worth University, whose entrance requirement is nominal; from the University of Oregon, College of Physicians and Surgeons, San Francisco, Keokuk, Denver and Gross. At the same time, it deals severely with its own student body, for it refuses promotion annually to a large number, who emigrate chiefly to Baltimore.

[2] Mississippi Medical College, Meridian, was similarly recruited.

[3] Among other schools guilty of advancing students to whom promotion had been refused by their own schools may be mentioned: College of Physicians and Surgeons, Atlanta, Georgetown University (Washington, D. C.), Denver and Gross, University of Colorado, George Washington University, Milwaukee Medical College.

[4] The former secretary of the Southern Medical College Association calculated that 300 would suffice.

[5] For these figures we are indebted to a painstaking census conducted by the secondary school inspectors maintained in these states by the General Education Board.

ginia and Texas; there were in the previous year 5877 male students in the academic departments of the southern state universities, and 1653 more in endowed institutions of similar grade;[1] a population of over 23,000[2] bordering on high school graduation and widely distributed over the entire area. Our question is thus already answered. The best material for the making of a few hundred southern doctors annually does not have to be torn from the plough.

But these figures convey by no means the whole truth. The south is in the midst of a genuine educational renaissance. Within the last few years every southern state under the leadership of the state university, the state department of education, and certain endowed institutions like Vanderbilt University, has set enthusiastically to work to develop its common and secondary school systems after the admirable model furnished by the robust communities of the middle west. The professors of secondary education in the state universities are the evangelists of this auspicious movement. Young, intelligent, well trained, these sturdy leaders ceaselessly traverse the length and breadth of their respective states, stimulating, suggesting, guiding, organizing. It is an inspiring spectacle. Three years ago the high school had no legal standing in Virginia; to-day the state is dotted with two-year, three-year, and four-year high schools, created by local taxation, with a considerable subvention from the state treasury. There are already 2511 boys in fairly well equipped four-year high schools, and as many more in private institutions of equal value; and the two-year and three-year schools are growing rapidly into fuller high school stature. It needs no argument to prove that Virginia can at once procure its doctors from among the *bona-fide* graduates of such high schools and better. What is true of Virginia is true of every other southern state. In Alabama, for example, three years ago there was scarcely a public high school in the state; to-day there are 61 public four-year high schools,[3] 11 private four-year high schools, and 15 town and city three-year high schools. Of the 345 teachers employed in these schools, 184 are college graduates and 55 more have had at least two years of college work. Of course the situation is uneven; it lacks homogeneity. Standards are more or less confused; distinctions are not everywhere clear. The schools have frequently shot up like ungainly boys, who first get their height and fill up afterwards; their four years are not yet the four years of Boston or Indianapolis. But this is a phenomenon of hopeful omen; it provides the framework for a vigorous and imminent maturity. The universities and the professional schools have in this emergency a clear duty: to call things by their right names, to abandon the apologetic attitude, to cease from compromises which tempt the student from the high school and then set up the successful temptation as a sufficient excuse for their

[1] Compiled from the Report of the United States Commissioner of Education, 1908.

[2] Not including four-year high schools of Mississippi, Florida, North Carolina, Tennessee, Arkansas, and Kentucky, which would considerably increase these figures. They are omitted because equally reliable data are not at hand.

[3] Under legislative enactment approved August 7, 1907, the state contributes $2000 a year to aid any county that establishes its own high school.

own folly in so doing. Let them reinforce the high school by the opposite policy; they will soon perceive the needlessness of the exceptions which they still suggest, and often even require. How much longer will the southern people, generously spending themselves in the effort to create high school systems, continue to handicap their development by allowing medical education legally to rest on an ante-bellum basis?

The duty of the southern universities at this juncture is clear. They are equally bound to assist the development of the secondary school and to furnish the southern people an improved type of physician. They do both if, while actually enforcing the standard above advocated, they provide the best medical training obtainable at that level. As a matter of fact, a highly useful doctor can be trained on the high school basis if his defects, frankly admitted, are made the occasion for more, instead of less, efficient instruction. The weak southern schools apologize for their wretchedness by alleging the shortcomings of the student body. But the shortcomings of the students are a call for better, rather than an excuse for worse, teaching. On the whole, a southern university will for a time probably do best to put its strength unreservedly into the improved instruction of a larger body of students at the high school level, rather than to train a smaller body on a somewhat higher basis. What with the other influences working to discredit the proprietary medical school, if Tulane, Vanderbilt, and Texas furnish actual high school graduates with an education as good as that of Toronto or of McGill, they will soon get control of the field, they will educate the southern public to look to them for their physicians, and they will induce the state legislatures to support a position undeniably reasonable, so that when they at last make the upward move, there will be no low-grade medical schools to profit by the step and to make it a pretext for the continuance of commercialism in medical education.[1]

The state of Texas has taken a sound and yet conservative position. Beginning with 1909, it has decreed a gradual annual rise of standard that will shortly result in making its four-year high school the legal basis of medical education. Cautious elevation thus avoids all danger of breaking with the state school system. The statute is not free from defects, for it provides for the acceptance, at their face value, of the medical student certificates of reciprocating states; but the Texas state board, having dealt vigorously with the worst of the Texas schools, will in all probability make effective use of the power in its hands. Other southern states must inevitably follow. It is of course important that they should not move faster than their educational facilities; but it is equally important that they should not move any more slowly. Thus far, Texas alone has made an effort to keep pace.

The situation is even clearer, in so far as it touches the rest of the country. We estimate[2] that outside the south 1500 doctors annually graduated will provide for

[1] For more detailed consideration on this point, the reader is referred to the discussions in Part II of the various southern states.
[2] In chapter ix.

all the real and many imaginary needs. There are at this date something like 8000 public and over 1000 private high schools, so widely dispersed over the area under consideration that on the average few boys need go over five miles to school.[1] In the public high schools alone there are enrolled 300,000 boys.[2] What excuse exists for cutting under the high school? We can indeed do better than to accept as the basis of a medical education the high school "flat." In the colleges, universities, and technical schools of the north and west, exclusive of preparatory and professional departments, there were in 1908, 120,000[3] male students. The number swells with unprecedented rapidity; long before the country has digested the number of doctors now struggling for a livelihood, it will have doubled. Already in 1907, 903 of the doctors graduated in that year held academic degrees; that is to say, fully one-half of the number the country actually needed could conform to the standard that has been urged, or better. There is at this moment absolutely nothing in the educational situation outside the south that countenances the least departure from the scientific basis necessary to the successful pursuit of modern medicine.

For whose sake is it permitted? Not really for the remote mountain districts of the south, for example, whence the "yarb doctor," unschooled and unlicensed, can in no event be dislodged; nor yet for that twilight zone, on the hither edge of which so many low-grade doctors huddle that there is no decent living for those already there and no tempting prospect for anybody better: ostensibly, "for the poor boy." For his sake, the terms of entrance upon a medical career must be kept low and easy. We have no right, it is urged, to set up standards which will close the profession to "poor boys."

What are the merits of this contention? The medical profession is a social organ, created not for the purpose of gratifying the inclinations or preferences of certain individuals, but as a means of promoting health, physical vigor, happiness — and the economic independence and efficiency immediately connected with these factors. Whether most men support themselves or become charges on the community depends on their keeping well, or if ill, promptly getting well. Now, can anyone seriously contend that in the midst of abundant educational resources, a congenial or profitable career in medicine is to be made for an individual regardless of his capacity to satisfy the purpose for which the profession exists? It is right to sympathize with those who lack only opportunity; still better to assist them in surmounting obstacles; but not at the price of certain injury to the common weal. Commiseration for the hand-spinner was not suffered for one moment to defeat the general economic advantage procurable through machine-made cloth. Yet the hand-spinner had a sort of vested right: society had tacitly induced him to enter the trade; he had grown up in it on that assurance; and he was now good for nothing else. Your "poor boy"

[1] Wilgus, *Legal Education in the United States*, p. 29.
[2] There are 33,000 more in the preparatory departments of colleges and universities.
[3] We are indebted for these statistics to the United States Commissioner of Education.

has no right, natural, indefeasible, or acquired, to enter upon the practice of medicine unless it is best for society that he should.

As a matter of fact, the attainments required by our entire argument are not, as a rule, beyond the reach of the earnest poor boy. He need only take thought in good season, lay his plans, be prudent, and stick to his purpose. Without these qualities, medicine is no calling for him; with them, poverty will rarely block his way. Besides, if poverty is to be a factor in determining entrance standards, just where does poverty cease to excuse ignorance? Apparently the inexcusable degree of ignorance begins just where the ability to pay fees leaves off. For the schools that maintain "equivalents" for the sake of the "poor boy" are not cheap, and the student who can pay his expenses in them can also pay for something better, and pay his fees the student must; for it is precisely the proprietary and independent schools, avowedly solicitous for the "poor boy," that do the least for him by way of scholarship or other exemption.[1] They exact a complete settlement in cash or notes. Thus a four-year medical education in Baltimore, Philadelphia, or Chicago schools, on the "equivalent" basis, costs a boy in tuition fees and board about $1420. The same student can go to Ann Arbor, get there two years of college work in the pre-medical sciences and modern languages, and four years in medicine, besides, for an expenditure of $1466, covering the same items. Thus six years at Ann Arbor are not appreciably more expensive than four years in Baltimore, Philadelphia, or Chicago. Or, if a large city be preferred, he can get his two years in the admirable pre-medical laboratories of the University of Minnesota, at Minneapolis, followed by his four-year medical work there, for very little more. Low entrance requirements flourish, then, for the benefit of the poor school, not of the poor boy. Meanwhile, opportunities exist, in a measure during the school year, still more during vacation, to earn part, perhaps all, of the required sum.[2] Doubtless in the near future, the problem will be still further simplified in the interest of the better training by increased scholarship and other endowments, as in Germany. Meanwhile, it is dubious educational philanthropy to interrupt a poor boy's struggle upwards by inviting him into a medical school where there are excessively large chances of failure, escaping which he is at once exposed to a disadvantageous competition with men better trained by far.

So much from the standpoint of the individual. The proper method of calculating cost is, however, social. Society defrays the expense of training and maintaining the medical corps. In the long run which imposes the greater burden on the community,—

[1] Three scholarships, amounting to tuition fees for one year, are, however, annually awarded at the University of Maryland.

[2] It is stated that at the University of Chicago "the opportunities for taking work are more numerous than the number of students desiring to take advantage of them. . . . There is ample opportunity for the energetic student to earn his way, either in whole or in part, and opportunities usually outnumber those seeking them." *School Review*, January, 1910 (Notes and News). It must, of course, be remembered that only the vigorous and talented can afford to undertake the study of medicine under such conditions. The others are barred just as effectively from the low-grade as from the high-grade school. Students are found "working their way through" at the medical departments of Harvard, Michigan, Toronto, McGill, etc.

the training of a needlessly vast body of inferior men, a large proportion of whom break down, or that of a smaller body of competent men who actually achieve their purpose? When to the direct waste here in question there is added the indirect loss due to incompetency, it is clear that the more expensive type is decidedly the cheaper. Aside from interest on investment, from loss by withdrawal of the student body from productive occupations, the cost of our present system of medical education is annually about $3,000,000, as paid in tuition fees alone. The number of high-grade physicians really required could be educated for much less; the others would be profitably employed elsewhere; and society would be still further enriched by efficient medical service.

The argument is apt to shift at this point. If we refuse to be moved by the "poor boy," pity the small towns; for it is speciously argued that the well trained, college-bred student will scorn them. Not sympathy for the poor boy requires us now to sacrifice the small town to him, but sympathy for the small town requires us to sacrifice the poor boy to it. Two vital considerations are overlooked in this plea. In the first place, the small town needs the best and not the worst doctor procurable. For the country doctor has only himself to rely on: he cannot in every pinch hail specialist, expert, and nurse. On his own skill, knowledge, resourcefulness, the welfare of his patient altogether depends. The rural district is therefore entitled to the best trained physician that can be induced to go there. But, we are told, the well trained man will not go; he will not pay for a high-grade medical education and then content himself with a modest return on his investment. Now the six-year medical education (that based on two college years) and the four-year medical education (that based on the high school or equivalent) may, as we saw above, be made to cost the same sum. As far as cost is concerned, then, the better sort of four-year medical education must have precisely the same effect on distribution of doctors as the six-year training furnished by the state universities. If a Jefferson graduate is not deterred by the cost of his education from seeking a livelihood in the country, the Ann Arbor or Minnesota man will not be deterred, either. But a deeper question may be raised. What is the financial inducement that persuades men scientifically inclined to do what they really like?—for a man who does not like medicine has no business in it. How far does the investment point of view actually control? Complete and reliable data are at hand. The college professor has procured for himself an even more elaborate and expensive training than has here been advocated for the prospective physician. Did he require the assurance of large dividends on his investment? "The full professor in the one hundred institutions in the United States and Canada which are financially strongest receives on the average an annual compensation of approximately $2500."[1] But the scholar does not usually advance beyond the assistant professorship: what figure has financial reward cut with him? "At the age of twenty-six or twenty-seven, after seven years of collegiate and graduate study, involving not only considerable outlay,

[1] "The Financial Status of the Professor in America and in Germany," *Carnegie Foundation for the Advancement of Teaching*, Bulletin II., p. vi.

but also the important item of the foregoing of earning during this period, he is the proud possessor of his Ph. D. and is ready to enter his profession. The next five years he spends as instructor. In his thirty-second year he reaches assistant professorship. He is now in his thirty-seventh year, having been an assistant professor for five years. His average salary for the ten years has been $1325. . . . At thirty-seven he is married, has one child, and a salary of $1800."[1] In Germany "the road to a professorship involves a period of training and of self-denial far longer and more exacting than that to which the American professor submits;"[2] in France "there are no pecuniary prizes whatever in their calling for even those who attain its highest posts."[3] What is even more to the point,—the posts of instructor and assistant in small colleges situated in out-of-the-way places can be readily filled at slender salaries with expensively trained men. Of course there are compensations. But the point is that a large financial inducement is not indispensable, provided a man is doing what he likes. In most sections the country doctor has better worldly prospects. The fact stands out that it is not income but taste that primarily attracts men into scholarly or professional life. That granted, the prospect of a modest income does not effectually deter; and not infrequently the charm of living away from large cities may even attract.

Our limited experience with physicians trained at a high level sustains this view. We have thus far produced relatively few college-bred physicians; large cities have bid high for them, without, however, bagging all. Johns Hopkins graduates in medicine, to take the highest quality the country has produced, are already scattered through thirty-two states and territories. As if to prove that money is not the sole deciding consideration, a dozen have gone as missionaries to the Orient and several into the army and navy. In this country there is a Johns Hopkins man practising at Clayton, Alabama, with 1000 inhabitants; at Fort Egbert, Alaska, with 458; at Gorham, Colorado, with 364; at Chattahoochee, Florida, with 460; at Fort Bayard, New Mexico, with 724; at Sonyea, New York, with 300; at Blue Ridge Summit, Pennsylvania, with 50; at Wells River, Vermont, with 660; at Fairfax, Virginia, with 200; at Fort Casey, Washington, with 300; at Kimball, West Virginia, with 2000; at Mazomanie, Wisconsin, with 900. They have scattered to the four winds, and inevitably.[4] No single influence controls: home, money, taste, opportunity, all figure. When we have produced as large a number of well trained doctors as Germany, they will be found in our villages, just as one finds them over there. Minnesota, closed after 1912 to all low-grade graduates, Kansas and North and South Dakota, agricultural states, Con-

---

[1] Statistics from twenty leading universities, discussed by Guido H. Marx in address, *The Problem of the Assistant Professor*, before Association of American Universities, January, 1910.

[2] *Carnegie Foundation*, Bulletin II., p. vii.

[3] Bodley: *France*, vol. i. p. 54.

[4] Western Reserve men (three years of college required for entrance) are to be found in Cochranton, Pennsylvania (population, 724); Solon Springs, Wisconsin (population, 400); Kinsman, Ohio (population, 824); Rawson, Ohio (population, 552).

necticut, Indiana, Colorado, look forward confidently to the high standard basis. Is there any reason founded in consideration for public welfare which holds back Illinois, New York, Pennsylvania, from similar action?

There is, however, still another standpoint from which the question under discussion ought to be viewed. We have been endeavoring to combat the argument in favor of admittedly inferior schools dependent on fees on the ground that in the east, north, and west, these schools have already outlived their usefulness; that, even in the south, the need, greatly exaggerated, will gradually disappear. Let us, however, for the moment concede that the south, and perhaps other parts of the country, still require some medical schools operating on the high school basis, or a little less. Does it follow that the proprietary or independent unendowed medical school has thereby established its place? By no means. It is precisely the inferior medical student who requires the superior medical school. His responsibilities are going to be as heavy as those of his better trained fellow practitioner : to be equally trustworthy, his instruction must be better, not worse. The less he brings to the school, the more the school must do for him. The necessity of recruiting the medical school with high school boys is therefore the final argument in favor of fewer schools, with better equipment, conducted by skilful professional teachers.

The truth is that existing conditions are defended only by way of keeping unnecessary medical schools alive. The change to a higher standard could be fatal to many of them without in the least threatening social needs. Momentarily there would be a sharp shrinkage. But forethought would be thus effectively stimulated; trained men would be attracted into the field; readjustment would be complete long before any community felt the pinch.[1] Despite prevailing confusion—legal, popular, and educational—as to what good training in medicine demands, the enrolment in the five schools which have during the last four years required two or more years of college work is already 1186 students, and is increasing rapidly.[2] When the Johns Hopkins plans were under discussion in the middle seventies, Dr. John S. Billings, the adviser of the trustees in things medical, suggested that the graduating class be limited to twenty-five. "I think it will be many years before the number of twenty-five for the graduating class can be reached," he said.[3] The school opened in 1893; the first class, graduated in 1897, numbered 15; the third, graduated in 1899, numbered 32: so promptly did the country respond. Institutions that have switched from the high

[1] It has been calculated that in the supply of doctors the country is now "about thirty-five years in advance of the requirements"! Benedict : *Journal of American Medical Association*, vol. lii., no. 5, pp. 378, 379.

[2] In the sixteen schools on the two-year college basis there were (1908-9) 1850 students who had entered at that level. The total enrolment in these sixteen institutions was much greater, because the upper classes in several had entered on a lower basis. These figures are far from the total number of college men in medical schools. The pity is that they are scattered through institutions in which they lose the advantage which their education should give them.

[3] *Medical Education: Extracts from Lectures before the Johns Hopkins University*, 1877-8, p. 22 (Baltimore, 1878).

school to the college standard after due notice given[1] have thus far lost only one-half or less of their former enrolment. The only thing that falls in proportion is the income from fees; the percentage of graduates is reduced much less. At the University of Minnesota, there used to be an average first-year attendance of 80 on the high school basis; on the two-year college basis it is now 40; at Harvard on the former basis, 160 new matriculants; now, on a college basis, 79. Western Reserve, with 34 on the high school basis, advanced suddenly in 1901 to a three-year college requirement; the enrolment fell to 12, but by 1908 the loss was practically recovered. Most significant is the demonstration that the greatest loss is due to the transition from the high school or equivalent to the one-year college basis; the rise from one to two years of college has relatively little effect on enrolment. It would appear that the college requirement compels deliberation. Once decided, the student is not seriously hampered by the effort or the expense of an additional year.

It does not follow, however, that if schools generally rose to the college requirement, their losses would be only one-half and the recovery therefrom ultimately assured. For the schools that came off thus lightly were previously attended by a large proportion of high-grade men.[2] A much greater loss would undoubtedly take place in the lower-grade schools; many of them would be practically annihilated. For the tendency of elevated standards and ideals is to reduce the number of students to something like parity with the demand, and to concentrate this reduced student body in fewer institutions, adequately supported.

The basis which we have urged for medical education gives an undoubted advantage to the university medical departments. We shall see in subsequent chapters that other equally important factors are at work tending to restore medical education to the university status; but for the moment the difficulty of procuring anywhere else the necessary educational foundation is perhaps most cogent. A countermove, by way of avoiding this tendency, has recently emanated from certain Philadelphia schools,[3] in the form of a suggested five-year course, the first year to be devoted to the pre-medical sciences.

Several serious objections to this proposition may be urged: (1) a single year is insufficient for three laboratory sciences, and makes no provision for modern languages; the very best medical schools could with difficulty give one year's pre-medi-

---

[1] Cornell changed from the high school to the three-year college requirement with less than a year's notice. There was, of course, no chance to readjust matters; the next first-year class (1908) numbered 15; in 1909, this increased to 23.

[2] In these schools standards were elevated in advance of the operation of the formal declaration to that effect. For example, Columbia (College of Physicians and Surgeons, New York) goes to the two-year college basis 1910–11; but the entering class 1909–10 contained among its 86 matriculates 48 students with degrees, and 11 more who had had two years of college work.

[3] These schools have no endowments; and the pre-medical sciences cannot be properly taught out of fees, as will become evident in chapter viii., "The Financial Aspects of Medical Education." Hence the work must be mainly make-believe. It would have to be given by already overburdened science teachers or, still worse, by practitioners. The Medico-Chirurgical College of Philadelphia offers these courses "in conjunction with classes in the sister department of pharmacy." This is absurd.

cal work,—they cannot possibly give two; as for anything more liberal, there is no chance at all. Hence the step would shortly prove an obstruction to further progress. (2) Unquestionably, the day is coming when the medical school proper will want a fifth or hospital year,—a culmination that will be indefinitely postponed if the year in question is prefixed to the course and assigned to preliminary training. (3) Finally, the arrangement protracts our present educational disorganization. It proposes that the medical school should do the work of the college, just as it is either doing—or doing without—the work of the high school. Now the strength of an educational system is wholly a question of the competent performance of differentiated function by each of its organic parts. Our tardily awakened educational conscience and intelligence find themselves confronted with several independent and detached educational agencies,—high schools, colleges, professional schools. Obviously, they are not indifferent to each other; they belong in a definite order and relation. We now know perfectly well what that order, what that relation, is. And the solidity of our educational and scientific progress depends on our success in making it prevail. To no inconsiderable extent, inefficiency has been due to irresponsibility resulting from just this lack of organized relationships; and the cure for evils due to lack of responsibility is not less responsibility, but more; not less differentiation, but more.

The reconstruction of our medical education on the basis of two years of required college work is not, however, going to end matters once and for all. It leaves untouched certain outlying problems that will all the more surely come into focus when the professional training of the physician is once securely established on a scientific basis. At that moment the social rôle of the physician will generally expand, and to support such expansion, he will crave a more liberal and disinterested educational experience. The question of age—not thus far important because hitherto our demands have been well within the limits of adolescence—will then require to be reckoned with. The college freshman averages nineteen years of age; two years of college work permit him to begin the study of medicine at twenty-one, to be graduated at twenty-five, to get a hospital year and begin practice at twenty-six or twenty-seven. No one familiar with the American college can lightly ask that this age be raised two years for everybody, for the sake of the additional results to be secured from non-professional college work. There is, however, little question that compression in the elementary school, closer articulation between and more effective instruction within secondary school and college, can effect economies that will give the youth of twenty-one the advantage of a complete college education. The basis of medical education will thus have been broadened without deferring the actual start. Meanwhile we are so far from endeavoring to force a single iron-clad standard on the entire country that our proposition explicitly recognizes at least three concurrent levels for the time being: (1) the state university entrance standard in the south, (2) the two-year college basis as legal minimum in the rest of the country, (3) the degree standard in a small number of institutions.

The practical problem remains. How is the existing situation to be handled? The higher standard is alike necessary and feasible. How long is it to be postponed because it threatens the existence of this school or of that? In general, our medical schools, like our colleges, are local institutions; their students come mainly from their own vicinity. The ratio of physicians to population in a given state is therefore a fair indication of the number of medical schools needed. Where physicians are superabundant, and high schools and colleges at least not lacking, the medical schools cannot effectively plead for mercy on the ground that elevated standards will be their death. New York has two schools on the two-year college basis or better; nine others rest on a lower basis. They would improve if they could "afford it."[1] But with one doctor for every 600 people in the state, with accessible high schools, with cheap—and in New York City, at least, free—colleges, it is absolutely immaterial to the public whether they can afford it or not. The public interest demands the change. We may therefore at once assume (what everybody grants) that the problem is insoluble on the basis of the survival of all or most of our present medical schools. To live, they must get students; they must get them far in excess of the number they will graduate; they must graduate them far in excess of the number of doctors needed. They will therefore require their clientele of ill prepared, discontented, drifting boys, accessible to successful solicitation on commercial lines. Inevitably, then, the way to better medical education lies through fewer medical schools; but legal enactments on the subject of medical education and practice will be required before the medical schools will either give up or relate themselves soundly to the educational resources of their respective states. No general legislation is at the moment feasible. The south, for instance, may well rest for a time, if every state will at once restrict examinations for license to candidates actually possessing the M.D. degree, and require after, say, January 1, 1911, that every such degree shall emanate from a medical school whose entrance standards are at least those of the state university. Such legislation would suppress the schools that now demoralize the situation; it would concentrate the better students in a few solvent institutions to which the next moves may safely be left. Elsewhere, every available agency should be employed to bring examining boards to reinterpret the word "equivalent" and to adopt efficient machinery for the enforcement of the intended standard. Equivalent means "equal in force, quality, and effect." The only authorities competent to pass on such values are trained experts. The entire matter would be in their hands if the state boards should in every state delegate the function of evaluating entrance credentials to a competently organized institution of learning. In many states, the state university

---

[1] The dean of a superfluous southern medical school writes : "Our faculty gets only what's left after all expenses are paid, and that averages $400 per session of seven months. This we will cheerfully forego, and teach gratis, if only a class, or endowment, will pay cost of running the college. We will advance to the highest requirements just as soon as the conditions will admit, and are ready now to open next session under highest requirements if the wherewith to pay expenses is in sight." Observe that there is small consideration here for the "poor boy" or the "back country;" it is simply a question of college survival.

could very properly perform this duty; elsewhere, an equally satisfactory arrangement could be made with an endowed institution. Whatever the standard fixed, it would thus be intelligently enforced. The school catalogues would then announce that no student can be matriculated whose credentials are not filed within ten days of the opening of the session, and that no M. D. degree can be conferred until at least four years subsequent to complete satisfaction of the preliminary requirement. These credentials, sent at once to the secretary of the state board, would be by him turned over to the registrar of the state or other university, whose verdict would be final. A state that desired to enforce a four-year high school requirement could specify as satisfying its requirements:

(1) Certificate of admission to a state university requiring a four-year high school education;

(2) Certificate of admission to any institution that is a member of the Association of American Universities;

(3) Medical Student Certificate of the Regents of the University of the State of New York;

(4) Certificates issued by the College Entrance Examination Board for 14 units.

In exchange for such credentials, or for high school diplomas acceptable to the academic authorities acting for the state board, a medical student certificate would be issued; in default thereof, the student must by examination earn one of the aforesaid credentials, in its turn to be made the basis of his medical student certificate. In the southern states, the legal minimum would be necessarily below the four-year high school; in Minnesota, above it. But the same sort of machinery would work. The schools would have nothing to do with it except to keep systematically registered the name of the student and the number of his certificate; the state board or the university acting for it would keep everything else, open to inspection.

This is substantially what takes place in New York, where the State Education Department superintends the process. What is wanted in other states is an agency similarly qualified. For the present nothing can so well perform the office within a given state as its state university, or, in default thereof, the best of its endowed institutions. This suggestion is perfectly fair to all medical schools, for the credentials would pass through the hands of the state board to the reviewing authority without information as to the purpose of the applicant. The directions required would take up less space in the medical school catalogues than the complicated details they now contain. It should be further provided that the original credentials of every student be kept on file in the office of the state board or the reviewing university, and that they shall be open to inspection, without notice, by properly accredited representatives of medical and educational organizations. These simple measures would introduce intelligence and sincerity where subterfuge and disorder now prevail. The beneficial results to the high school and the medical school would be incalculable. Nor would the poor boy be subjected to the least hardship; for by exercising forethought, he could accumulate genuine scholastic credits by examination or otherwise, *pari passu*, during the time he is accumulating the money for his medical education. So much actually accomplished, the rest will be easier. The reduced number of schools will not resist the forces making for a higher legal minimum. The state universities of the west will doubtless lead this movement; for once established on the two-year college basis, they will induce the states to protect their own sons and the public health against the lower-grade doctors made elsewhere. The University of Minnesota, having by statesmanlike action got rid of all other medical schools in the state, is thus backed up by the legislature and the state board. North Dakota and Indiana have taken the same stand. Michigan and Iowa will probably soon follow. "The adjustment is perhaps difficult, but not too difficult for American strength."[1]

[1] Adapted from Billroth: *Ueber das Lehren und Lernen der medicinischen Wissenschaft*, quoted by Lewis, *loc. cit.*

CHAPTER IV

THE COURSE OF STUDY: THE LABORATORY BRANCHES

(A) FIRST AND SECOND YEARS

THREE characteristic stages are to be discerned in the evolution of medical teaching.[1] The first and longest was the era of dogma. Its landmarks are Hippocrates (B.C. 460–377) and Galen (A.D. 130–200), whose writings were for centuries transmitted as an authoritative canon. Observation and experience had indeed figured considerably in their composition,[2] but increasingly remote disciples in accepting the tradition lost all interest in its source. The Galenic system took its place in the medieval university with Euclid and Aristotle,—a thing to be pondered, expounded and learned; facts had no chance if pitted against the word of the master. So completely was medicine dominated by scholasticism that surgery, employing such base tools as sight and touch, was held to be something less than a trade and accordingly excluded from intellectual company.

The second era is that of the empiric. It began with the introduction of anatomy in the sixteenth century, but did not reach its zenith until some two hundred years later. At its best it leaned upon experience, but its means of analyzing, classifying, and interpreting phenomena were painfully limited. Medical art was still under the sway of preconceived and preternatural principles of explanation; and rigorous therapeutic measures were not uncommonly deduced from purely metaphysical assumptions. The debility of yellow fever, for example, Rush explained by "the oppressed state of the system;" and on the basis of a gratuitous abstraction, resorted freely to purging and bleeding. His first four patients recovered; there is no telling how many lives were subsequently sacrificed to this conclusive demonstration. The fact is that the empiric lacked a technique with which to distinguish between apparently similar phenomena, to organize facts, and to check up observation; the art of differentiation through controlled experimentation was as yet in its infancy. Under vague labels like rheumatism, biliousness, malaria, or congestion, a hodgepodge of dissimilar and unrelated conditions were uncritically classed; the names meant nothing, but they answered as explanation, and even sanctioned severe and nauseous medication. Ignorant of causes, the shrewdest empiric thus continued to confound totally unlike conditions on the basis of superficial symptomatic resemblance; and with amazing assurance undertook to employ in all a therapeutic procedure of doubtful value in any. He combined the vehemence of the partisan with something of the credulity of

[1] Nothing would do more to orient the student intelligently than a knowledge of the history of medical science and teaching. It is a great pity that some effort is not made in the better medical schools to interest the student in the subject. A proper historical perspective would render impossible such opposition to improved medical teaching as is now based on conscientious but mistaken devotion to outgrown conditions.

[2] "The correct inductive method was borne in on the triumph of Hippocrates." Gomperz's *Greek Thinkers* (translated by Magnus, vol. i. p. 308).

a child, persuading too often by ardent insistence rather than by logical proof. His students were thus passive learners, even where the teaching was demonstrative. They studied anatomy by watching a teacher dissect; they studied therapeutics by taking the word of the lecturer or of the text-book for the efficacy of particular remedies in certain affections.

The third era is dominated by the knowledge that medicine is part and parcel of modern science. The human body belongs to the animal world. It is put together of tissues and organs, in their structure, origin, and development not essentially unlike what the biologist is otherwise familiar with; it grows, reproduces itself, decays, according to general laws. It is liable to attack by hostile physical and biological agencies; now struck with a weapon, again ravaged by parasites. The normal course of bodily activity is a matter of observation and experience; the best methods of combating interference must be learned in much the same way. Gratuitous speculation is at every stage foreign to the scientific attitude of mind.

We may then fairly describe modern medicine as characterized by a severely critical handling of experience. It is at once more skeptical and more assured than mere empiricism. For though it takes nothing on faith, the fact which it accepts does not fear the hottest fire. Scientific medicine is, however, as yet by no means all of one piece; uniform exactitude is still indefinitely remote; fortunately, scientific integrity does not depend on the perfect homogeneity of all its data and conclusions. Modern medicine deals, then, like empiricism, not only with certainties, but also with probabilities, surmises, theories. It differs from empiricism, however, in actually knowing at the moment the logical quality of the material which it handles. It knows, as empiricism never knows, where certainties stop and risks begin. Now it acts confidently, because it has facts; again cautiously, because it merely surmises; then tentatively, because it hardly more than hopes. The empiric and the scientist both theorize, but logically to very different ends. The theories of the empiric set up some unverifiable existence back of and independent of facts,—a vital essence, for example; the scientific theory is in the facts,—summing them up economically and suggesting practical measures by whose outcome it stands or falls. Scientific medicine, therefore, has its eyes open; it takes its risks consciously; it does not cure defects of knowledge by partisan heat; it is free of dogmatism and open-armed to demonstration from whatever quarter.

On the pedagogic side, modern medicine, like all scientific teaching, is characterized by activity. The student no longer merely watches, listens, memorizes; he *does*. His own activities in the laboratory and in the clinic are the main factors in his instruction and discipline. An education in medicine nowadays involves both learning and learning how; the student cannot effectively know, unless he knows how.

Two circumstances have mediated the transformation from empirical to scientific medicine: the development of physics, chemistry, and biology; the elaboration out of them of a method just as applicable to practice as to research. The essential dependence of modern medicine on the physical and biological sciences, already adverted to,[1] will hereafter become increasingly obvious in the wealth of the curricula based upon them, and no less in the poverty of those constructed without them. But the practical importance of scientific method as such to the general practitioner is by no means so generally conceded. Its function in investigation is granted: there it is justified by its own fruits. But what has this to do with the education or the daily routine of the family doctor?

The question raised is fundamental; the answer decides the sort of medical education that we shall seek generally to provide. If, in a word, scientific method and interest are of slight or no importance to the ordinary practitioner of medicine,[2] we shall permanently establish two types of school,—the scientific type, in which enlightened and progressive men may be trained; the routine type, in which "family doctors" may be ground out wholesale. If, on the other hand, scientific method is just as valuable to the practitioner as to the investigator, it may indeed be expedient partly, or even in some instances altogether, to set aside gifted individuals as teachers or investigators and to guard the undergraduate student against original work prematurely undertaken. But this will not be construed to involve the abrupt and total segregation of medical education from medical research. Much of the educator's duty may consist in traversing a well known path; but if otherwise he is progressively busy, the well known path will never look exactly the same twice. The medical school will in that case be more than the undergraduate curriculum. Activities will be in progress that at every point run beyond the undergraduate's capacity and interest at the moment. But the undergraduate curriculum will not differ in spirit, method, or aspiration from the interests that transcend it.

The conservative in medical education makes much of what he conceives to be a fundamental opposition between medical practice and medical science; occasionally a despairing progressive accepts it. The family doctor represents the former type. One can ask of him—so the conservative thinks—only that he be more or less well grounded in things as they are when he gets his degree. The momentum with which he is propelled from the medical school must carry him to the end of his days,—on a gradually declining curve; but that cannot be helped. The other type—the scientific doctor—either himself "investigates," or has a turn for picking up increases due to others. How profound is the opposition here depicted? Opposition of course there is between all things in respect to time and energy. The doctor who puts on his hat and goes out to see a sick baby cannot just then be making an autopsy on a guinea-pig dead of experimental dysentery. But does the opposition go any deeper? Is there any logical incompatibility between the science and the practice of medicine?

[1] Chapter ii. p. 24.
[2] This is the common contention of the routine schools that run on low admission requirements and employ practitioner teachers.

The main intellectual tool of the investigator is the working hypothesis, or theory, as it is more commonly called. The scientist is confronted by a definite situation; he observes it for the purpose of taking in all the facts. These suggest to him a line of action. He constructs a hypothesis, as we say. Upon this he acts, and the practical outcome of his procedure refutes, confirms, or modifies his theory. Between theory and fact his mind flies like a shuttle; and theory is helpful and important just to the degree in which it enables him to understand, relate, and control phenomena.

This is essentially the technique of research: wherein is it irrelevant to bedside practice? The physician, too, is confronted by a definite situation. He must needs seize its details, and only powers of observation trained in actual experimentation will enable him to do so. The patient's history, conditions, symptoms, form his data. Thereupon he, too, frames his working hypothesis, now called a diagnosis. It suggests a line of action. Is he right or wrong? Has he actually amassed all the significant facts? Does his working hypothesis properly put them together? The sick man's progress is nature's comment and criticism. The professional competency of the physician is in proportion to his ability to heed the response which nature thus makes to his ministrations. The progress of science and the scientific or intelligent practice of medicine employ, therefore, exactly the same technique. To use it, whether in investigation or in practice, the student must be trained to the positive exercise of his faculties; and if so trained, the medical school begins rather than completes his medical education. It cannot in any event transmit to him more than a fraction of the actual treasures of the science; but it can at least put him in the way of steadily increasing his holdings. A professional habit definitely formed upon scientific method will convert every detail of his practising experience into an additional factor in his effective education.

From the standpoint of the young student, the school is, of course, concerned chiefly with his acquisition of the proper knowledge, attitude, and technique. Once more, it matters not at that stage whether his destination is to be investigation or practice. In either case, as beginner, he learns chiefly what is old, known, understood. But the old, known, and understood are all alike new to him; and the teacher in presenting it to his apprehension seeks to evoke the attitude, and to carry him through the processes, of the thinker and not of the parrot.

The fact that disease is only in part accurately known does not invalidate the scientific method in practice. In the twilight region probabilities are substituted for certainties. There the physician may indeed only surmise, but, most important of all, he knows that he surmises. His procedure is tentative, observant, heedful, responsive. Meanwhile the logic of the process has not changed. The scientific physician still keeps his advantage over the empiric. He studies the actual situation with keener attention; he is freer of prejudiced prepossession; he is more conscious of liability to error. Whatever the patient may have to endure from a baffling disease, he is not further handicapped by reckless medication. In the end the scientist alone draws the line accurately between the known, the partly known, and the unknown. The empiricist fares forth with an indiscriminate confidence which sharp lines do not disturb.

Investigation and practice are thus one in spirit, method, and object. What is apt to be regarded as a logical, is really but a practical, difficulty, due to the necessity for a division of labor. "The golden nuggets at or near the surface of things have been for the greater part discovered, it seems safe to say. We must dig deeper to find new ones of equal value, and we must often dig circuitously, with mere hints for guides."[1] If, then, we differentiate investigator and practitioner, it is because in the former case action is leisurely and indirect, in the latter case, immediate and anxious. The investigator swings around by a larger loop. But the mental qualities involved are the same. They employ the same method, the same sort of intelligence. And as they get their method and develop their intelligence in the first place at school, it follows that the modern medical school will be a productive as well as a transmitting agency. An exacting discipline cannot be imparted except in a keen atmosphere by men who are themselves "in training." Of course the business of the medical school is the making of doctors; nine-tenths of its graduates will, as Dr. Osler holds, never be anything else. But practitioners of modern medicine must be alert, systematic, thorough, critically open-minded; they will get no such training from perfunctory teachers. Educationally, then, research is required of the medical faculty because only research will keep the teachers in condition. A non-productive school, conceivably up to date to-day, would be out of date to-morrow; its dead atmosphere would soon breed a careless and unenlightened dogmatism.

Teachers of modern medicine, clinical as well as scientific, must, then, be men of active, progressive temper, with definite ideals, exacting habits in thought and work, and with still some margin for growth. No inconsiderable part of their energy and time is indeed absorbed in what is after all routine instruction; for their situation differs vastly from that of workers in non-teaching institutions devoted wholly to investigation. Their practical success depends, therefore, on their ability to carry into routine the rigor and the vigor of their research moments. A happy adjustment is in this matter by no means easy; nor has it been as yet invariably reached. Investigators, impressed with the practical importance of scientific method to the practising physician, tend perhaps to believe that it is to be acquired only in original research. A certain impatience therefore develops, and ill equipped student barks venture prematurely into uncharted seas. But the truth is that an instructor, devoting part of his day under adequate protection to investigation, can teach even the elements of his subject on rigorously scientific lines. On the other hand, it will never happen that every professor in either the medical school or the university faculty is a genuinely productive scientist. There is room for men of another type,—the

[1] C. A. Herter: "Imagination and Idealism in the Medical Sciences," *Columbia Univ. Quart.*, vol. xii., no. 11, p. 16.

non-productive, assimilative teacher of wide learning, continuous receptivity, critical sense, and responsive interest. Not infrequently these men, catholic in their sympathies, scholarly in spirit and method, prove the purveyors and distributors through whom new ideas are harmonized and made current. They preserve balance and make connections. The one person for whom there is no place in the medical school, the university, or the college, is precisely he who has hitherto generally usurped the medical field,—the scientifically dead practitioner, whose knowledge has long since come to a standstill and whose lectures, composed when he first took his chair, like pebbles rolling in a brook get smoother and smoother as the stream of time washes over them.

The student is throughout to be kept on his mettle. He does not have to be a passive learner, just because it is too early for him to be an original explorer. He can actively master and securely fix scientific technique and method in the process of acquiring the already known. From time to time a novel turn may indeed give zest to routine; but the undergraduate student of medicine will for the most part acquire the methods, standards, and habits of science by working over territory which has been traversed before, in an atmosphere freshened by the search for truth.

For purposes of convenience, the medical curriculum may be divided into two parts, according as the work is carried on mainly in laboratories or mainly in the hospital; but the distinction is only superficial, for the hospital is itself in the fullest sense a laboratory. In general, the four-year curriculum falls into two fairly equal sections: the first two years are devoted mainly[1] to laboratory sciences,—anatomy, physiology, pharmacology, pathology; the last two to clinical work in medicine, surgery, and obstetrics. The former are concerned with the study of normal and abnormal phenomena as such; the latter are busy with their practical treatment as manifested in disease. How far the earlier years should be at all conscious of the latter is a mooted question. Anatomy and physiology are ultimately biological sciences. Do the professional purposes of the medical school modify the strict biological point of view? Should the teaching of anatomy and physiology be affected by the fact that these subjects are parts of a medical curriculum? Or ought they be presented exactly as they would be presented to students of biology not intending to be physicians? A layman hesitates to offer an opinion where the doctors disagree, but the purely pedagogical standpoint may assist a determination of the issue. Perhaps a certain misconception of what is actually at stake is in a measure responsible for the issue. Scientific rigor and thoroughness are not in question. Whatever the point of view—whether purely biological or medical—scientific method is equally feasible and essential; a verdict favorable to recognition of the explicitly medical standpoint would not derogate from scientific rigor. There is no doubt that the sciences in question can be properly cultivated only in the university in their entirety

[1] An introductory course in physical diagnosis is given in the second year; occasionally clinical work is begun in its latter half.

and in close association with contiguous, contributory, or overlapping sciences. No one of them is sharply demarcated; at any moment a lucky stroke may transfer a problem from pathology to chemistry or biology. There are indeed no problems in pathology which are not simultaneously problems of chemistry and biology as well. So far the rigorously and disinterestedly scientific viewpoint is valid. These considerations, however, still omit one highly important fact: medical education is a technical or professional discipline; it calls for the possession of certain portions of many sciences arranged and organized with a distinct practical purpose in view. That is what makes it a "profession." Its point of view is not that of any one of the sciences as such. It is difficult to see how separate acquisitions in several fields can be organically combined, can be brought to play upon each other, in the realization of a controlling purpose, unless this purpose is consciously present in the selection and manipulation of the material. Pathology, for example, is a study of abnormal structure and function; the pathologist as such works intensively within a circumscribed field. For the time being, it pays him to ignore bearings and complications outside his immediate territory. Undoubtedly, the progressive pathologist will always be at work upon certain problems, thus temporarily, but only temporarily, isolated. But in the undergraduate class-room he is from time to time under necessity of escaping these limitations: there he is engaged in presenting things in their relations. The autopsy, the clinical history, will be utilized in presenting to the student, even if incidentally, the total picture of disease. Similarly, the anatomist can score many a point for the physiologist without actually forestalling him. He views the body not as a mosaic to be broken up, but as a machine to be taken to pieces, the more perfectly to comprehend how it works. The pharmacologist is in a similar relation to the clinician. The principles of bacteriology lose nothing in scientific exactitude because, taught as a part of the medical curriculum, they are enforced with illustrations from the bacterial diseases of man rather than from those of animals and plants; and histology is not the less histology because tissues from the human body are preferably employed.[1] In

[1] The following quotations from "An Outline of the Course in Normal Histology," by L. F. Barker and C. R. Bardeen (*Johns Hopkins Hospital Bulletin*, vol. vii., nos. 62, 63, p. 100, etc.), forcibly illustrate the above contention.

"In deciding as to the plan to be adopted we have been much influenced, too, by the fact that our students are students of medicine. Thus it will be noticed that in the selection of tissues, those from the human body make up a large part of the material used; and when animal tissues are employed, special care has been taken to point out how they differ from the human. Moreover, in deciding what to exclude from the course thought was given to the bearing of the specimens on the practical work in medicine which was to follow, and stress was laid upon those portions of human histology which previous experience has taught us are of the most importance in the appreciation and interpretation of the pathological alterations in disease. In the present status of pathological histology a knowledge of certain details is of much greater value than that of others; and for the student entering medicine, a judicious selection of what shall be given and what shall be left out should be made by some one who has had a more or less wide training in pathological histology.

"Further bearing in mind the life-work for which the student is preparing himself, we have not always chosen the method which would show the finest structural details of the tissues. While the most delicate methods have been introduced in places, we have endeavored to familiarize the students with a large number of different modes of preparation. The student who has been brought up entirely on 'gilt-edged' histological methods will find himself sadly at a loss in battling with the 'rough and ready' world in which the pathologist has to live." (Somewhat abridged.)

short, research, untrammeled by near reference to practical ends, will go on in every properly organized medical school; its critical method will dominate all teaching whatsoever; but undergraduate instruction will be throughout explicitly conscious of its professional end and aim. In no other way can all the sciences belonging to the medical curriculum be thoroughly kneaded. An active apperceptive relation must be established and maintained between laboratory and clinical experience. Such a relation cannot be one-sided; it will not spontaneously set itself up in the last two years if it is deliberately suppressed in the first two. There is no cement like interest, no stimulus like the hint of a coming practical application.[1]

Medical reference, in the sense that the laboratory sciences should, while freely presented, be kept conscious of their membership in the medical curriculum, has been discredited in this country, because it had so long meant a mechanical drill in an inert outline of the several sciences by untrained and busy practitioners. In the effort to teach the modicum of chemistry or physiology or pathology that "the family doctor needs to know," they neglected to teach anything of permanent scientific value at all. A revulsion was inevitable. It was supposed that the harm was due to the simple fact of medical reference. Such was not really the case. The sciences were badly taught, not merely because they were made prematurely and excessively conscious of medical application,—though such had indeed been the case,—but because the teachers lacked abundant scientific knowledge and spirit. Had they had these, the medical reference would neither have dominated nor impoverished their presentation. Our experience then furnishes a conclusive argument against delegating the teaching function to essentially unscientific practising physicians; it does not recommend the isolation of the laboratory sciences, locally or scientifically, from the clinical work. If it meant that, then institutions like the Johns Hopkins Medical School, in which laboratories and hospital are compactly organized from the standpoint of a scientific education in medicine, would labor under a positive disadvantage as compared with schools that, by reason of their situation, must in the scientific years forego the bedside and the autopsy altogether. In sober truth, four years are none too many thoroughly to saturate the student with medical enthusiasm and to give him the physician's standpoint; nor will laboratory and clinical ends make a genuine whole unless they have throughout a speaking acquaintance with each other.

Physiology and pathology belong, then, in the university, because there is much more to them as sciences than the medical school has time for. In so far, however, as they figure in medical education, they cannot be allowed to be indifferent to this definite function. "There must be an outlying division of workers who will keep the

[1] "An individual mind appropriates those new points of view and those fragments of knowledge that find in the mind fitting points of contact; but others that fail to meet with suitable receptors, to borrow a term from the modern theory of immunity, remain unattached and alien. The more thoroughly we can utilize existing interests and established relations, the more likely is our teaching to be real training." Letter from Professor Edwin O. Jordan, University of Chicago.

subject in touch with practical medicine, though the flower of the army, the imperial guard, are busy elsewhere."[1] This same consideration would appear conclusive as to the wisdom of crediting the medical student with such subjects when pursued in a college of liberal arts. Physiology, for instance, as an element of a liberal education, sweeps the whole horizon impartially, interested in genetic processes, searching for general laws. It works to best advantage with simple forms,—with jellyfish and cats in preference to man: an admirable introduction to medical physiology, but not really the same thing. It does not follow, therefore, that because professional studies are now freely counted toward the bachelor's degree, ordinary college work in physiology is equally satisfactory to the medical school. The academic purpose is vague; the professional purpose, distinct; and a medical education is more than the sum of its constituent courses taken separately and without reference to their ultimate object.[2]

So much for the point of view; certain general considerations affect equally instruction in all these laboratory sciences. The medical laboratories must be manned, equipped, and organized like university laboratories devoted to non-medical subjects. The laboratory staff consists necessarily of a chief—the professor in charge—with a corps of paid assistants, coöperating with him in the work of teaching, busy at other times with their problems, as he is with his, and with at least one intelligent departmental helper (*Diener*) who will relieve the staff of the care and handling of apparatus and material. The needs of pharmacology are in these respects not different from those of physics; and the pharmacologist can as little make the teaching of pharmacology a side issue to the practice of medicine or the conduct of a drug store as the physicist can subordinate his academic duties to the operation of a trolley line. Hardly less urgent is an adequate material equipment: class-rooms, laboratories for class use, private rooms adapted to the independent work of the staff, a reference library in regular receipt of important publications, and proper quarters for caring for an abundant and varied supply of animals.[3]

In methods of instruction there is, once more, nothing to distinguish medical from other sciences. Out-and-out didactic treatment is hopelessly antequated; it belongs

[1] W. H. Howell: "The Present Problems of Physiology," *Congress of Arts and Sciences*, vol. v. p. 434. More concretely, Professor F. S. Lee (Columbia University), in discussing the medical curriculum, wrote: "Many experiments of merely technical physiological interest should be omitted, especially those that have only a remote connection with human physiology.... [In physiological chemistry] pathological constituents [of tissues and secretions] and changes should be touched upon." Professor Matthews (University of Chicago) took the opposite position. "As soon as possible these sciences should follow the example of physics, botany, and chemistry and leave the medical faculty and be regarded as subjects prerequisite to the study of medicine." The analogy seems hardly valid; physics and chemistry are, from the standpoint of medicine, of merely instrumental value. The medical sciences are not simply instrumental; they deal with the actual phenomena and material which the physician handles. Professor Lee employs pathological cases to illustrate and enrich his course in physiology at Columbia. The contrast between normal and abnormal deepens the student's impression of both.

[2] The same problem presents itself in the German university. See Paulsen, *loc. cit.*, pp. 411, 412.

[3] An utterly mistaken notion prevails as to the extent to which animal experimentation is practised in this country. Only a very small minority of our medical schools use animals at all; as a matter of fact, ordinary medical teaching suffers seriously from the failure to employ them.

to an age of accepted dogma or supposedly complete information, when the professor "knew" and the students "learned." The lecture indeed continues of limited use. It may be employed in beginning a subject to orient the student, to indicate relations, to forecast a line of study in its practical bearings; from time to time, too, a lecture may profitably sum up, interpret, and relate results experimentally ascertained. Text-books, atlases, charts, occupy a similar position. They are not, in the first place, a substitute for sense experience, but they may well guide and fill out the student's laboratory findings. In general, the value of the recitation and of the quiz is in proportion to their concreteness and informality. Outside the workshop there is danger of detachment and rote.

The curriculum of a medical school, requiring for admission at least a competent knowledge of physics, chemistry, and biology, offers in the first two years systematic instruction in the following subjects:

First year: anatomy, including histology and embryology; physiology, including bio-chemistry..

Second year: pharmacology, pathology, bacteriology, physical diagnosis.

A brief discussion will show the relations of these subjects to each other and to the clinical work occupying the third and fourth years.

The order in which subjects are taken up is largely determined by considerations inherent in the subjects themselves. Anatomy—the study of the architecture of the body—comes logically first. It is indeed the oldest of laboratory sciences,[1] and so fundamental in medical study that for a time the student may well defer all other subjects whatsoever. For several centuries it was taught simply by professorial demonstration. During the first half of the nineteenth century, gross dissection by the students themselves was in vogue. The subject, long almost a closed book, has tremendously expanded in recent years. Embryology, histology, physiology, and pathology have given it back its youth; it is once more a green and flourishing science.[2] The anatomist carries a steadily increasing load. The surgeon, embarking on hitherto undreamed-of ventures; the clinician, guiding himself by physical indications involving the most delicate structural discrimination; the physiologist, the pharmacologist, the pathologist,—all lean upon him. With an eye to varied uses, the student must gain a picture of the body as a working whole; of its parts, taken severally and in their relations; and finally of the microscopic structure of tissues and organs. The teacher of anatomy may take one of two roads. He may attempt to forecast literally the special requirements of each of the above branches, confining his instruc-

[1] " For over six huⁿdred years there has been at least some practical instruction in anatomy, and for over three hundreⁿ years there have existed anatomical laboratories for purposes of teaching and investigation, although only those constructed during the present century (nineteenth) meet our ideas of what an anatomical laboratory should be." Welch : *The Evolution of Modern Scientific Laboratories: an Address delivered at the Opening of the William Pepper Laboratory, University of Pennsylvania,* Dec. 4, 1895.

[2] For an extremely readable account of the development of the science and teaching of anatomy, see "Anatomy in America," by C. R. Bardeen, *Bulletin of the University of Wisconsin,* no. 115.

tion to the indispensably useful thus arrived at; or he may handle his subject freely —not unmindful of its practical value, but with broad scientific background and sympathy. It needs no argument at this point to vindicate the latter policy. Dissection has therefore ceased to be synonymous with anatomy; for no one way of looking at or of dealing with the cadaver will enable the student to grasp even its gross structure. It is one thing to take the body to pieces; it is something else to conceive these severed and dissociated elements in stereoscopic relation; and it is a still further task to unravel the tissues themselves: hence, on the macroscopic side, the prominence now given to reconstruction through drawing and modeling, and the close study of charts and of cross-sections, of models and of special preparations that form the indispensable teaching museum. Courses in histology and embryology, closely correlated with gross anatomy, furnish the accompanying microscopical discipline. Something like one-fifth of all the available time of the entire medical curriculum[1] is commonly absorbed by the various branches constituting a modern department of anatomy. How much of this may be profitably spent in the lecture-room is yet under discussion. It needs perhaps still to be emphasized that description is no substitute for tactile and visual experience, and that such experience, if intelligently controlled, both records and organizes itself with surprisingly little formal revamping.

Outside of anatomy, the laboratory method in medicine is considerably less than a century old. Its rapid spread has been in conservative quarters decried as a fad; but the facts suggest a nobler view. For the century which has developed medical laboratories has seen the death-rate reduced by one-half and the average expectation of life increased by ten or twelve years.[2] Of these laboratories, physiology had the first, that of Purkinje, at Breslau, established in 1824. In general, the experimental physiologist has proceeded upon the hypothesis that physiology is the physics and chemistry of living matter. He employs the apparatus and procedure of the physical laboratory to study the mechanical properties of tissue and the physical conditions to which these properties respond. The mechanism of the nervous system, the circulation, respiration, assimilation, muscular activity, lend themselves more or less readily to description and interpretation from the physical point of view. The apparatus and procedure of the chemical laboratory have been brought to bear in the analysis of bodily tissues, fluids, and secretions, and in the experimental reproduction of digestive and other processes. Not infrequently the subject is presented in two divisions, the former called physiology, the latter physiological- or bio-chemistry. That the mechanical standpoint has richly justified itself is indisputable; nevertheless, so far as concerns medical education, it is not yet ready wholly to absorb the functional point of view. An unbridged gap exists. Whether the physical sciences will ever so far refine their procedure as altogether to resolve function in mechanical

[1] Between 3600 and 4000 hours of instruction make up the entire curriculum.
[2] Welch: *University of Chicago Record*, vol. xii., no. 3, p. 79.

terms, it is needless here to discuss. Such an outcome is at any rate more distant than the early investigators, in the first flush of their splendid successes, supposed:

"*For long the way appears which seemed so short
To the less practised eye of early youth.*"

Meanwhile, whatever its limitations, the physiological laboratory is of immense educational importance to the prospective physician. Physiology is, in a sense, the central discipline of the medical school.[1] It is the business of the physician to restore normal functioning: normal functioning is thus his starting-point in thought, his goal in action. The physiological laboratory enables the beginner to observe the functions of the body in operation and to ascertain how they are affected by varying conditions, —a wholesome discipline for two reasons: it banishes from his mind metaphysical principles, such as vital force, depression, etc.; it tends, in exhibiting the infinite sublety and complexity of the physiological mechanism, to emphasize normal conditions rather than medication as ultimately responsible for its orderly working. The student who has been successfully trained to regard the body as an infinitely complex machine learns to doubt his capacity to mend it summarily. It is true he lacks time to master any considerable part of the field which experimentation has covered from this point of view; but characteristic and pregnant illustrations at least insure his sanity. He may do ever so little, yet for that little he cannot take anyone's word. His actual contact with facts puts him squarely on his feet and cures him once for all of mystical and empiric vagaries.

Anatomy and physiology form but the vestibule of medical education. They teach the normal structure of the body, the normal function of the parts, fluids, organs, and the conditions under which they operate. The next step carries the student *in medias res;* he begins pharmacology,[2]—the experimental study of the response of the body to medication.

The science got its problem in the first place from the credulity of which the traditional pharmacopoeia is the encyclopedic expression. It undertook to question the complacency and vagueness of the empiric. How far was his reliance upon specific agents justified? If at all, was it possible to ascertain the source of their efficiency and its limits?

Pharmacology was thus originally negative and critical. It rapidly pruned away exaggeration and superstition, leaving, however, a vigorous growth behind. It ascertained, for example, that quinine was administered in vain nine times out of ten; but that in the single condition in which it was applicable—malaria—it struck at the root of the disease by actually destroying in the blood the obnoxious parasite. The limits of the effectiveness of digitalis, atropine, strychnine, have been discovered and explained; and similarly, the utter uselessness of dozens of concoctions with which

[1] About 450 hours of instruction are devoted to it on the average, in the best schools.
[2] The first laboratory of experimental pharmacology was that of Rudolph Buchheim in Dorpat, 1849.

the digestive capacity of the race has long been taxed. Intelligence has thus been introduced into a realm for ages unguardedly open to ignorance and recklessness.

The science did not long remain merely critical: the development of chemistry and experimental physiology created a positive opportunity. Given, in a word, this or that condition,—a disease, a symptom, or pain itself,—cannot an agent be devised capable of combating it? Cocaine, the antipyretics, the various glandular preparations, and serum therapy are among the affirmative replies that witness the constructive possibilities of pharmacodynamics. The strictly experimental science, thus richly rewarded, has reinforced physiological conceptions independently at work in the effort to rationalize materia medica and therapeutics. Instead of naïve reliance upon poly-pharmacy, diseases and their attendant symptoms have now been divided into some half-dozen provisional classes, subject to continuous revision, according to the method of attack to which they are at the moment most accessible. There are those that drugs actually combat,—syphilis and malaria, for example; next, the self-limited diseases, in the course of which therapeutic measures may be used to avert dangerous symptomatic consequences,—as bathing reduces the temperature in typhoid, as chloroform checks convulsions in strychnine poisoning, as morphine relieves mere pain. There are those in which the body's natural methods of defense may be hastened or strengthened, as through serum therapy; those in which our only reliance thus far is on environment or suggestion; and finally, those in which summary relief may be had through the surgeon. A great change, this, from indiscriminate and largely ignorant dosing! The body diseased is indeed like a city besieged. No single form of military manœuvre can be prescribed as a sure defense; now a sally from the main gate discomfits the enemy; again, a diversion from some unexpected quarter; sometimes the inhabitants conserve their strength in the hope of wearing the enemy out, feeding the soldiers at the expense of all the others; and sometimes, as in tuberculosis, there is no hope except by actually decamping, leaving a vacant Moscow to a cheated foe.

In the university, pharmacology has critically an extensive, creatively an apparently boundless, opportunity. The medical student can at best browse the field here and there. But as was found to be the case with experimental physiology, he cannot forego that opportunity, limited though it be. The young doctor's therapeutic environment is still distinctly unfavorable. He is exposed to danger, front and rear. The traditions of the profession are in the main crudely empiric; they embody a "pop-gun pharmacy, hitting now the malady and again the patient, the doctor himself not knowing which."[1] Besides, the practitioner is subjected, year in, year out, to the steady bombardment of the unscrupulous manufacturer, persuasive to the uncritical, on the principle that "what I tell you three times is true."[2] Against bad

[1] Osler, *Aequanimitas*, p. 127.
[2] "On a basis of 5000 prescriptions examined, 47 per cent are for proprietary medicines." M. G. Motter, in *Bull. Amer. Acad. Med.*, vol. ix., no. 1.

example and persistent asseveration, only precise scientific concepts and a critical appreciation of the nature and limits of actual demonstration can protect the young physician. The laity has in this matter more to fear from credulous doctors than from advertisements themselves: for a nostrum containing dangerous drugs is doubly dangerous if introduced into the household by the prescription of a physician who knows nothing of its composition and is misled as to its effect.[1] Experimental physiology and pharmacology must train the student both to doubt unwarranted claims and to be open to really authoritative suggestion: for it is equally important to reject humbug and to accept truth. Fortunately, even a brief concrete experience may teach one to be wary in weighing evidence.

The course in pharmacology need include, therefore, actual experimental determination by the student himself of the effect on animals of a relatively small number of carefully selected agents; demonstration of others by the instructor; and a critical survey of the rest by means of lectures and recitations.[2] Materia medica, now much shrunken, need concern itself only with the pharmaceutical side, aiming to familiarize the student with drugs of proved power and the most agreeable and effective forms in which these may be administered. Therapeutics subsequently adds to these agents whatever other resources the clinician has accumulated,—baths, electricity, massage, psychic suggestion, dietetics, etc.,—approaching the subject from the standpoint of disease, as opposed to the pharmacological approach from the standpoint of the drug itself.

The last division of the medical sciences—and the most extensive—includes pathology and bacteriology. The three subdivisions of pathology are symmetrical with anatomy, physiology, and physiological chemistry. To the first corresponds pathological anatomy; to the second, pathological physiology; to the third, chemical pathology.

In its modern form the study began on a comprehensive basis when Virchow, called from Würzburg, established the first pathological institute in Berlin in 1856. His plans went far beyond the gross morbid anatomy then current. He conceived pathology not only as a descriptive but as an experimental science, whose laws are the laws of general biology. The pathological is not, in this view, an anarchic, extralegal freak; it is the product of agencies and forces, operating on regular and inevitable lines. The problem of the pathologist is through observation and experiment to get the key to the pathological process, in order that he may understand its origin and significance, and, if necessary, avert or control it. The pathological is abnormal from the standpoint, not of biological law, but of the human interests that it sometimes thwarts—sometimes, only; for not infrequently it is a beneficent, compensa-

---

[1] See *The Propaganda for Reform in Proprietary Medicines*, published by the American Medical Association, Chicago, Ill.

[2] On the average, about 150 hours are devoted to instruction in pharmacology; something more than half of these can be given to the laboratory, the remainder to recitations.

tory adjustment, actually favorable to the individual. Experimental pathology has developed along both biological and chemical lines: the former, accentuating the life-history of the abnormal growth, the latter, endeavoring to trace back the changes observed to the chemical activities involved in the life-process. Somewhat recently, a shifting of emphasis has made the physiological point of view more prominent,— a wholesome development, medically speaking. The physician is constantly in contact with disease processes that he is unable to correlate with the accompanying structural modifications. Occasionally the surgeon throws a stream of light upon such a situation; too often, all is dark until the autopsy reveals the truth. Pathological physiology aims to study structural change from the standpoint of function. It asks primarily not what is the history of the structural modification itself, but what are its progressive consequences to the functional routine of the organism. It reproduces disease experimentally, interrupting its course at significant stages, in order, having observed the functional disturbance, to ascertain exactly the structural readjustment that corresponds. "In animals," says Professor Hektoen, "the course of disease may be cut short at any time for the purpose of investigation. The disease may be studied in all its phases. Comparative pathology became the refuge of the investigator, blocked by the necessary restrictions governing the study of human diseases. The great influence of the comparative method is shown in the relatively advanced state of our knowledge in regard to human diseases readily communicable to animals, as compared with our ignorance in regard to other human diseases which, so far as we know, are not transferable to animals."[1] For the prospective physician the value of such a course depends, of course, on the opportunity to compare the laboratory findings with the symptoms shown by patients in the hospital wards.

In general, the effective teaching of pathology is dependent on ease and frequency of access to the autopsy-room. It would be difficult just now to over-emphasize that point. We shall soon see that the post-mortem is in this country relatively rare and precarious; that not infrequently pathological courses are organized and given whose illustrative material is limited to models, to a small number of preserved specimens, or even to bits of material already cut into microscopic sections or just lacking that last touch. Such instruction may do justice to the subject on the histological side, but it leaves much to the already overburdened third and fourth years. And it is surely a serious disadvantage to the teacher of pathology to find himself year after year teaching the subject without access to the post-mortem room.

Specimens alone—whether gross or microscopic—are inadequate for several reasons. In the first place, gross fresh specimens are too perishable: they change quickly after removal from the body and in consequence of handling during transportation; refrigeration avoids softening and putrefaction only at the cost of destroying the blood,—a most important link in the chain. More important still, however, is the consideration that disease is not an affair of a single organ or tissue, still less, of a

[1] *Congress of Arts and Sciences*, vol. vi. pp. 112, 113 (slightly abridged).

microscopic portion of such organ or tissue. Even an acute disease—pneumonia, diphtheria—involves the body as a whole; chronic defects—such as heart lesion or cancer—affect the organism likewise in its entire extent. The pathologist, then, seeking to convey to the student an objective conception of the nature and effects of disease as a process, needs the entire body in order to do so. Pathology is taught for that purpose; it fails of its object just so far as the lack of autopsies makes it impossible. Cancer, for example, is not a local disturbance involving this or that organ. The student who is expected to grasp its character cannot do so if all he does is to see a cross-section put up in gelatine, or to handle a papier-maché reproduction, or to observe the cell changes on a small slide. These things are well enough as far as they go, but they go only a short distance. The cancerous process is complicated and extensive. Other organs, far from the original site of the disease, are involved; nay, the original site itself may be in question. The vastness of the involvements, the relationships of affected locations to each other, the response of the bodily mechanism fighting to achieve a readjustment—only the autopsy can disclose these; and without them, the student cannot attain an intelligent conception of the subject he is studying.

Pathology's greatest contribution to the comprehension and mastery of disease has been by way of illuminating its causation,—or etiology. The student who is to comprehend the significance of disease must not only make the inventory of results disclosed by the post-mortem: he should be allowed to observe the process from the very start. To this end, a demonstrative course, using living animals, must be provided. Tuberculosis, for example, should be exhibited through the inoculation of a few guinea pigs with different varieties of the tubercle bacilli, showing the various ways in which the bacilli enter and are distributed, and the variety of lesions that they produce.

We thus cross the threshold of still another science, bacteriology, developed in late years in close sympathy with pathology. It presents the same two sides,—biological and chemical; the former investigating the life-history of the microscopic organism, the latter isolating and resolving its toxic or other products. The search of the pathologist for the original causation of abnormal structural change has been immensely facilitated by the bacteriologist. He can now account for as well as describe the ravaged tissues that mark the path of a diphtheritic, typhoid, or tuberculous infection. Out of the life-history of the parasites in question has sprung the serum therapy, which has already stripped tetanus, diphtheria, and meningitis of much of their horror.

Perhaps even more important than its services to curative, have been the suggestions of bacteriology to preventive, medicine. It is hardly too much to say that modern hygiene, largely the outcome of bacteriology, has elevated the physician from a mainly personal to a mainly social status. Directly or indirectly, disease has been found to depend largely on unpropitious environment. A bad water-supply, defective drainage, impure food, unfavorable occupational surroundings,—matters, all of them, for social regulation,—at once harbor our parasitic enemies and reduce our powers of resisting them. To the intelligent and conscientious physician, a typhoid patient is not only a case, but a warning: his office it is equally to heal the sick and to protect the well. The public health laboratory belongs, then, under the wing of the medical school. It is the clearing-house into which data from an entire state should pour. Tax-supported institutions are most favorably circumstanced in this respect. The material which they readily accumulate is at once a basis for teaching, for investigation, and for practical sanitation. Thus the laboratory sciences all culminate and come together in the hygienic laboratory; out of which emerges the young physician, equipped with sound views as to the nature, causation, spread, prevention, and cure of disease, and with an exalted conception of his own duty to promote social conditions that conduce to physical well-being.

From the standpoint of medical education, a detached academic or scientific treatment of pathology and bacteriology would sacrifice needlessly much of their value. Both subjects are, indeed, full-grown biological sciences,—university subjects, capable of cultivation only in special laboratories, closely affiliated with general biology and chemistry. But the medical student in the brief five hundred hours which he can at most secure for them gains the clearest insight into their philosophy and their bearing by following out their principles mainly in the small group of phenomena illustrated in human disease. Experimental pathology concerns him because it enables him later to conceive his clinical problems intelligently. From an early hour in his pathological work, the student may then begin in the autopsy-room to saturate himself with the clinical spirit. This is not to be confused with the premature "cutting" or the impatient "prescribing" to which the old-fashioned medical student was addicted. "Cutting" and "prescribing" may still be two years distant; but meanwhile it is both possible and "important to keep ever before the student the part which the work he is doing plays in leading to a more complete comprehension of disease."[1]

One closes a brief review of the medical sciences with a feeling akin to dismay. So much remains to find out, so much is already known,—how futile to orient the student from either standpoint! Practically, however, there is no ground for despair. Enough can be achieved to give him precise conceptions in each of the realms touched upon; and the actual value of these conceptions and of the habits grounded on them depends less on the extent of his acquisitions than on his sense of their reality.[2] Didactic information, like mere hearsay, leaves this sense pale and ineffective; a first-

[1] Report of Committee on Pathology, Council on Education, Amer. Med. Assn., *Bulletin of Amer. Med. Assn.*, Sept. 15, 1909, p. 47.

[2] That method rather than any particular content is the very essence of scientific discipline is admirably pointed out by Professor Dewey in his address "Science as Subject-matter and as Method," *Science*, xxxi., no. 787, p. 122. "Science has been taught too much as an accumulation of ready-made material, with which students are to be made familiar, not enough as a method of thinking, an attitude of mind, after the pattern of which mental habits are to be transformed."

hand experience, be it ever so fragmentary, renders it vivid. After a strenuous laboratory discipline, the student will still be ignorant of many things, but at any rate he will respect facts: he will have learned how to obtain them and what to do with them when he has them.

NOTE

For the details of a course of study, framed on the lines above described, the reader is referred to the following:

A. GENERAL

1. Report of Curriculum Committee, Council on Education, American Medical Association, *Bulletin of the Amer. Med. Assn.*, September, 1909.
2. *What Constitutes a Medical Curriculum?* Issued by Association of American Medical Colleges.
3. COLWELL, N. P.: In *Bulletin of American Academy of Medicine*, vol. x., no. 3.
4. BILLROTH, T.: *Ueber Lehren und Lernen in Medicin.*
5. BICKEL, ADOLF: *Wie Studiert man Medizin?* (Stuttgart, 1906).

B. SPECIAL SUBJECTS

1. *Anatomy.*

BARKER, L. F., and BARDEEN, C. R.: Outline of Course in Normal Histology and Microscopic Anatomy, *Johns Hopkins Hospital Bulletin*, vol. xii., nos. 62, 63.

BARKER, L. F., and KYES, P.: On Teaching of Normal Anatomy of Central Nervous System to Large Classes of Medical Students, *Proc. Assn. Amer. Anat.*, 1900.

BARKER, L. F.: Study of Anatomy, *Journal Amer. Med. Assn.*, March, 1901.

DWIGHT, T.: Methods of Teaching Anatomy at Harvard Medical School, *Boston Med. and Surg. Journal*, vol. cxxiv. pp. 457–77.

HUNTINGTON, G. S.: The Teaching of Anatomy, *Columbia University Bulletin*, 1898.

KEILLER, W.: On Preservation of Subjects for Dissection, etc., *Amer. Jour. Anat.*, 1902–3, vol. ii.

McMURRICK, J. P.: Conservatism in Anatomy, *Anat. Record*, vol. iii., no. 1.

MALL, F. P.: The Anatomical Course and Laboratory at Johns Hopkins University, *Johns Hopkins Hospital Bulletin*, vol. vii., nos. 62, 63.

MALL, F. P.: On Teaching Anatomy, etc., *Ibid.*, vol. xvi., no. 167.

MALL, F. P.: On the Teaching of Anatomy, *Anat. Record*, vol. ii., no. 8.

MOODY, R. C.: On the Use of Clay Modelling in the Study of Osteology, *Johns Hopkins Hospital Bulletin*, 1903, vol. xiv.

2. *Physiology.*

PORTER, W. T.: The Teaching of Physiology in Medical Schools, *Boston Med. and Surg. Journal*, December 29, 1898.

CHITTENDEN, R. H.: The Importance of Physiological Chemistry as a Part of Medical Education, *N. Y. Med. Journal*, September 30, 1898.

BOWDITCH, H. P.: The Study of Physiology, *Univ. Pa. Med. Bulletin*, June, 1904.

HOWELL, W. H.: Instruction in Physiology in Med. Schools, *The Michigan Alumnus*, January, 1900.

LEE, F. S.: Physiology (Series: Lectures on Science, Philosophy and Art, Columbia Univ. Press, 1909).

3. Pharmacology.

ABEL, J. J.: On the Teaching of Pharmacology, Materia Medica, and Therapeutics, *Phila. Med. Jour.*, September 1, 1900.

SOLLMAN, T.: The Teaching of Therapeutics and Pharmacology from the Experimental Standpoint, *Jour. Amer. Med. Assn.*, September 6, 1902.

4. Pathology and Bacteriology.

ADAMI, J. G.: On the Teaching of Pathology, *Phila. Med. Jour.*, 1900, pp. 399–402.

DELEPINE, A. S.: On the Place of Pathology in Medical Education, *Brit. Med. Jour.*, 1896, vol. ii.

JORDAN, E. O.: Place of Pathology in the University, *Jour. Amer. Med. Assn.*, 1907, vol. xlviii. p. 917.

BARKER, L. F.: On Methods of Studying Pathology, *Amer. Text-Book of Path.*, Philadelphia, 1901.

5. Hygiene.

DITMAN, N. E.: Education and its Economic Value in the Field of Preventive Medicine, *Columbia University Quarterly*, vol. x., supplement to no. 3, June, 1908.

WINSLOW, C. E. A.: Teaching of Biology and Sanitary Science in the Massachusetts Institute of Technology, *Tech. Quarterly*, vol. xix., no. 4, December, 1906.

WESBROOK, F. F.: The Laboratory in Public Health Work, *Twelfth Biennial Report of Iowa State Board of Health*.

WESBROOK, F. F.: The Public Health Laboratory, *Jour. Amer. Med.*, vol. xi., no. 9.

CHAPTER V

THE COURSE OF STUDY: THE LABORATORY BRANCHES

(B) First and Second Years (continued)

With the preceding characterization, the schools included in our first division [1] on the whole agree. They are all organic parts of full-fledged universities; their medical courses are as a rule constructed upon the basis of adequate pre-medical scientific training. In general, the laboratories of institutions upon a college basis reflect university ideals in equipment, management, and appearance.[2] As a rule these institutions have at least four separate laboratories, for anatomy, physiology and bio-chemistry, pharmacology, pathology and bacteriology. As their resources have grown, the departments have tended to increase by subdivision: histology, physiological chemistry, clinical pathology, bacteriology, attain departmental stature. Hygiene is especially prominent at the state universities, where effective departments of public health bring the laboratories of pathology and bacteriology into fruitful relation with local authorities and the local profession throughout the state; and endowed schools are making determined efforts to develop departments of preventive medicine. In some cases abundant, in several others increasing, facilities are offered in all branches for both teaching and research; and teaching and research permeate each other. The various departments, in intimate communication with each other and with the general science work of the institution, are officered each by its own full-time professor, in most instances with a more or less satisfactory corps of paid assistants. Within these active hives of scientific interest a thoroughly charming relation prevails: a vigorous, stimulating, and appreciative chief, on the one hand, enjoying the coöperation of enthusiastic young disciples on the other. It is difficult to realize that so substantial an organization is so recent,—hardly more than a half-century old in Germany, less than twenty years old in America. In this brief period the earlier subordinates have themselves become departmental heads in their own schools, or have gone forth to found or to reconstruct distant institutions. Laboratories have increased in number so rapidly that the rewards of early promise or of early performance have been alike great and prompt. It is unlikely that this pace will permanently keep up.

In anatomy and physiology it occasionally occurs that the departmental head is not himself a graduate in medicine.[3] This innovation arises out of a dual motive: it

---

[1] i.e., those requiring for entrance two or more years of college work; a list of them is given on page 28.

[2] A few of these, formerly on a lower basis, have elevated their entrance requirements, while leaving facilities as they were. Several schools are pledged to higher entrance requirements, though quite unable to improve their facilities. Indeed, as higher standards mean fewer students and reduced income, their facilities may suffer deterioration.

[3] Occasionally the dean of a medical school is a non-medical man. In such cases it is extremely important that he be in close sympathy with the clinical side and well acquainted with modern developments in clinical teaching. Even more dangerous is the expedient of making a professor in the academic department dean of the medical department.

represents a reaction from the superficial methods of the practitioner professor, as well as a realization of the essential continuity of medical with biological science. The non-medical professor is not necessarily indifferent to explicit medical reference; his department need not lack sympathy with medicine merely because he has no M.D. degree; and his disinterested attitude is in any event indispensable. But the experiment is not free from danger, and its outcome will be watched with interest. Meanwhile, there is no question that these posts cannot be satisfactorily filled by active physicians. The practitioner usually lacks impartial and eager scientific spirit; he can at best give set hours to teaching, and these are not infrequently interrupted by a patient's superior claim; of course he has little or no time and rarely any zest for research. Western Reserve and the New York City department of Cornell, alone of schools of this rank, continue an active surgeon in the chair of anatomy.

Of the twenty-five institutions either now, or by the fall of 1910 to be, on the two-year college basis, or more, fourteen[1] offer the entire four-year course in one organized institution; five[2] are divided, offering the laboratory branches in one place and the clinical branches, more or less independently organized, in another, sometimes close by, at other times widely separated; six[3] are half-schools, offering only the work of the first and second years. The complete school in touch with the rest of the university represents the normal and correct form. The study of medicine must center around disease in concrete, individual forms. The ease with which the clinics and the laboratories may there illuminate each other is an incontestable advantage to both. It is difficult to imagine effective teaching of pathology, for example, under conditions where the operating-room, the medical clinic, and the autopsy do not constantly contribute specimens and propound queries to the laboratory; and assuredly the teaching of medicine and surgery cannot proceed intelligently without constant intercourse with the laboratories. Any disintegration of hospitals and laboratories is harmful to both, — and to the student, in shaping whom they must coöperate. So important is organic wholeness that the remote department, if entire, is from all points of view preferable to division. The initial difficulty — that of sharing the university ideals — may be met by liberal provision for intercourse with the academic body and by redoubled efforts to maintain creative activity, as Cornell, for example, has done at New York. Fortunately, our needs in respect to medical

[1] Johns Hopkins, Harvard, Western Reserve, Minnesota, Cornell (New York City department), Yale, Michigan, Indiana (Indianapolis department), Iowa, Pennsylvania, Syracuse, Columbia, Dartmouth, Colorado. Of these, two are not located in the same town as the university, — Cornell (New York City), Indiana (Indianapolis).

[2] Rush Medical College (of which, though both parts are in Chicago, the first two years belong to the University of Chicago, and the last two, given elsewhere in the city, are only affiliated with it), California (first and second years at Berkeley, third and fourth at San Francisco and Los Angeles), Nebraska (first and second years at Lincoln, third and fourth at Omaha), Kansas (first and second years at Lawrence, third and fourth at Rosedale), Stanford (first and second years at Palo Alto, third and fourth at San Francisco).

[3] Wisconsin, Missouri, South Dakota, North Dakota, Utah, Wake Forest. Cornell repeats the first year at Ithaca; Indiana duplicates the first and second years at Bloomington.

schools can be met without considerable resort to either the divided or the remote department.[1]

The divided school begins by inheriting a serious problem. Its laboratory end, situated at the university, has been recently constituted of modern men; the clinical end, situated in a city at some distance, is usually what is left of the old-fashioned school which the university adopted in taking on its medical department.[2] In such cases, there are practically two schools with a formal connection; such is essentially the situation in California, Kansas, and Nebraska. In course of time these clinical faculties will be reconstituted of men of more modern stamp. But the separation of the clinical branch, with the increasing absorption of the teachers in practice, involves constant danger of fresh alienation. The clinical professor of the university is very apt to be a busy physician; and if so, pedagogical and scientific ideals are all the more easily crowded into a narrow corner, when he does not breathe the bracing atmosphere of adjacent laboratories. In time, a more exacting pedagogical code and increased sensitiveness to real scientific distinction may to some extent correct the tendency. Meanwhile, these institutions, so long as they continue, require much more vigorous administrative supervision than they have anywhere received. A dean, moving freely between the two branches, and frequent opportunities for social and scientific intercourse between scientific and clinical faculties, may throw a more or less unsteady bridge across the gap. But there is little reason to believe that the divided school will ever function as an organic whole, though it may be tolerable as a halfway stage on the road from the proprietary school to the complete university department. "I cannot help wondering," said President Pritchett,[3] "how it would affect the pedagogic and professional ideals of an engineering school if its first two years were given in one place and the last two years in a place two hundred miles away. My impression is that there would be two separate schools with very little more reaction, the one upon the other, than exists between any other two schools so located." Thus far the difficulty seems hardly to have been suspected: the dean of Nebraska at Lincoln is a busy professor who has no real hold on the clinical men at Omaha; the dean of California is superintendent of the hospital in San Francisco, with no real control of what goes on at Berkeley, and surely without any possible control over the second clinical department at Los Angeles; Kansas practically accepts the split by setting up a dean at each of the two ends, though they are only an hour and a half apart; Mississippi, with even better reason, does the same, for the journey from Oxford to Vicksburg, not great when measured in miles, takes the better part of a day even if one is lucky enough to make the necessary railroad connections.

The problem of the half-school is different. The two-year school originated in

[1] See chapter ix.

[2] In a measure, also still true of some of the complete schools; but the constant contact of laboratory and clinical men tends gradually to bring the edges together.

[3] Address : "The Obligations of the University to Medical Education," before Council on Education, American Medical Association, Feb. 28, 1910 (*Journal A. M. A.*, vol. liv. p. 1109).

institutional expediency; but it may prove of actual pedagogical importance. When Columbia and Michigan arranged that the four years of the A.B. course might contain two years of the M.D. course, institutions lacking medical departments were impelled to offer just enough of the medical curriculum to meet the competition. The half-school thus avoids loss of time to the student and loss of students to the university. The arrangement took advantage of the break in the middle between the laboratory and the clinical years; but a deeper reason made the experiment feasible.

The bachelor's course has under modern conditions a double aim: it is simultaneously cultural and vocational. The sciences fundamental to medicine have obviously both characters: they are vocational to the extent that they are instrumentally indispensable; they are cultural, as is all enlarging and releasing experience, whether of men, books, or travel. Culture is indeed in this aspect an incidental value of all novel experience. So far, then, the combined course may be fairly said to be feasible, because it enriches the college curriculum; and the college may do well to offer the opportunity.

Is the scheme equally sound from the standpoint of medical education? The professional and cultural standpoints, though obviously overlapping, are not identical. The professional purpose involves greater concentration, is on the lookout for definite correlations, and steers towards an evident practical goal. The medical curriculum possesses a certain organic unity in virtue of the fact that each of its parts does this same thing. The college as college is indifferent to the ultimate practical bearing; the medical school cannot afford to forget it. As to certain subjects, indeed, there is perhaps little to choose. The college has already taken chemistry wholly out of the medical curriculum; it may be allowed to take bio-chemistry, too. In reference, however, to other subjects, pathology, physiology, etc., it is important—once more from the standpoint of medical education—to distinguish between two forms which the combined course assumes. To take advantage of it at Columbia or Michigan—complete four-year schools—the student goes over into the medical department, which is compactly organized with laboratories and clinics interwoven. He spends the entire period of four years there. The college has nothing to do with it beyond registering his credits for the first two years towards his A.B. degree. That fact makes absolutely no difference to the medical teachers. The student is trained for four years just as he would be trained if he had his A.B. degree to start with. The combined course in this form exacts no sacrifice from the medical school.

In the case of the half-school or the divided school the situation is different: the medical subjects are apt to be parceled out among the general scientific laboratories, and there are no clinics or clinicians at all. The professors themselves may lack medical training. There is no observable goal to steady or beckon the teacher.[1] Counting

[1] The medical department of the University of Wisconsin, a half-school, combats the difficulty by appointing a professor of clinical medicine.

the two years' work as the latter half of the A.B. course may, under these circumstances, distinctly weaken it from the medical standpoint. It is, of course, true that the German medical schools are without the sort of organization we are now emphasizing; but they have what we lack, ideals and traditions. Dispersion does not cost them their point of view. When our ideals are as sound, we too may be capable of dispensing with a more or less formal organization. Some of our schools may already be.[1] Would it, however, be equally safe even in Germany, if there were no clinics at all?

Take, for instance, the subject of pathology. The two-year school, remote from hospitals and autopsies, can provide museum specimens, models, and microscopic mounts. Under favorable conditions, animal experimentation can still further supplement its resources. But the pathologist will suffer from isolation; he is part of the college, but not part of a hospital, and what is hurtful to him cannot be helpful to his students. For them much depends on the arrangement of courses in the institution to which they emigrate for their third and fourth years. Meanwhile, in any case, at the fateful moment of their introduction to the subject, however admirably they may have been drilled in the specific content of the course, little advantage can be taken of their general absorptive power. For even a fair student, while learning his lessons in pathological histology, might assimilate incidentally much that goes beyond. Not infrequently what is most stimulating in his experience would be thus obtained. It would appear, then, that, while the college will surely gain, it is not certain that the medical curriculum may not lose when the first and second years are separated or detached.

There would be the less necessity for the cautious attitude here taken in reference to the two-year school if these departments were everywhere organized, as they have been by Wisconsin, Cornell, Missouri, and Indiana, with a keen appreciation of the difficulties to be surmounted and with financial resources capable of coping with them. Apparatus, books, animals, laboratory material, must be provided in abundance. In the institutions above mentioned they are. Too frequently, however, apparatus is limited, books are scarce, animals hard to get, running expenses reduced to a mere pittance. Skilled assistants and competent helpers may also be lacking. The teachers are young and well trained; but their professorial salaries are paid to them in part for menial labor. They care for apparatus, get it out, put it away, prepare all demonstrations and experiments, and clean up after class. Be the students ever so few, routine drudgery and isolation will wear out the enthusiasm of their instructors. The men will grow stale, the department sterile. As the two-year schools now generally require two years of college work for entrance, they cannot be parsimoniously organized. Yet their rapid spread seems to indicate a mistaken notion that the laboratory years can safely be conducted on a small scale at comparatively slight expense.

[1] For an extremely lucid and able discussion from this point of view see the *Harvard Bulletin*, Nov. 3, 1909: "Education in Medicine: The Relations of the Medical School to the College."

A uniform or fixed apportionment between various subjects is in schools of the highest grade neither feasible nor desirable. The endeavor to improve medical education through iron-clad prescription of curriculum or hours is a wholly mistaken effort; while mechanical regulation cannot essentially improve the poorer schools, it may very seriously hamper competent institutions. There is no one way to study medicine, still less one way to advance it. If the teaching is in inferior hands, printed directions will not save it. The prescribed curriculum is a staff upon which those lean who have not strength to walk alone.

Fortunately, current practice varies widely. The Johns Hopkins, for example, offers 700 hours' instruction in anatomy, of which about 400 are required, Harvard 427; Rush gives 108 hours to histology, Cornell 265; Columbia requires 490 hours in anatomy, embryology, and histology; Harvard gives 513 hours to pathology, Western Reserve 304. These discrepancies are of slight importance, for the medical curriculum is throughout constituted of overlapping parts: apparent deficiencies in one subject are supplied in another. Physiology revises and mends anatomy, and the clinical years may be safely relied on to build out here and there the details of pathology. A certain carefully selected, irreducible minimum in each subject must of course be common throughout these institutions; the rest may be left open, to vary from school to school, and within each school to vary to some extent with different individuals. The medical school is above collegiate grade; it is a professional school on a college basis. Its students are presumably mature and will doubtless prove increasingly well trained. They are fit to be trusted with a certain degree of discretion, in a field within which selection between alternatives of equal importance must in any event take place. The fourth year at Harvard is left open to choice; at Johns Hopkins one-fourth of each year is subject to election; intensive study at certain points is encouraged without endangering the fundamentals common to all. The problem of medical education and orientation is not otherwise manageable. In the effort to force every important subject as it has developed into the common curriculum — be it ever so inadequately — the average curriculum now calls for something like 4000 hours of prescribed work. The demand is an impossible one.[1] It originates partly in the effort to make the medical school repair the omissions of preliminary education; higher standards will relegate something at least to the high school and college, and so far relieve congestion. As for the rest, we require a modified conception of what any sort of school can and ought to attempt. The mature student, competently guided, needs not to be policed like the "breeching scholar in the schools." His every moment must not be preëmpted by an assigned task. Von Strümpell rebukes the same tendency in Germany: "Somewhat more rarely in the first, very often, however, in the later semesters, many students hear lectures for eight to ten hours a day. From morning to night their time is taken up with classes; they rush out of one lecture hall into another, hearing a huge mass of facts and theories put forward. One can readily imagine the condition inside their

[1] A large percentage of students are making up preliminary "conditions" besides.

heads by the time night comes. The actual outcome of this absurd overcrowding is that only a small amount of what is heard is retained. One can profitably listen only when one can take in readily and follow up systematically with work at home."[1]

The maturity of the student body at this level makes possible another innovation. The low standard or immature type of medical student must have his medical knowledge carefully administered in homeopathic doses. He carries a half-dozen studies simultaneously because his untutored interest fatigues easily and his assimilative ability in any one direction is relatively slight. Time and energy are of course lost in hourly breaking off one connection and making another. But it is unavoidable; the practitioner teacher must leave at the close of his "hour" anyhow. At the university studies may be concentrated. The laboratories are open all day; the professors are there at work.[2] The first months of the medical curriculum are then given over to anatomy alone; for it is clearly illogical to begin even physiology till the anatomist has made some headway. Concentration[3] is economical of time and energy, and stimulates the student to push on beyond definitely prescribed limits. How far it can wisely be carried is a point to be determined by experiment.

The schools of our second division — those requiring for admission high school graduation or the "equivalent" — move within narrower limits. Two factors are at work. Most schools of this class live on their fees; McGill, Toronto, Tulane, are among the few that are enabled by additional resources to provide a complete laboratory outfit. The strongest of the others, Jefferson and Northwestern University, for example, relying practically altogether on income from students, can at best develop highly a department or two;[4] the rest are necessarily restricted. The quality of the student body is likewise a limitation. Laboratory courses, following the lines that we have marked out, are impossible to boys whose preliminary training in science has barely begun. At best the students have an elementary acquaintance with physics or chemistry; frequently not even that. Those that have and those that have not sit side by side on the same benches. A difficult dilemma is thus presented. It is impossible to teach the medical without the pre-medical sciences; the medical course, already crowded, cannot be either cut or compressed sufficiently to accommodate them. The situation cannot, therefore, be wholly retrieved within the medical school. Makeshifts vary somewhat from school to school. A rigid medical curriculum, clipped to the quick, leaves perhaps a few hundred hours available for pre-medical work. Chemistry as a rule absorbs them all; nothing is attempted in biology; occasionally physics gets a slight opportunity, as at Tulane, where first-year students hear one lecture a week,

---

[1] *Ueber den Medizinisch-Klinischen Unterricht,* p. 11 (Leipzig, 1901). To the same effect, Professor T. Clifford Albutt: *On Professional Education,* p. 49 (Macmillan, 1906).

[2] "Die Studierenden sollen jederzeit eintreten dürfen," Virchow's laboratory motto, quoted by Orth: *Berliner Med. Woch. Sch.* vol. xliii. p. 890.

[3] See "The Concentration Plan of Teaching Medicine," by H. A. Christian, *Proceed. Assn. Amer. Med. Colleges, March, 1910.*

[4] See p. 133.

"abundantly illustrated," or at St. Louis University, where sixty-four hours of didactic instruction are devoted to the subject.[1]

After all, however, there are different ways of meeting even a desperate condition; and in this instance the variations are within limits amazingly wide.[2] There are schools that sink ignominiously without a struggle; others that take advantage of the student's plight to palm off cheap instruction at a profit; and a small number that by valiant effort minimize, and to no slight degree surmount, the difficulty. According as an institution reacts in one or another of these ways, we make out three main varieties among schools on the high school basis:

1. Those that by careful selection of students and extraordinary pains in teaching make the very most of the situation;

2. Those that, content to operate on a lower plane, are still commercially effective;

3. Those that are frankly mercenary.

We shall briefly consider these three types in succession.

(1) These schools form a small minority. They are straining hard to get from the high school to the college basis; in equipment, organization, and scientific spirit they are to greater or less degree already there. They have usually four scientific departments,[3] already in most instances well equipped, each in charge of a full-time professor, for whom private quarters and more or less free time[4] procure some opportunity to push ahead. Energy, sincerity, and intelligence are abundantly in evidence throughout these institutions. In resources they vary greatly, but in spirit they are alike; and all are admirable. Every possible point is scored: the more difficult the contest, the keener the play. However scant the resources, something is put into books; however hard pressed the instructor, a museum, carefully catalogued and labeled, has been painfully assembled.

Of schools of this type, two Canadian institutions—McGill and Toronto—deserve especial attention. In point of laboratory equipment they equal Minnesota and Michigan; their lower entrance requirement, minimized by conscientious adherence to a strict interpretation of their announced standards, is now compensated by the addition of a fifth year to the curriculum.[5] At Toronto the teaching is wholly in

---

[1] Sometimes the provision is sheer make-believe. At Denver and Gross College of Medicine (Denver, Col.) the physics is thus described: "One hour each week in practical chemistry as applied to medicine. The first year's work will include medical physics, chemic philosophy, and organic compounds." *Catalogue, 1908–9*, p. 22.

[2] See table at close of this chapter.

[3] Anatomy, chemistry, physiology (including pharmacology), pathology (including bacteriology and hygiene).

[4] How much, depends on the quality of the assistants furnished. There is great variation in this respect.

[5] This is a very different thing from adding a year devoted to pre-medical sciences taught by the medical faculty of a proprietary school,—a makeshift without possibility of development. The Canadian year is a year in the university, where teachers of science are in position to do their subjects justice; eventually a second year will be demanded. The optional fifth year offered by our proprietary schools is commercially profitable and educationally futile. See page 47.

charge of full-time instructors, for whose original work splendid provision has been made in laboratories of ideal construction and admirable equipment. McGill is in respect to full-time teachers somewhat less fortunate; but its great museum, recently much damaged by fire, proves that genuine enthusiasm may succeed contrary to all the established rules of the game. In both institutions the shortcomings of the student body, instead of excusing perfunctory work, have rather been regarded as an obstacle to be overcome, a condition to be met. The students have had little high school science: all the more reason, then, to provide excellent laboratories, skilful teachers, abundant assistants. In keeping with effective performance are their modesty and candor. The number of "greatest anatomists" and "greatest pathologists" teaching on small salaries in obscure places in the United States, and of laboratories "as good as Johns Hopkins," is nothing less than staggering. Nor is a boastful pride in mediocrity lacking even in institutions of some real merit. At Toronto and McGill one hears in the medical schools no such bravado. There they deprecate the defects, which they hasten to show for fear they may escape notice. The absence of competition[1]—be it business competition between schools conducted for profit, or academic competition between endowed or tax-supported institutions, mad to "make a showing"—may perhaps be responsible for their more guarded utterance and more assured ideals.

Perhaps a dozen institutions in the United States belong with greater or less right to the category under consideration. Regard being had to the quality of the student body, to the number of full-time teachers and assistants, and to the adequacy of laboratories, museum, and library, the best of them, in respect to the first and second years, are New York University, Syracuse,[2] Northwestern University, Jefferson Medical College (Philadelphia), Tulane University (New Orleans), St. Louis University, the University of Texas, handicapped though some of them are in one respect or another by resources inadequate to the ambition and competency of their faculties and by a student body of somewhat uneven composition. St. Louis University affords an excellent example of a brave, uphill contest, by no means barren of result. Unable for the moment to do all it wishes, it has, like a good general, concentrated its effort at critical points. It secures a pervasive scientific atmosphere in the first two years through the intensive cultivation of anatomy and physiology. The departmental head of the former subject stipulated that his routine work be kept in close bounds; with wise liberality he has been provided with an assistant professor, a draughtsman, and a competent helper; the productive department thus created has invigorated the entire school on the laboratory side.

To the schools just described we must look for such further facilities in high-grade medical education as the country still requires. Their ideals are correct; they lack only the means; and these they have already in comparative poverty shown the ca-

[1] There are eight medical schools in British America.
[2] Already requiring more than four-year high school education.

pacity to use. Once the necessary resources have been bestowed upon them, the remaining task will be merely the absorption or the suppression of the various types of medical school yet to be discussed. It is surely significant that with but a single exception, these schools are also, like those of the first division, *bona-fide* university departments.

So much for the best type of medical school on the high school basis. We consider next (2) the schools that on the same basis are shrewdly and more or less outspokenly commercial. A few of them—those at Chicago, Philadelphia, and Baltimore—have accumulated extensive and, in one or two departments, elaborate plants.[1] They are on a routine level and, within the limits marked out by state board examinations, pedagogically effective. They drill their students energetically in the elements of such of the sciences as they touch at all, but the atmosphere is at best that of a successful factory. There is no free scientific spirit. The teaching of chemistry at the Medico-Chirurgical College of Philadelphia is an extreme case in point. The course is subdivided into fixed lessons, each of them so much raw material, for which the student receives a voucher, to be returned in proper shape before he can get the voucher for the succeeding task. The vouchers returned constitute an automatic record of attendance and form the basis of an oral quiz by an instructor. "The whole system is an imitation of the business system in vogue in the better organized business offices."[2] Mechanically admirable, no doubt; but what convincing evidence the system itself affords of the unfitness of the students for the study of modern medicine!

Two schools of this group—the Long Island College Hospital (Brooklyn) and the Albany Medical School—are closely affiliated with laboratories which provide good teaching in certain branches: the Hoagland Laboratory at Brooklyn relieves the school of histology, pathology, and bacteriology; the Bender Laboratory at Albany carries the laboratory work in the same subjects. It will be noted that physiology and pharmacology are not properly provided by either; neither are they by the school. One might suppose that the school, relieved at one point, would become more effective at another. Not at all. Both schools pay in dividends to prosperous practitioners the sums that should be used in completing their fundamental instruction.

Scientifically, then, these schools may be called inert. They rarely cultivate any research at all; their faculties are generally composed of active practitioners whose training has rarely been modern. By way of exception Louisville has four full-time professors in the fundamental branches, the Medico-Chirurgical three, Creighton one. But very rarely has the full-time teacher opportunity to work ahead. His time and energies are bespoken by heavy routine, unlightened by a competent or organized force of assistants and helpers. In general, school positions are valued as professional

[1] Preëminently the Medico-Chirurgical (Philadelphia), University of Maryland and College of Physicians and Surgeons (Baltimore), and College of Physicians and Surgeons, Chicago.
[2] From a description by the head of the department.
[3] Strictly speaking, even these are not full-time men in the medical school, since they also teach in pharmacy and dental departments.

stepping-stones, not as scientific opportunities; laboratories are often slovenly and, except during class hours, entirely abandoned. Strange professorial combinations are found: anatomy and surgery, very commonly; clinical medicine and physiology, at the University of Maryland; orthopaedic surgery and pathology, at the Baltimore Medical College; medicine and pathology, at the Chicago College of Medicine and Surgery (Valparaiso University); pathology and the physical directorship of the academic department, at Bowdoin. Scientific chairs are held by non-residents at the Universities of Colorado[1] and Vermont[2] and at the Medical School of Maine (Bowdoin);[3] and itinerant teachers, giving the same branches at several schools, are to be found in Philadelphia, New York, and Chicago. If the larger institutions under consideration chance to contain a full-time teacher, his time usually belongs equally to dental and pharmacy departments, developed as "business propositions" to keep the plant constantly going; despite the manifest incongruity, dental or pharmacy students mingle in the same classes with medical students at the Medico-Chirurgical College (Philadelphia), Temple University (Philadelphia), and the Creighton Medical College (Omaha).[4] Occasionally a non-practising teacher will be found who is simultaneously holder of a municipal office, to which he devotes his main thought. The medical school gets the few brief hours that it pays for. Thus the non-practising professor of chemistry at the Creighton school is the city gas inspector; the professor of bacteriology at Denver and Gross is city bacteriologist,[5] with his laboratory at the City Hall. In the few cases where a non-practising full-time professor is found,[6] he is swamped with work; for he has as a rule only student assistants to aid him in coping with several hundred pupils utterly inexperienced in laboratory manipulation.

For many years a school of this sort was a veritable gold mine to its owners. Fees were divided outright, or invested in buildings which the faculty owned. Once in a while the income was split: a large share went to the teachers, the rest was devoted to carrying mortgaged buildings held by the trustees. These structures themselves were not infrequently erected in pursuance of business policy. Recent agitation has forced increased expenditure on buildings and equipment. The schools

[1] Anatomy, by a non-resident surgeon.

[2] Physiology, pathology, and hygiene.

[3] Anatomy and physiology.

[4] Likewise at University of Maryland, Valparaiso University, College of Physicians and Surgeons (Chicago), Georgetown University, College of Physicians and Surgeons (Baltimore), Baylor University, College of Physicians and Surgeons (San Francisco), Barnes (St. Louis), Starling-Ohio, University of Texas, Toledo Medical College, Medical College of the State of South Carolina, Milwaukee Medical College, College of Physicians and Surgeons (Boston), Wisconsin College of Physicians and Surgeons. Even at Harvard, dental and medical students are mixed in some classes, though it is admitted that "the Dentals don't do as well and are harder to teach." Students are admitted to the Harvard Dental School on the basis of a four-year high school education. The discrepancy is therefore considerable.

[5] The same is true at the University of Oregon (Portland), though in this case the laboratory is in the medical college; it is also the only real laboratory there.

[6] Physiology, College of Physicians and Surgeons (Chicago); pathology, Creighton; chemistry, Baltimore Medical College.

have been willing enough to build; but in the matter of equipment they have usually yielded as little as they could. The conclusive evidence of lack of educational conscience or pride is the general absence of a decent museum.[1] Material, of course, abounds, the expense involved is slight; but the practitioner simply will not take the trouble. The College of Physicians and Surgeons (Baltimore), Georgetown University (Washington), Long Island College Hospital (Brooklyn), the medical department of Valparaiso University, the Chicago Hahnemann, Ensworth (St. Joseph, Missouri), are among the schools that have little or nothing in the way of a museum at all. Such specimens as one meets are often putrid, rarely labeled properly, and still more rarely catalogued. But a few exceptions may be fortunately noted: the great anatomical and pathological museum at McGill has already been mentioned. To the same class belong the excellent collections made by Souchon at Tulane and by Keiller at Galveston (University of Texas). A small but beautifully mounted collection at Boston University is once more an evidence of what conscience and intelligence will achieve despite slender financial resources.

Practically the same may be said on the subject of books. The College of Physicians and Surgeons of Chicago and the Medical College of Virginia have small working libraries; but in general no funds are set aside for the purchase of books. The school grind is merrily independent of medical literature. The University of Maryland possesses indeed a large library under a separate roof, but the building was unheated when visited in midwinter, and at best it is open only two hours a day. Denver and Gross (Denver, Colorado) and the Medico-Chirurgical College of Philadelphia have limited accumulations of textbooks and cheap medical periodicals;[2] Long Island and Albany have no books at all. In the College of Physicians and Surgeons, Los Angeles, the word "Library" is prominently painted on a door which, on being opened, reveals a class-room innocent of a single volume. Once more it is pleasant to record exceptions: a good library, excellently administered, is to be found at Jefferson, at Buffalo, and at Galveston.

In the matter of laboratory equipment and work, our progress may be facilitated by simple elimination. None of these schools has laboratories of pharmacology; in consequence, their teaching of materia medica and therapeutics is wholly on didactic lines. Only a few of them — the Medico-Chirurgical (Philadelphia), University of Maryland (Baltimore), the College of Physicians and Surgeons, Chicago — are well equipped to do either demonstrative or experimental work in physiology; as a rule, physiology is still didactically presented with a varying amount of experimental demonstration. The general laboratory equipment is therefore limited to chemistry, anatomy, pathology, and bacteriology.

[1] The Hahnemann (Philadelphia), University of Maryland (Baltimore), Oakland College of Medicine and Surgery (California), each has a small museum.

[2] The former behind a counter in the business office, — practically inaccessible; the latter at the College Club House.

As a rule, chemistry advances little beyond the high school level; at the best, elementary organic chemistry is included.[1] The equipment is ordinary; there is nowhere the faintest evidence of independent scientific interest, nowhere any interplay between the chemical and other laboratories. The ground covered satisfies the state board prescription, enabling the student to pass the state board examination. Nothing more is intended; the teaching is accordingly in large measure didactic and quiz drill. It cannot be otherwise; for even in the cases where sufficient desk space is provided, competent assistants are lacking. The instruction therefore quickly deteriorates into demonstration and drill.

The teaching of anatomy clings to thoroughly conventional lines. Embryology is practically unknown; osteology is taught by lectures instead of by practical methods, such as modeling, or the like; histology is relegated to pathology because the anatomical department possesses no microscopes, in the first place, and because the practitioner teacher rarely understands their use, in the second. The laboratory is a mere dissecting-room, in which the student is required to dissect part of a cadaver under the guidance of upper-class students or recent graduates. Into none of the schools mentioned have modern ideas as to the conduct of this department permeated. Well conducted anatomical laboratories are in these days clean, attractive, sweet-smelling places; the cadavers, neatly covered when not in use, are moist, thoroughly well preserved, and not repulsive even to a layman. The dissecting-rooms under discussion are rarely clean, always unattractive, and not infrequently unpleasant. They contain tables, cadavers, and a vat; usually nothing more. Not infrequently the school skeleton is defective, as at Creighton, the College of Physicians and Surgeons, Milwaukee, and at the Kansas City Hahnemann. The models, charts, cross-sections, bone-sets,[2] drawings, microscopes, that complete the outfit of the modern anatomist, are conspicuously absent. Large and financially prosperous schools, such as the Medico-Chirurgical (Philadelphia), the University of Maryland (Baltimore), in immediate proximity to institutions like the University of Pennsylvania and the Johns Hopkins, where the subject is properly conducted, have profited nothing by opportunities to modernize their teaching. Of course it could not be otherwise. The professor is a busy physician or surgeon. He lectures to ill prepared students for one hour a few times weekly, in a huge amphitheater, showing a bone between his

---

[1] The Medico-Chirurgical College of Philadephia offers decidedly more. The instruction there occupies part of three years and requires 544 hours of work. Nothing could better illustrate our contention that, with medical students on the high school or equivalent basis, anything like a thorough treatment of the pre-medical sciences within the medical curriculum is fatal to the medical curriculum itself. Chemistry here takes up over one-eighth of the entire medical curriculum. Of course physics and biology deserve something too, though they get practically nothing. What would happen to the medical curriculum if a similar effort were made to teach them thoroughly? For the time being, the instruction limps along without them. When their necessity is generally recognized, as that of chemistry is now recognized, it will be impossible to attempt them within the medical school, and the battle for the preliminary scientific training will have been won.

[2] At Cornell (Ithaca) a complete set of bones is given out to each student. There are over 100 complete skeletons. This makes a striking contrast with numerous schools that do not possess a single complete skeleton.

finger-tips or eloquently describing an organ which no one but the prosector distinctly sees; at the close of which oratorical performance he snatches his hat and, amid mingled applause and cat-calls, makes for his automobile to begin his round of daily visits. In the afternoons "demonstrators" supervise the dissecting, where eight or ten inexpert boys hack away at a cadaver until it is reduced to shreds. The actual emphasis falls on the didactic teaching and the quiz-drills; something like half the student's time is spent in the lecture-room: 220 out of 450 hours at Louisville, 360 out of 684 at the College of Physicians and Surgeons (University of Illinois), Chicago. The really effective work is not infrequently done by quiz-masters, who drill hundreds of students in memorizing minute details which they would be unable to recognize if the objects were before them. This is a flourishing industry in "great medical centers" like Chicago[1] and Philadelphia.

Pathology is practically in the same condition. The best of these schools are well supplied with microscopes, microtomes, and material. But the teaching is usually uninspired routine drill. Sections are cut, stained, mounted, and observed. At the close of the year the student will perhaps have accumulated a box of several dozen slides, which he may carry home with him. But the work has been largely histological, — devoid of experimental features, on the one hand, and but feebly articulated with clinic and autopsy, on the other. The autopsy is indeed the indispensable adjunct of an effective department of pathology. "A course in pathology without autopsy work and fresh material is like a course in systematic botany without field work."[2] The facilities of all but a few of our best schools are in this respect unduly limited; at no other point is the lack of a hospital under school control more acutely felt. Makeshifts of various kinds are invoked by way of remedy: in New York, for example, Columbia and Cornell have attached the two coroner's physicians who serve in the autopsy-room of the great Bellevue Hospital, thus procuring fresh material from a large number of cases. The arrangement still leaves the professor of pathology himself out of account. Of the schools belonging to the class under consideration few have even fair opportunities of this character; some of them rely altogether on a friendly coroner's cursory performance in the rear room of an undertaker's establishment.[3] The classes at the University of Maryland witness "perhaps ten [autopsies] a year;" the College of Physicians and Surgeons, Baltimore, describes its opportunities as "restricted;" Georgetown University (Washington) gets a "few," Hahnemann (Chicago), "four or five a year;" at Northwestern they are "scanty, the students do none;" at Cooper (San Francisco) they are scarce. For the most part, the student has merely made the microscopic rounds of the typical abnormal growths; his fundamental ignorance of biology, which no serious attempt is made to cure, comes

---

[1] A Chicago drill-master is reported as having classes of 300.

[2] Letter from Richard M. Pearce, professor of pathology, University and Bellevue Hospital Medical College (New York University).

[3] e.g., University of Oregon, Portland.

between him and a really intelligent grasp of the principles and bearing of pathology. One is not surprised to find the instruction once more heavily inclined to the didactic side: 72 out of 144 hours at the College of Physicians and Surgeons, Chicago; 90 out of 140 at the College of Physicians and Surgeons, Baltimore.[1]

Bacteriology—the last of the sciences concerning which there is even a pretense —fares in general rather worse. At the Medico-Chirurgical of Philadelphia the subject is the best developed of all the scientific branches; elsewhere it is a mere tag to pathology. Sterilizers, incubators, and culture-tubes are of course common enough; this is the orthodox equipment, stipulated by the state boards. But the subject cannot be intelligently studied without animals,—cats, rabbits, or guinea pigs. In general, one finds no arrangements to care for animals either before or during experimentation.[2] As a rule, "they are too difficult to keep;" at Creighton, Oakland (California), the Cleveland College of Physicians and Surgeons, the University of Vermont, Georgetown University (Washington), they are "got as needed,"—elsewhere, often not even then. "I think I am not violating any confidence," says Dr. Victor C. Vaughan,[3] "when I say that there are certain men who teach bacteriology who start at the beginning of their lectures with a lot of tubes already made. They do not know enough about bacteriology to make cultures. They hold up these tubes and say, 'This is a diphtheria culture; this is a culture of tubercle bacillus,' and if by any chance a culture goes bad, they send and get another."

(3) There yet remains for our consideration the third variety of school on the high school or equivalent basis, namely, those described as basely mercenary. In point of equipment and teaching methods these schools are not substantially different from institutions on a still lower basis.[4] Some of the latter institutions show, indeed, a better spirit: the University of Alabama, at Mobile, the College of Physicians and Surgeons and the School of Medicine, at Atlanta, the Medical College of the State of South Carolina, at Charleston, are not without traditions and a certain present dignity. Educationally, however, subject to certain exceptions to be specified from time to time, they may without violence be considered together; for limitations of one kind or another—now of equipment, now of intention, again of both—make the effective teaching of any of the laboratory sciences frankly impossible. They are for the most part cramming establishments, in many of which it is freely admitted that the students do not even own the regular textbooks. Their main weapon is the quiz-compend. Such laboratories as they have cannot be effectively used; of teaching accessories—books, museum, modern charts, or models—they are generally devoid.

[1] At the Johns Hopkins, out of a total of 400 hours, 40 are didactic; at Minnesota, out of 456, 146; at Wake Forest, out of 195, 50.

[2] The College of Physicians and Surgeons, Baltimore, operates a Pasteur plant, but animals are only slightly used in teaching.

[3] *Third Annual Conference, Council on American Medical Education, American Medical Association, held in Chicago, April 29, 1907*, p. 59.

[4] Those in the south and elsewhere asking two years of a high school, or less.

It is indeed stretching terms to speak of laboratory teaching in connection with them at all.[1] It is hardly more than make-believe; in the better schools, a futile imitation, without actual bearing on the subsequent clinical work; in others, a grudging compliance with the state board behest; occasionally there is nothing at all. The Mississippi Medical College (Meridian) did not, when visited,[2] own a dollar's worth of apparatus of any description whatsoever; the pathological laboratories of the Chattanooga Medical College and the College of Physicians and Surgeons, San Francisco, rejoice in the possession of one microscope apiece; Halifax Medical College provides one utterly wretched laboratory for bacteriology and pathology; the Toledo school has a meager equipment in one or two branches, but for the rest is bare; the Detroit Homeopathic College has a dirty and disorderly room, with a few dozen wet specimens, that is called the pathological laboratory; at the Milwaukee Medical College, bacteriology is represented mainly by several wire baskets of dirty test tubes; Temple University (Philadelphia) has no individual outfit for students in any science at all; the Chicago National Medical University is practically as bare as the Meridian school; the eclectic school at Lincoln, Nebraska, pretends to give clinical instruction in Lincoln, laboratory instruction at Cotner University, a few miles from town. When questions are asked in Lincoln regarding physiology or pathology, the answer is made: "That is given at Cotner;" when the same question is asked at Cotner, it is answered: "That is given at Lincoln." A quick transit from one to the other failed to find anything at either. Prestidigitation is, however, familiar enough in schools of this grade. Entrance credentials in the college safe frequently vanish as it is being opened: why should not equipment similarly resent inspection? At the College of Physicians and Surgeons, Denver, the outfit in pathology and bacteriology was mostly stored in a certain compartment under a table. There was some difficulty and delay in opening it; by the time the key was found, everything had disappeared except an empty demijohn and some jugs, obviously too clumsy to whisk themselves away in such airy fashion. At Willamette University (Salem, Oregon) "physiology is taught experimentally." The apparatus? "That is kept in a physician's office downtown." At the Eclectic Medical College of New York an inquiry was made as to the teaching of experimental physiology, no outfit for which had been noticed in the course of the inspection. A mere oversight! A messenger was despatched to fetch it, and did—a single small black box, of about the size and appearance of a safety-razor case, containing a small sphygmograph. "Good standing" requires the schools of St. Louis and Chicago to own a certain equipment in experimental physiology. They do; it is displayed prominently on tables, brand-new, like samples shown for sale on a counter; the various parts had never been put together or connected at the College of Physicians and Surgeons or at the Hippo-

[1] *e.g.*, Western University (London, Ont.), Halifax Medical College, University of Arkansas, Southwestern University (Dallas, Texas), Fort Worth University, Epworth University (Oklahoma City). Other examples are given in the text.

[2] January 12, 1909. It was then in its third year.

cratean, both of St. Louis, at the Western Eclectic (Kansas City), or at the College of Physicians and Surgeons (Denver). The Littlejohn School of Osteopathy (Chicago) was in the throes of rebuilding to accommodate the growing classes that seek its superior advantages: every "laboratory" but that of chemistry was dismantled; there was no prospect that they could be again set up for months, but the teaching of "science" went on just the same.[1]

Chemistry is the "star" laboratory course of these schools—"medical chemistry," of course. It never rises above a fair high school level and often falls far below it. At Chattanooga the students could not follow the subject, however simply presented. The laboratories are of the most elementary description,—sometimes active and in good order, as at Mobile and Augusta, at the Illinois Medical College, and at the Eclectic Medical College of New York; oftener in utter disorder, as at the Maryland Medical College (Baltimore). At the University of Oregon (Portland) and Willamette (Salem, Oregon) there is no running water at the desks; at the North Carolina Medical College (Charlotte) a single set of reagents is provided for the entire class; at the University Medical College, Kansas City (Missouri), instead of individual reagent sets, huge bottles are provided for general use.

Almost, but not quite all the schools dissect. At Meridian (Mississippi), for example, anatomical material is too difficult to get. In Chicago they have learned how to teach anatomy practically without dissection. At the National Medical University the teacher dictates, the students learn; this process is kept on, night after night, from October until the middle of April. So far there had been no dissection at all, but there would be ultimately, in "May or June," though there were no cadavers at hand as yet. At the Jenner Medical College—also a Chicago night school—a similarly enlightened pedagogy was employed: "the subject is taught by lectures, with dissection from May 15 until the close of the session." The same methods are practised at Pulte— the Cincinnati homeopathic school—where dissection had not yet begun on December 14: "the anatomy teaching goes on independent of dissecting." At Kirksville, Missouri, in the American School of Osteopathy, anatomy is taught with a textbook the first year; lectures, demonstrating, and dissecting are postponed to the second year,—and the whole course takes but three years, all told. The Central College of Osteopathy, Kansas City, Missouri, holds that the student should know anatomy before he dissects: "he will get more out of it." On November 8 there was no cadaver in the school: they already had had one and "will get another in February." At the Bennett Medical College, Chicago, there was witnessed a quiz in anatomy in a room without a skeleton, bone, or chart. At the College of Physicians and Surgeons, Denver, it was impossible to find any evidence of active dissecting; and it was admitted that material was scarce: "there had been two bodies this year, ten men on each."

[1] These schools are generally quite devoid of teaching aids,—charts, modern models, etc. The rooms are bare. What they have is out of reach of the students: "if it were not locked up, it would disappear,"—a significant indication of the sort of students gathered in by low standards.

Elsewhere, dissecting-rooms are indeed found, but the conditions in them defy description. The smell is intolerable; the cadavers now putrid, as at Temple University (Philadelphia), the Philadelphia College of Osteopathy, the Halifax Medical School, and in many of the southern schools,[1] including Vanderbilt; again, dry as tanned leather, —at the University of Tennessee, Bennett (Chicago), Denver and Gross (Denver), Creighton (Omaha), College of Physicians and Surgeons, St. Louis, for example. At the Barnes Medical College (St. Louis) the first-year students listen to lectures only in the last "semestry;" they are not permitted to dissect because first-year men only "hack and butcher." The dissecting-room of the Kansas Medical College, Topeka (the medical department of Washburn College), did duty incidentally as a chicken yard: corn was scattered over the floor—along with other things—and poultry fed placidly in the long intervals before instruction in anatomy began.

A few of these schools have the apparatus requisite to teach pathology and bacteriology in routine fashion: the Atlanta College of Physicians and Surgeons, for one. But in general they own an inadequate and at times decreasing supply of microscopes—for everywhere one hears theft assigned in extenuation of a short supply or defective instruments. Post-mortems are practically nil. None are claimed at Chattanooga, Atlanta, Charlotte (North Carolina), or Dallas (Baylor and Southwestern Universities); two in six years were remembered at the medical department of the University of Georgia (Augusta). In default of post-mortems, material is sometimes obtained from the surgeons; but not all the schools can even then prepare it properly. To cut matters short, hardened material and sometimes sections are bought "in the east." The student at most stains and mounts them. Too frequently he does no more than look at them through the microscope. Whether he sees anything, remains a problem; for he rarely makes a drawing. In many cases it is impossible to believe that even this is done. At the College of Physicians and Surgeons, St. Louis, individual lockers are provided; on examination they prove to be empty. An explanation is offered: "the boys bring slides and cover-glasses along; they furnish their own and keep them at home."

It is, of course, not to be supposed that these schools would be materially better even if well equipped and decently cared for. It makes very little difference to the student body that they assemble whether microscopes and incubators are provided or not. The poor fellow who in an unguarded moment is caught by advertisements, premiums, or canvassing agents[2] cannot be taught modern medicine, no matter what investments in apparatus the state boards force. Meanwhile the sole beneficiaries of the traffic are the teachers—as a rule, the small group that constitutes the "faculty;" in some instances, however, only the dean, who "owns" or "runs" the school. His associates profit indirectly by what is technically known as the "reflex." Their pro-

---

[1] An exception must be recorded in favor of the Memphis College of Physicians and Surgeons, where excellent rooms with hot and cold water are provided.
[2] Employed at Jefferson Park College, feeder to the Bennett Medical College, Chicago.

fessorial dignity impresses the crude boys who will be likely to require with their first cases the aid of a "consultant." The "dean" of one such institution was frankly explaining his methods. "What do you give your teachers?" he was asked. "Titles," he replied.

The less obviously commercial schools allege not infrequently that medical education no longer pays, that it is kept up for the sake of the "back districts." We have already shown that the back districts deserve and can get something better. Meanwhile the statement does not persuade. Hundreds of thousands of dollars annually pour into these institutions; in many cases, this has been going on for years. What becomes of the money? There is in general nothing to show for it; a few hundred dollars would replace the fixtures and equipment of most of them.[1]

The discreditable showing made by our commercial medical schools must not, however, be permitted to obscure the fact that we have at this date perhaps thirty institutions well equipped to teach the medical sciences in laboratories usually of modern construction, invariably of modern equipment. Twenty years ago we had not one. Our immediate problem has therefore two aspects: on the one hand, to strengthen these institutions, increasing their number only as actual need requires; on the other, with all the force that law and public opinion can wield to crush out the mercenary concerns that trade on ignorance and disease.

[1] In a few places there is a considerable investment: Atlanta College of Physicians and Surgeons, Atlanta School of Medicine, the two Richmond schools, for example. See for detailed discussion, chapter viii.

COMPARATIVE SCHEDULE, FIRST AND SECOND YEARS

SHOWING BEARING OF ENTRANCE REQUIREMENT ON CURRICULUM*

FIRST YEAR

Western Reserve University, 32 weeks per year (College basis)	Did.	Lab.	New York University, 32 weeks per year (Four-year high school basis)	Hrs.	Medico-Chirurgical College, 32 weeks per year (High school equivalent basis)	Hrs.	University of Alabama, 32 weeks per year (Nominal requirement)	Hrs.
Anatomy			Anatomy		Anatomy		Anatomy	
Comparative anatomy	24	48	Lectures & recitations	96	Lectures	96	Lectures	56
Descriptive anatomy	84		Demonstrations	96	Demonstrations	96	Recitations	56
Splanchnology		32	Practical work	360	Recitations	32	Comparative osteology	120
Neurology		72	Histology and Embryology		Dissections	98-144	Practical anatomy[1]	144
Dissections		216	Laboratory work	128	Histology and Embryology		(all practical)	
Microscopical technique		16	Lectures and recitations	64	Didactic	64	Inorganic Chemistry	
Histology	24	32	Physiology		Laboratory	96	Chemical physics	112
Microscopical anatomy	40	80	Lectures	48	Physiology		Chemical laboratory	168
Embryology	40	80	Recitations	32	Didactic	96	Physiology	
Physiology and Bio-chemistry			Chemistry and Physics		Laboratory	128	(none in first year)	
Experimental physiology	16	64	Lectures		Chemistry		Physiological Chemistry	32
			Inorganic chemistry (¾)		Didactic	160	(part practical)	
Bio-chemistry	16	64	Organic chemistry (¼)	96	Laboratory	96	Biology, Embryology, & Histology	
Organic chemistry	64	112	Recitations	32	General Pathology		Laboratory work	196
			Laboratory work	112	Didactic	64	Pharmacy	
			Bacteriology		Hygiene		Didactic	28
			Practical work	64	Lectures	32		
					Recitations	?		
					Materia Medica			
					Lectures	64		
					Recitations	?		
					Pharmacy			
					Lectures	32		
					Laboratory	64		
					Recitations	?		
					Bandaging and Surgical Dressings			
					Practical	32		

New York University note: Note page 29 says: For freshmen — Total lectures 128 hrs.; Total recitations 64 hrs.; Total laboratory work 112 hrs.

University of Alabama notes:
[1] 2 to 5 p.m., 6 days per week, for 8 weeks.
Hours figured out from announcement and the class schedule. See inspection report.

SECOND YEAR

Western Reserve University	Did.	Lab.	New York University	Hrs.	Medico-Chirurgical College	Hrs.	University of Alabama	Hrs.
Anatomy			Anatomy		Anatomy		Anatomy	
Descriptive anatomy	84		Lectures and recitations	96	Lectures	96	Lectures	56
Dissections		144	Demonstrations	64	Demonstrations	64	Recitations	56
Applied anatomy	64		Practical work	360	Recitations	32	Practical anatomy[1]	144
Physiology and Bio-chemistry			Physiology		Dissections	216	Chemistry	
Advanced experimental physiology	6	106	Lectures and recitations	96	Physiology		Lectures	56
Advanced bio-chemistry		32	Practical work	96	Lectures	64	Physiology	
Lectures and recitations	72		Chemistry		Recitations	48	Lectures and demonstrations	86
Pathology and Preventive Medicine			Lectures		Demonstrations	?	Laboratory work[2]	64
Bacteriology	40	32	Organic chemistry		Laboratory	48	Materia Medica	
Protozoology	14	28	Physiological chemistry		Chemistry		Lectures[3]	28
General pathology and pathological histology	75	145	Toxicology	48	Didactic	48	Histology	
Gross pathological anatomy		32	Recitations	16	Laboratory	128	Lectures	14
Pharmacology, Materia Medica & Therapeutics			Laboratory work	96	General Pathology		Laboratory	112
Pharmacology, toxicology, and prescription writing	19	38	Materia Medica and Pharmacology		Lectures	64	Bacteriology	
Experimental pharmacodynamics	24	60	Lectures	64	Laboratory	192	Lectures	11
Systematic pharmacology	12	6	Recitations	32	Bacteriology		Laboratory	88
Physical Diagnosis		24	Laboratory work	63	Laboratory	96		
Minor Surgery and Bandaging	30		Pathology		Hygiene			
Surgical Recitations	60		Lectures	16	Didactic	64		
			Recitations	16	Laboratory	16		
			Laboratory work	128	Pharmacology and Therapeutics			
			Lantern demonstration	16	Didactic	96		
			Elementary Clinic		Physical Diagnosis: Normal			
			Physical diagnosis	30	Practical	64		
			Surgery		Physical Diagnosis: Pathological			
			Practical work	16	Lectures	32		
			Clinic	32	Demonstrations	?		
					General Etiology and Symptomatology			
					Lectures	32		
					Surgical Pathology			
					Didactic	16		
					Laboratory	32		
					Surgical Fevers and Inflammations			
					Lectures	16		

University of Alabama notes:
[1] 2 to 5 p.m., 6 days per week, for 8 weeks.
[2] 2 weeks of 8 hours per week (4 periods per week).
[3] Only one hour (lecture) per week. See schedule.

CHAPTER VI

THE COURSE OF STUDY
THE HOSPITAL AND THE MEDICAL SCHOOL

THE THIRD AND FOURTH YEARS (A)

LET us make an inventory of the presumptive acquirements of the well trained medical student at the threshold of his third year. He knows the normal structure of the human body, the normal composition of the bodily fluids, the normal functioning of tissues and organs, the physiological action of ordinary drugs, the main departures from normal structure, and in a limited fashion the significance of such departures both to the organs and tissues immediately involved and to the general economy of the organism. He will have had his first lessons in physical diagnosis, learning, perhaps in the class-room through examination of his fellow students, the use of the stethoscope, the arts of palpation, auscultation, and percussion, accustoming his ear to the normal sounds, his fingers to the normal "feel," of the chest and abdomen in health. His studies in pathology will have introduced him further to the essential clinical terminology, obviating the necessity of a separate detached course in "elementary medicine."[1]

It remains, then, in the first place to teach the student how to get from the direct study of the patient himself whatsoever data remain to be collected. He will then possess two sets of facts: one in a way indirectly obtained, through microscopic or other study of excretions, secretions, tissues, etc.; the other set procured directly at the bedside. He must learn the art of combining them; he must see them together as the total picture of the situation with which he is called on to deal. Upon this inductive process all intelligent therapeutic procedure is based: hence his final task —to learn through an extension of the elementary discipline that began in the pharmacological laboratory, the therapeutic measures calculated to meet the more or less precisely ascertained and inferred conditions, responsible for the disturbance he is trying to quell.

A somewhat absurd controversy has at times raged as to which is of the higher scientific quality or diagnostic value—the laboratory disclosures or the bedside observations. Occasionally champions of the laboratory prejudge the issue by calling pathology a real or pure or more or less accurate science, as against the presumably unreal or impure or inaccurate data secured from the patient himself. It becomes

---

[1] The place of pathology in the American medical curriculum—if the instruction takes advantage of it—saves us from the difficulty encountered in Germany, where pathology and clinical medicine begin together. "According to current use the study of general pathology and pathological anatomy begin simultaneously with attendance on the clinic. For that reason the first semester of the clinic is of very slight value.... We ought first to procure for the student clear pathological conceptions: only then will it be easy for him to follow the clinical instruction intelligently and profitably. I consider it absolutely necessary that the instruction in general pathology and pathological anatomy should precede the clinic." Von Strümpell, *loc. cit.*, pp. 16, 17.

a serious question of professional etiquette, who should speak first or loudest,—the pathologist, armed with his microscope, or the clinician, brandishing his stethoscope. To parallel the dispute, one must go back to the two knights who, meeting at a cross-road, disputed at the hazard of their lives as to the color of a shield which, as neither had stopped to reflect, had two sides. It is as profitable to discuss which was the right side of the shield as to raise the question of precedence between the laboratory and the bedside. Both supply indispensable data of coördinate importance. The central fact may be disclosed now by one, now by the other, but in either case it must be interpreted in the light of all other pertinent facts in hand. The scientific character of the procedure depends not on where or by what means facts are procured, but altogether on the degree of caution and thoroughness with which observations are made, inferences drawn, and results heeded. The essence of science is method,—the painstaking collection of all relevant data, the severe effort to read their significance in connection. These objects are promoted in some directions by the laboratory appliances that eke out our defective senses; even so, however, we do not escape or rise superior to these same senses; for with them we use the implements in question. Whatsoever, then, the senses actually ascertain, pertinent to the matter in hand, is scientific datum. The way to be unscientific is to be partial,— whether to the laboratory or to the hospital, it matters not. The test of a good education in medicine is the thorough interpenetration of both standpoints in their product, the young graduate.

If, then, a laboratory is a place constructed for the express purpose of facilitating the collection of data bearing on definite problems and the initiation of practical measures looking to their solution, the hospital and the dispensary are laboratories in the strictest sense of the term. And just as it makes no difference to science whether usable data be obtained from a slide beneath a microscope or from a sick man stretched out on a cot, so the precise nature of the act or experiment is equally immaterial: it matters not in the slightest, from the standpoint of scientific logic, whether the step take the form of administering a dose of calomel, operating for appendicitis, or stimulating a particular convolution of a frog's brain with an electric current. The logical position is in all three cases identical. In each a supposition,— whether expressed or implied, whether called theory or diagnosis,—based on supposedly adequate observation, submits itself to the test of an experiment. If proper weight has been given to correct and sufficient facts, the experiment wins; otherwise not, and a second effort, profiting by previous failure, is demanded. The practising physician and the "theoretical" scientist are thus engaged in doing the same sort of thing, even while one is seeking to correct Mr. Smith's digestive aberration and the other to localize the cerebral functions of the frog.

Certain conclusions as to clinical teaching follow. The student is to collect and evaluate facts. The facts are locked up in the patient. To the patient, therefore, he must go. Waiving the personal factor, always important, that method of clinical teaching will be excellent which brings the student into close and active relation with the patient: close, by removing all hindrance to immediate investigation; active, in the sense, not merely of offering opportunities, but of imposing responsibilities.

Clinical teaching has had substantially the same history as anatomical teaching. It was first didactic: the student was told what he would find and what he should do when he found it.[1] It was next demonstrative: things were pointed out in the amphitheater or the wards, those who got the front seats[2] seeing them more or less well. Latterly it has become scientific: the student brings his own faculties into play at close range,—gathering his own data, making his own construction, proposing his own course, and taking the consequences when the instructor who has worked through exactly the same process calls him to account: the instructor, no longer a fountain pouring forth a full stream of knowledge, nor a showman exhibiting marvelous sights, but by turns an aid or an antagonist in a strenuous contest with disease.

The backbone of the structure is the clinic in internal medicine.[3] This central fact cannot in America be too strongly emphasized. The sufficiency of the school's clinical resources depends at bottom on its medical clinic; the value of its training depends on the systematic thoroughness with which it is in position to use an adequate supply of medical cases. To sample a school on its clinical side, one makes in the first place straight for its medical clinic, seeking to learn the number of patients available for teaching, the variety of conditions which they illustrate, and the hospital regu-

[1] The reader must not suppose, however, that this method of teaching or practising medicine is extinct. The following is quoted from the *Chicago Night University Bulletin*, vol. iii., no. 24, p. 169:

"A young married man, wife and babe recently returned from Arkansas. They were all loaded with so-called malaria. . . . The old mother came in to tell me of the cases and get some 'chill medicine.' She said they were all chilling three times a day. . . . I sent the little tot ipecac 1M. She said the mother chilled every morning about ten o'clock, and that during the chill she had a very severe cough which hurt her right side. . . . I sent the mother bryonia 200. She said the husband and father chilled at various times. Great thirst during fever, severe cough before and during the chill, with drenching sweat following the fever. I sent him rhus tox, 75M. The prescriptions proved to be rifle-shots for the mother and babe, for they never chilled again; but only a glancing shot for the husband. He missed his chill for a few days, when it returned with new symptoms and more severe and with which no medicine seemed to correspond. I saw him then personally. Found he still had cough during chill, but not before; that he wanted to be covered during fever just the same as during the chill, like nux v. and rhus t.; he had other symptoms which ruled these out. *After searching several hours with repertory in hand, I decided that this was a mixed case and agreed with no medicine in the book.* Hence, following Hahnemann's advice, I gave him cinchona (1M) to clear up his case. After twenty-four hours he chilled again. This time the most peculiar thing noticed was that he was very thirsty during the chill, but in no other stage. He drank large quantities, but during the heat and sweat, not a drop. Also that during the chill the coldness was relieved by the heat of a hot stove. He wanted to get near the hot stove. Remembering . . . that for a chill with thirst for large drinks of cold water, and no thirst in any other stage, ignatia stands alone, I gave him ignatia 1M. to be taken every two hours until he missed his chill—then to be discontinued. Well, he missed the next chill and also every one which has been due him from that day to this."

[2] This method, too, survives in both medical and surgical clinics. It is in process of abandonment in medical teaching, just as rapidly as proper arrangements for ward and bedside work can be made. But it is still favored by surgeons, despite its very slight practical value.

[3] "For clinical studies proper, internal medicine forms the center at German universities. Medical education there follows the principle that medicine is a scientific whole; . . . all its varied disciplines must play upon each other; and from this point of view internal medicine is regarded as the mother of all other clinical divisions." W. Lexis, *Das Unterrichtswesen im Deutschen Reich*, vol. i. pp. 138, 139 (Berlin, 1904).

lations in so far, at least, as they determine (1) continuity of service on the part of
the teachers of medicine, (2) the closeness with which the student may follow the
progress of individual patients, and (3) the access of the student to the clinical laboratory. It matters much less what else a school has by way of clinical opportunity if it
has this, though, of course, the school that has it will have whatever else it needs too.
The main point is that there is no substitute for a good clinic in internal medicine;
the school sampled and found wanting there suffers from a fatal organic lesion. Excellent didactic instruction is no compensation; successful passing of written state
board or other examinations is no proof that the school has managed to do without.
A large surgical service with amphitheater operations every day in the week, a dispensary crowded with eye, ear, and throat cases,—these are all very well in their way.
But one comes back to the medical clinic: that is the really important item. Until
practical state board examinations can be trusted to disclose defective school facilities on the clinical side, it is thrice important to scrutinize carefully the situation
of every medical school in this respect. For proper provision rests at this moment
on the conscientiousness and intelligence of medical educators. Thus far the states
have not adopted an examination procedure that will destroy schools not able to do
their duty in regard to the medical clinic.

The student's clinical work is classified under four heads: (1) medicine, in which
pediatrics and infectious diseases may be included, (2) surgery, (3) obstetrics, (4) the
specialties, such as diseases of the eye, ear, skin, etc. A teaching hospital consists
essentially of a series of wards, accommodating patients belonging to these several
departments, each ward systematically organized with a permanent staff; of a clinical
laboratory, similarly organized and in close organic relation with the wards; and of
an autopsy-room. The clinical laboratory of the hospital is not the same as the
pathological laboratory of the medical school. "A clinic of medicine needs a laboratory equipped with apparatus for chemical, physiological, pathological, and bacteriological work, not so completely equipped as is the laboratory of these respective
departments in the medical school, but specially equipped for certain needs of the
work."[1] On the value of the data thus obtainable it is unnecessary longer to dwell.
The clinical laboratory is the connecting link between the two parts of the medical
school; and it must be immediately accessible. The clinical teacher cannot stop for
data that he must perhaps cross town to get; the student responsible for a particular case will not include in the facts on the basis of which he is making up his
mind the results of an examination of blood, sputum, and feces, if these must be
transported for study much beyond the hospital walls. Nor will the interne or the
young practitioner require the knowledge in question before coming to a conclusion,
unless he has formed at school the habit of so doing.[2] In this laboratory a theoreti-

[1] Henry A. Christian: "The Clinical Laboratory," in *Columbia University Quarterly*, vol. xi., no. 3,
p. 339.
[2] "We see the necessity of laboratories with room for each clinical student, each with his work-place

cal course in clinical microscopy will precede the period when the student is specifically charged with responsibility for the laboratory facts in his own "cases," shortly to be described. Of equally essential importance to the rounding out of the medical curriculum is the autopsy-room, where the wise are brought to book. "Successful knowledge of the infinite variations of disease can only be obtained by a prolonged study of morbid anatomy. While of special value in training the physician in diagnosis, it also enables him to correct his mistakes, and if he reads its lessons aright, it may serve to keep him humble."[1]

The teaching dispensary follows the same lines as the teaching hospital in respect to both organization and equipment, and must be constructed with its pedagogical use in view. It consists essentially of a commodious receiving-room, leading from which are separate rooms, sufficiently large, clean, well lighted, each assigned to a separate department. The several rooms are appropriately equipped with instruments, apparatus, etc., and with a recording system which enables the workers to keep track of each patient and to collate readily all cases of the same general character. Each department must have an organized teaching staff; the receiving-room must be in charge of a physician, who will assign patients to the departments to which they severally belong. The clinical laboratory must be at hand so that the necessary microscopical examinations can be made without loss of time.

From the teaching point of view, the hospital and the dispensary differ in certain respects; certain classes of cases do not usually enter the hospital wards at all: minor surgery, trivial medical ailments, numerous afflictions involving eye, ear, nose, throat, skin, etc. Ambulatory patients are also under less satisfactory control; a large proportion never come a second time. The dispensary is therefore excellently adapted to show a large variety of conditions; it is a relatively poor place to watch their development. In the dispensary the student can become expert in initial physical examination; but only the hospital wards enable him to study progress, to observe nature's comment on therapeutic moves. The dispensary corresponds to the "office hour,"—so important an item in the physician's early progress; the hospital ward represents the sick-room. Clearly, a huge dispensary does not wholly offset a defective hospital.

Between dispensary and hospital, clinical instruction in the third and fourth years is variously apportioned.[2] But apportioned they must be; for the mingling of third

properly equipped. In building this well arranged laboratory the university has by no means erected something superfluous. . . . It has simply met a positive need. In putting the laboratories in such intimate relations with the hospital, and especially with the dispensaries, it has provided means for an immense increase of its facilities. It is a place for practice, for doing as an undergraduate the things that must be done afterward in carrying on the profession of medicine." George Dock, "Address at Opening of Clinical Laboratory of the University of Pennsylvania Hospital," *University of Pennsylvania Medical Bulletin*, Aug., 1909 (slightly abridged).

[1] Osler, *loc. cit.*, p. 144.

[2] Taking a four-year curriculum of 4100 hours as a basis, the pattern curriculum worked out by the Council on Education of the American Medical Association allowed 1970 hours to anatomy, physiology, physiological chemistry, pathology, bacteriology, pharmacology, toxicology, and therapeutics, —or, in other words, the scientific subjects included in the first two years. Clinical instruction gets 2130 hours, distributed as follows:

and fourth year students in clinical work is severely reprehensible,—an infallible indication of deficient clinical material, imperfect teaching organization, or of both. As for the rest, there can be no fixed rule. Important, mainly, is it that the student be brought into immediate and increasingly responsible contact with the disordered machine.

Let us consider briefly the dispensary first. The classes are divided into small rotating sections, each with regular appointments in every one of the dispensary departments. The sections, in charge of separate instructors, should not contain more than ten students apiece—rather fewer would be even better. The student is trained at once to take the patient's history, to make the physical examination, to examine blood, sputum, etc., and on the basis of all the facts thus amassed to make a diagnosis and suggest a course of treatment. The instructor stands by, to correct and to stimulate by question, criticism, or suggestion. Everything is a matter of record, and the student's work is thus part of, in a sense the basis of, the complete dispensary records. In the surgical out-patient department, bandaging, stitching up a wound, administering anesthetics, quickly fall to his lot. Schools favorably located in large cities are able to develop considerable out-patient obstetrical work. Thus the student not only amplifies his experience, but learns to combat the conditions under which he will subsequently be called upon to work. He should, of course, in justice to his charge, be accompanied by an instructor, though in the weaker schools this is by no means always arranged. Even so, however, out-patient obstetrical work, though an experience, is not a discipline: it does not dispense with the necessity of careful training in method under ideal hospital conditions. The young physician will never learn technique and the importance of technique properly except in the maternity hospital; having learned them there, his problem in practice is to secure the essentials even amidst the most unpromising environment. In certain of the specialties— dermatology, ophthalmology—the bulk of the direct instruction received is in the dispensary service. To some extent, of course, the conditions observed in them come under repeated observation in the medical clinics of both third and fourth years; full mastery of a specialty belongs of course to the postgraduate years. But the student must be sufficiently at home to help himself in emergencies and to know when and whence to seek further assistance.

The fourth year is spent in the hospital under precisely the same conditions. The class is again broken up into small groups. Each student gets by assignment a succession of cases, for a full report upon each of which he is responsible; he must take the history, conduct the physical examination, do the microscopical and other clinical laboratory work, propound a diagnosis, suggest the treatment. For this

Medicine (including clinical pathology and pediatrics),	890 hours
Surgery	650 "
Obstetrics and gynecology	240 "
Diseases of the eye, ear, nose, and throat	140 "
Dermatology and syphilis	90 "
Hygiene and medical jurisprudence	120 "

purpose he has easy access to the hospital wards. His "beds" are under his continuous observation from the day his "patient" is admitted until the day of discharge; or, in the event of death, he and the physician ultimately responsible for the steps taken in treatment repair with others to the autopsy-room to bring their knowledge to the test, as Thomas Bond quaintly phrased it. Meanwhile, the clinical teaching has closely followed the development of the case. At brief and regular intervals its status is reviewed. All other members of his group, and the patient too, are at hand when the student presents his report, which forms, once more, part of the permanent record of the case. At every point he has been checked up; the instructor in charge of the clinical laboratory inspects and verifies his work there; the clinical instructor, here. The latter officer reviews everything, pointing out omissions, errors, misinterpretation. The student has always an appeal. He may on second trial convince himself of his blunder. He may, however, be only the more convinced he was right, whereupon another look may persuade the instructor that it is he who errs! Subject to this control, complete, of course, from the standpoint of treatment followed, the student is a physician practising the technique which, it is to be hoped, may become his fixed professional habit; learning through experience, as indeed he will continue to learn, long after he has left school,—a controlled, systematized, criticized experience, however, not the blundering, helpless "experience" upon which the didactically or demonstratively taught student of medicine has hitherto relied for a slow and costly initiation into the art of medicine.

In the surgical ward, a similar arrangement is feasible. The student assists in the operation of his own "case" and follows the after-treatment. Obstetrical training pursues analogous lines. After preliminary drill with the manikin, the student first assists, then has charge under an instructor, of the cases in question. He learns in the hospital wards the proper care and manipulations, his experience supplemented, as we have pointed out, by a regularly organized out-patient department, which brings him in the home, in contact with the trying conditions that he will encounter in practice. Pediatrics and infectious diseases are likewise scheduled and organized. A simple method of rotation carries the student in this intimate and responsible fashion through all departments in the course of two years.

Demonstrative teaching necessarily accompanies the method described: in each group of five, only one student personally explores each case.[1] At the next bed a new protagonist comes to the front; and so on, until each man has had his turn. Always, then, four of the five men are getting demonstrative teaching, though of a somewhat intimate kind. The demonstrative method must, for lack of time, also be more widely employed: large sections are sent on ward rounds, in the course of which the instructor demonstrates the salient features of a considerable number and variety of cases. The defects of the method are manifest: it is not sufficiently direct, accountable, and systematic to constitute the sole lasting discipline. At best, the student becomes in

[1] In some schools two students have charge of each case, the principle remaining the same.

this way familiar with conditions singly and in their combination and interconnection. He gets cross-sections of disease—a most important experience, but, once more, not the same thing as the continuous observation of the developing disease process and the influence thereon from day to day of whatever therapeutic procedure is adopted. In the same way, an instructor in physics might take his students through a large laboratory, showing them how electrical attraction or some other single factor produces a particular type of effect in each of a dozen different experiments,—a most valuable method to impress upon them the specific tendency or effect of the force under discussion; but no substitute for experiments performed by the student himself from beginning to end, in which electrical attraction and much besides come into play. Under any but the most vigorous teaching, the demonstrative method may fail to stimulate sufficiently: the student looks and listens,—a passive attitude that may relapse into something more deeply negative. Finally, the ease with which an expert passes from case to case, the necessity of confining attention to decisive features which he selects, may, if not elsewhere corrected, tend to encourage the superficial examination and the hasty conclusions with which current practice may be justly reproached. Outside the wards there is a narrowly limited use for demonstrative instruction in the class-room or small amphitheater, where groups of cases can conveniently be shown; but the value of demonstration increases apace, as it approaches the intimacy of the individual experiment. Remoteness is quickly fatal. "The larger the circle of listeners, the more difficult for the teacher to hold the interest of them all; as soon as those sitting some distance off no longer see and hear exactly what is to be seen and heard, their thoughts run wild, they lose the logical thread of the diagnostic process."[1] This is especially true of spectacular amphitheater surgery, which is of meager educational value, though as a rule prominently exploited.

Other methods have their uses also; even the didactic lecture may not perhaps be wholly dispensed with. Case work is discrete; students rarely possess sufficient generalizing power to redeem it from scrappiness. At the bedside not much time is available for comprehensive or philosophical elucidation. The lecture—hugging as closely as may be the solid ground of experienced fact—may therefore from time to time be employed to summarize, amplify, and systematize. In time, the student's sense of reality will be sufficiently pronounced to enable him to grasp a rare condition that he knows only through exposition. The wards may have failed to supply an example. But however used—whether to classify first-hand knowledge or to fill up a gap—the didactic lecture would appear to be pedagogically sound only at a relatively late stage of the student's discipline. It has no right to forestall experience, filling the student with ill comprehended notions of what he is going some time to perceive.

Some ingenious Harvard men, profiting by the experience of the Harvard law school, have evolved an effective discipline in the art of inference. Just as a preliminary course in physical diagnosis, teaching the student how to gather his facts, is

[1] Von Strümpell, loc. cit., p. 23.

valuable, so, it is urged, a formal training in the inductive handling of ascertained data may be of use to students whose logical habit has been none too strictly formed. "Let us assume such and such data: what do they mean? What would you do?" This is the essence of the case method,—a method, by the way, excellently adapted to class use, calculated there to develop the friction, competition, and interest which are powerful pedagogical stimulants. It is, moreover, economical, for it brings considerable numbers in touch with fertile teachers, at a minimum expenditure of time and energy.

The class in medicine has another use: it may be made the means of training students to use the "literature;" once more, of course, only by way of amplifying an actual sense-experience. One's own experience always falls short; yet without a very vivid realization of just what one's own experience is and means, one is in no position to use a vicarious experience intelligently. The careful taking and keeping of records is in the first instance the means of clarifying the student's own experience; the instructor's comments raise the questions which he may profitably investigate in the literature. The case record in full and an abstract of important publications on the same subject may well fill a regularly appointed hour given to informal conference and discussion. The student will thus get into the way of reading substantial journals and "running down" literature in the course of his actual practice.

It is a nice question as to how the student's time in the third and fourth year is to be apportioned between patient work, ward work, demonstrative and class exercises, and didactic lectures. The number of hours is itself necessarily elastic: for if the hospital is a laboratory, it is open at all hours, and, subject to the limitations fixed in each case by the condition of the patient, the wards may be used by students, even though no teaching is going on. The principle upon which division may be made has been, however, very clearly stated by Cabot and Locke. "Learning medicine is not fundamentally different from learning anything else. If one had one hundred hours in which to learn to ride a horse or to speak in public, one might profitably spend perhaps an hour (in divided doses) in being told how to do it, four hours in watching a teacher do it, and the remaining ninety-five hours in practice, at first with close supervision, later under general oversight."[1]

In what relation is the medical school to stand to its hospital if the methods above described are to be instituted? Exactly the relation which it occupies to its laboratories generally. One sort of laboratory may as well be borrowed as another. The university professor of physics can teach his subject in borrowed quarters quite as well as the university professor of clinical medicine. Courtesy and comity will go as far in one case as in the other: in both it keeps teaching to the demonstrative basis,—or worse, according to the limitations prescribed. The student can never be part of the organization in a hospital in which he is present on sufferance. A

[1] "The Organization of a Department of Clinical Medicine," by Richard C. Cabot and Edwin A. Locke, p. 9. (Reprinted from *Boston Med. and Surg. Journal*, Oct. 19, 1905.)

teaching hospital will not be controlled by the faculty in term-time only; it will not be a hospital in which any physician may attend his own cases. Centralized administration of wards, dispensary, and laboratories, as organically one, requires that the school relationship be continuous and unhampered. The patient's welfare is ever the first consideration; we shall see that it is promoted, not prejudiced, by the right kind of teaching. The superintendent must be intelligent and sympathetic; the faculty must be the staff, solely and alone, year in, year out. There will be one head to each department — a chief, with such aides as the size of the service, the degree of differentiation feasible, the number of students, suggest. The professor of medicine in the school is physician-in-chief to the hospital; the professor of surgery is surgeon-in-chief; the professor of pathology is hospital pathologist. School and hospital are thus interlocked. Assistants, internes, students, collaborate in amassing data and compiling case records. The student is part of the hospital machine; he can do no harm while all the pressure of its efficient and intelligent routine is used to train him in thorough and orderly method. There comes a time, indeed, in a physician's development when any opportunity to look on is helpful; but only after he is trained: his training he cannot get by looking on. That he gets by *doing:* in the medical school if he can; otherwise, in his early practice, which in that case furnishes his clinical schooling without a teacher to keep the beginner straight and to safeguard the welfare of the patient.

The relationship here indicated has not thus far, as a rule, proved attainable in the United States except through the separate creation of a university hospital. In Germany, where hospitals and universities belong to the same government, our problem does not arise; nor in England and Scotland, where hospital and school have grown up together. In the United States — outside, once more, the few fortunate institutions like Johns Hopkins, the University of Virginia, and the University of Michigan — the schools developed as detached faculties, craving, after a while, some sort of demonstrative teaching privilege in hospitals conducted by the municipality or by philanthropic associations as temporary homes for sick people. Political reasons in the former instance, prudential in the latter, generally forbade an exclusive relationship. Lack of funds interfered with the establishment of laboratories; competition between rival schools required that privileges be both divided and restricted; finally, the inferiority of the students was an insuperable obstacle to any teaching method which sought to use them in the wards in any responsible way whatsoever. More intelligent conceptions are becoming current: the student body improves; competition yields here and there to consolidation. Even so, there remain generally insuperable difficulties: purely philanthropic enterprises must be economically conducted, and they cannot in most places play favorites in the local profession. Adequate equipment, effective organization, and continuous staff service are therefore as a rule improbable. The hospital and dispensary which the medical school must provide to obtain these conditions need be large enough to furnish only the fundamental training of the student body in method and to afford the various members of the faculty their own several workshops. Each department needs beds and accompanying facilities enough to care for typical clinical cases for instruction and for such other cases as the teacher himself wants to study under the most favorable conditions. Beyond this requirement, other local hospitals may well provide supplementary illustrative material, particularly for advanced students. Once more, a long list of such supplementary opportunities scattered through the town is no substitute for the fundamental teaching and working hospital, on the existence of which even a fairly satisfactory use of additional and imperfectly controlled clinical material depends. Indeed, without such a teaching hospital, the school cannot even organize a clinical faculty in any proper sense of the term.

The control of the hospital by the medical school puts another face on its relations to its clinical faculty. What would one think of an institution that, requiring a professor of physics, began by seeking some one who had his own laboratory or had got leave to work a while daily in a laboratory belonging to some one else? That is the position of the medical school that, in order to gain even limited use of a hospital ward, has to cajole a staff physician with a professorial title! When the hospital belongs to the medical school, appointments are made on the basis of fitness, eminence, skill. A man is promoted if he deserves it; if a better man is available elsewhere, he is imported. Opportunities are his in virtue of the university's choice: it is absurd to reverse the order. The men thus freely selected will be professors in the ordinary acceptation of the term: they hold chairs in an institution resting on a collegiate basis,—a graduate institution, in other words. They will be simultaneously teachers and investigators. Non-progressive clinical teaching involves a contradiction in terms. The very cases which are exhibited to beginners have their unique features. New problems thus spring up. Every accepted line of treatment leaves something to be desired. Who is to improve matters, if not your university professor, with the hospital in which he controls conditions, with a dozen laboratories at his service for such aid as he summons, with a staff who will be eyes and ears and hands for him in his absence? These conditions exist in Germany, and clinical science has there thriven; they are lacking here, and clinical medicine droops in consequence. Undoubtedly, outright research institutions for clinical medicine are also necessary: the routine of the clinical teacher cuts into his time, to some extent limits the tasks he may essay, for the knotty problems of clinical medicine are excessively complicated and difficult. But the field abounds in questions for which the university hospital with its laboratories is the right place. Nor will the young doctor, for all his admirable technique, prove a progressive practitioner, even to the extent of keeping up his reading, unless his teachers have been so before him.

By the laboratories connected with the university hospital we do not mean merely the fundamental laboratories, described in a previous chapter, or the clinical laboratory, just mentioned: the former as such deal with the subject-matter of their respective sciences, in their general relations; the latter is part of the routine machinery of the hospital. To suffice for clinical investigation the laboratory staff must be so extended as to place, at the immediate service of the clinician, the experimental pathologist, experimental physiologist, and clinical chemist in position to bring all the resources of their several departments to bear on the solution of concrete clinical problems. Of these branches, experimental pathology and physiology have already won recognition; the next step in progress seems to lie in the field of clinical chemistry, thus far quite undeveloped in America.

It follows that in other respects, too, the clinical professors will be on the common university basis: salaried, as other professors are. Of course, their salaries will be inadequate, i.e., less than they can earn outside,—all academic salaries paid to the right men are. But there is no inherent reason why a professor of medicine should not make something of the financial sacrifice that the professor of physics makes: both give up something—less and less, let us hope, as time goes on—in order to teach and to investigate. The clinical teacher should indeed not arbitrarily restrict his experience: he may wisely develop—preferably in close connection with the hospital—a consulting practice, assured thus that his time will not be sacrificed to trivial ailments. On the same basis, other university facilities are at the service of those who require unusually skilful aid; for at all points only good can come of educational contact with unsolved problems,—practical or other. But a consulting practice—developed in a professional or commercial, rather than in a scientific spirit —may prove quite as fatal to scientific interest as general practice. University hospitals, academic salaries, etc., make the conditions in which clinical medicine may be productively cultivated. They do not create ideals; and without ideals, superabundant and highly paid consultations are perhaps as demoralizing as superabundant low-priced "calls."[1]

The financial resources at this moment available are far from adequate to provide hospitals exclusively and continuously the laboratory of the clinical departments of medical schools, and faculties composed in the first place of scientific teachers of clinical medicine. Twenty-five years ago as much would have been said in reply to a plea for thirty medical schools each equipped with a complete set of scientific laboratories. When the number of our medical schools is once reduced to our actual requirement, the sum involved in properly equipping them with hospitals will not appear impossibly formidable. Meanwhile, existing hospitals may well enlarge their teaching facilities, where such facilities are open to a high-grade student body. Nothing is clearer than that an intimate relation to medical education properly carried on is to the advantage of all concerned,—to the larger public, by producing better physicians, to the patient, by procuring for him more competent attention. On this point there is no room for doubt. "I speak after an experience of nearly forty years,"

[1] See, for example, Graham Lusk: "Medical Education," *Journal Amer. Med. Assn.*, April 17, 1909, pp. 1229, 1230, and S. J. Meltzer, "The Science of Clinical Medicine," *ibid.*, August 14, 1909, pp. 508-12.

says Dr. Keen, "as a surgeon to a half-dozen hospitals, and can confidently say that I have never known a single patient injured or his chances of recovery lessened by such teaching. Moreover, . . . who will be least slovenly and careless in his duties, —he who prescribes in the solitude of the sick-chamber and operates with two or three assistants only, or he whose every movement is eagerly watched by hundreds of eyes, alert to detect every false step? . . . I always feel at the Jefferson Hospital as if I were on the run, with a pack of lively dogs at my heels."[1] Miss Banfield, after an ample experience, looking at the question solely from the standpoint of patient and nurse, takes the same position: "As a matter of fact, in a properly administered hospital, medical schools are a protection to the patient rather than otherwise, for it usually means that the hospital is a very live one. . . . In teaching hospitals, I think that on the whole patients are generally better nursed, for every one is kept up to the mark, including the professors."[2] The committee appointed in 1905 to inquire into the financial relations between the hospitals and the medical schools of London, touch in their conclusions the point here in question: "We find," they say, "that the presence of a body of eager young men watching the proceedings of their teacher has the tendency to keep the medical man on the alert and to counteract the effects of the daily routine of duties."[3]

There is little difference of opinion as to the necessary size of a teaching hospital. Less than two or three hundred beds, in practically continuous occupation, can hardly supply either the number or the variety of cases required. It is held that a hospital of 400 beds will support a medical school of at least 500 students. It is highly important that the instructor should have the material that he needs when he needs it. The material must, moreover, be properly distributed: an abundant clinic in diseases of the eye is no substitute for defects in the departments of internal medicine and obstetrics; seventy-five cases of operated appendicitis do nothing to compensate for the lack of typhoid, pneumonia, or scarlet fever.

The size of the school has, of course, some bearing on the necessary size of the hospital, though the hospital cannot be allowed to shrink in exactly the same ratio as the number of students. Because two hundred beds may be made to suffice for one hundred students, it does not follow that twenty beds suffice for ten students. Twenty-five students require in general the same minimum as one hundred students. On the other hand, it is fair to weigh advantages and disadvantages against each other. A small number of students in a small but still fairly representative and completely controlled university hospital, through whose corridors fresh scientific breezes from the university and medical school laboratories blow, will get a better discipline in the

[1] W. W. Keen: "The Duties and Responsibilities of the Trustees of Public Medical Institutions," *Transactions Congress Amer. Physicians and Surgeons*, 1903.
[2] Maud Banfield: "Some Unsettled Questions in Hospital Administration in the United States," *Publications of Amer. Acad. Pol. and Soc. Science*, no. 351, pp. 46, 47 (slightly abridged).
[3] *Report of the Committee*. Published for King Edward's Hospital Fund for London, by George Barber, 23 Furnival Street, Holborn, E. C. p. v, 15 (B).

technique of modern medicine than a larger body, loosely supervised in an antiquated city hospital where "students" are eyed askance as interlopers. The defects of the former, due to somewhat circumscribed experience, a hospital year will quickly redeem, for he has, and knows how to use, the tools; the defects of the latter will as a rule never be repaired at all. Such a hospital year is in any event highly desirable. It is to be hoped that a more effective and economical organization of preliminary education and a more intelligent public opinion may presently make its exaction generally feasible.[1]

On the basis of the undergraduate instruction described, opportunities for advanced or graduate instruction must supervene. Such opportunities serve two quite different functions. In the first place, the various specialties must be systematically and thoroughly developed as graduate pursuits, resting on a thorough training and experience in general medicine. The number of these specialties is increasing, as more varied and more effective appliances suggest increased differentiation,—a safe tendency, in the interest of efficiency, provided the discipline required does not infringe upon undergraduate territory. In the next place, to these postgraduate institutions the hard-run intelligent practitioner in smaller towns will at intervals return, in order to be invigorated at the head-waters: he will want to get in touch with recent improvement, to see in a brief period a large variety of interesting material, handled by experts in his own field. To both these purposes, the larger hospitals of our great cities may freely lend themselves. Their abundant wards can be used to excellent advantage, even though they may continue to be governed by their present boards. It is probable that the obstacles to such use will largely disappear as the competitive and commercial exploitation of medical education is itself abandoned. For beyond all doubt, not the least serious of the deplorable consequences that have followed in the wake of mercenary medical education is the limitation of hospital opportunities, due to the rivalry of "faculties" and to the incompetent student body to which, largely because of such antagonisms, the intimacy of the ward privilege would have had to be extended.

[1] Our required medical course, prior to practice, now covers four years. In Germany five years must be spent at the university, a sixth in a hospital; in England, "official statistics published recently under the authority of the General Medical Council show that the mean length of the curriculum in the case of 1111 students investigated was three weeks less than seven years; only 14 per cent succeeded in obtaining a qualification in the minimum period of five years, 35 per cent obtained it in the sixth year, 18 per cent in the seventh year, 13 per cent in the eighth year. When the remaining 20 per cent obtained it does not appear, probably never. Looking at the figures in another way, we find that at the end of six years less than half had obtained a qualification for registration, and at the end of seven years only two-thirds." *British Medical Journal*, Sept. 5, 1908, p. 634.

CHAPTER VII

THE COURSE OF STUDY
THE HOSPITAL AND THE MEDICAL SCHOOL

The Third and Fourth Years (continued)

In the end the final test of a medical school is its outcome in the matter of clinicians. The battle may indeed be lost before a shot is fired: a low average of student intelligence and inferior laboratory training will fatally prejudice even excellent clinical opportunities, for they rule out certain essential features of clinical training on a modern basis. A serviceable type of doctor was doubtless once produced under conditions that we now pronounce highly unsatisfactory; again, students defectively trained sometimes meet with success in examination or other tests designed to ascertain the quality of their instruction. It is not necessary to investigate closely the merits of the test in order to refute the argument that it endeavors to sustain. The institutions that seek to establish the non-importance of facilities that they do not possess emphasize strongly the importance of those they do. And with good reason. Before undertaking the responsibility of instruction in chemistry or physics or biology, a competent teacher stipulates that he be provided with this, that, or the other. He is not to be put off with the assurance that some men have successfully mastered the subject without laboratory or tools. Very properly he takes the ground that whatever may be true of individuals, in general boys will be much better trained in a laboratory with the essentials than in a bare room practically without them. It is equally true of clinicians. Doctors have after a fashion been made by experience,— i. e., their patients paid the price; further, some graduates of every feeble clinical school in the country have passed state board examinations or obtained hospital appointments, at times after competitive examinations in which they defeated students from schools more highly favored; it still remains true that to do full duty by the young student of clinical medicine, his teachers need access to acute cases of disease in respectable number and variety; that the school which lacks such medical facilities is in no position to teach modern medicine.

In the matter of laboratories we discovered no slight cause for satisfaction. Within two decades the laboratory movement has gained such momentum that its future, even its immediate future, is in no doubt. A race of laboratory men has been trained and quite widely distributed. They know their place and function; they have educated the college administrator to accept them at their own valuation. Where deficient resources still force a compromise, the apologetic attitude is a sufficient promise of more liberal provision by and by. On the clinical side the outlook is less reassuring. The profession itself has in large measure still to be educated; the clinical faculty often stands between the university administrator and a sound conception of clinical training. It happens, therefore, not infrequently that a university president will hear with astonishment, if not with resentment, that facilities made up of insecure and disconnected privileges scattered here and there through the hospitals, public and private, of a community now large, now small, do not satisfy the fundamental requisites of clinical discipline surpervening upon modern laboratory work; or that a surgical clinic is no substitute for a clinic in internal medicine. The regeneration of clinical education is therefore apt to proceed somewhat slowly: the sources from which well trained clinical teachers can be drawn are few; the places in which they can be freely utilized are equally restricted. Students trained in the laboratories on modern lines enter clinical departments still more or less unconverted. The result is at best a half-result, yet upon it progressive amelioration in large measure depends.

Once more a few schools meet the specifications set forth in the preceding chapter. We there urged that the backbone of clinical instruction must be a pedagogically controlled hospital best developed on its medical side. The exact status of the hospital may indeed vary: a proper footing has been obtained now through coördinate and coöperative endowment,[1] again through state support in connection with the state university,[2] at times through a really effective affiliation.[3] The crucial points are these: (1) the hospital must be of sufficient size; (2) it must be equipped with teaching and working quarters closely interwoven in organization and conduct with the fundamental laboratories of the medical school; (3) the school faculty must be the sole and entire hospital staff, appointment to which follows automatically after appointment to the corresponding school position; (4) the teaching arrangements to be adopted must be left to the discretion and judgment of the teachers, subject only to such oversight as will protect the welfare of the individual patient.

As long ago as 1869 the department of medicine of the University of Michigan began in a remodeled dwelling-house, capable of accommodating twenty patients, the development of a university hospital on fundamentally sound lines. From this modest beginning a teaching hospital of two hundred beds has now grown up, every patient available for the purposes of instruction, in so far as his own welfare permits. The staff of the hospital is the faculty of the school; the ward service in his own department is the laboratory of the professor. Ward rounds and amphitheater clinics are used for demonstrative teaching; but, better still, students are assigned to individual cases, which they work up at the bedside and in the clinical laboratory. An isolation ward is provided for infectious diseases; a lying-in ward is administered by faculty obstetricians and senior students; recently a psychopathic hospital, thoroughly modern in construction and management, has been made available. Difficulties, of course, of a serious nature have been encountered; the state by a liberal policy has minimized them. Ann Arbor is a small residential town; it is necessary to attract or

[1] Johns Hopkins.
[2] Michigan; Iowa.
[3] Lakeside Hospital and Western Reserve (Cleveland). The newly endowed Barnes Hospital (St. Louis) will occupy a similar position in reference to Washington University.

to transport thither many cases from other parts of the state. The outcome practically formulates for us the terms upon which such an enterprise is feasible: a modern equipment, a salaried clinical faculty, clean-cut ideals, and careful husbandry will build up a substantial clinic in a small American as in a small German town. It can be supplemented by bringing the hospitals of the entire state into working relation with the medical department of the state university. The expense of the establishment is relatively great; but the advantages over a divided, perhaps even a remote department,[1] are on the whole cheap at the price. How many more such institutions we should, however, now undertake to create is of course quite another question.[2]

The Johns Hopkins Medical School has been even more highly favored. Its hospital endowment was, fortunately, sufficient to warrant a comprehensive design from the start. The general teaching hospital then provided has been recently supplemented by generous benefactions that add separate clinics for tuberculosis, pediatrics, and psychiatry; wards, dispensary, clinical and scientific laboratories, coöperate for both pedagogic and philanthropic purposes. The clinical departments are organized like any other. Nowhere else in the country has so consistent a scheme been so admirably realized. The student is made a factor in the conduct of the hospital: he assists on the clinical side as clerk, on the surgical side as dresser, following the admirable method long in vogue in the Scotch and English schools. In each department he serves an appointed novitiate, following his "cases" from start to finish,—now to recovery, again to autopsy.

There is no insuperable reason why several other medical schools should not take advantage of a fortunate relation to hospitals to bring about an equally effective organization. In one place lack of money, in another, hampering tradition, alone prevents. The organization above described cannot be perfected unless these two defects are simultaneously cured. If hospitals are to enter into exclusive and practically complete relationship with a single medical school, the university must on its side procure funds which enable it to be independent of the local profession. Unless these two conditions are coincidently fulfilled, the clinical situation cannot be thoroughly made over. Three Philadelphia schools (the University of Pennsylvania, the Jefferson Medical College, and the Medico-Chirurgical College), two Baltimore schools (the University of Maryland and the College of Physicians and Surgeons), and one Chicago school (Rush Medical College),[3] are in sole and complete control of excellent hospitals, more or less adequate in size. The same intimacy is equally desirable and equally feasible for both parties in interest between Wesley Hospital and North-

[1] The divided department is discussed from the laboratory side, page 74; from the clinical side, page 119. For an account of remote departments, see (Part II) University of Texas, University of Indiana, Cornell University.

[2] Similar hospitals, not as yet so well developed, are at present connected with several other state universities: the Universities of Iowa, Colorado, Minnesota, Texas. The details are given in Part II, under the several institutions.

[3] But in this instance the patient's consent must first be obtained.

western University,[1] between Roosevelt Hospital and Columbia University. The reluctance of the hospital to go the whole length is in these latter cases the most formidable obstacle to perfecting a relation that would be of incalculable advantage to all concerned. For assuredly the university medical schools just named, if offered complete teaching control, could cope with the problem of procuring means with which to reorganize their clinical faculties on a scientific and pedagogical basis. The enlightened action of its trustees is rapidly perfecting the same connection between the admirable Lakeside Hospital of Cleveland and Western Reserve University. The new Barnes and Children's Hospitals of St. Louis have engaged to do as much for the reconstructed medical department of Washington University. McGill, Toronto, the University of Manitoba (Winnipeg), and Tulane are in practically secure possession of clinical facilities that are adequate in respect alike to extent and control. It is to be noted that the schools above named do not own the hospitals in which their clinical teaching is given. Western Reserve and Lakeside thus prove the feasibility of a smooth working connection between a university department of medicine and a private hospital; Toronto proves the same as between a university medical school and a municipal hospital. Technically, neither set of trustees can renounce control; they must ratify appointments; but that act can either be reduced to a formality or expanded into meddlesome supervision, as the trustees choose. In the two instances cited, it has become a mere form; and two objects, both precious, are most effectively promoted in consequence. On the strength of these instances it is perhaps worth while to make one more plea for an understanding between existing hospitals and deserving medical schools. Cannot an arrangement be consummated by which the administration and financing of a private or a municipal hospital shall be left to the trustees and their appointed agents, while equally, even though not technically, complete and separate responsibility for the medical conduct of the hospital and for teaching within its wards is left to the medical faculty? As these functions are absolutely distinct from each other, there is no reason why two bodies of intelligent men, desirous of doing right in their respective spheres, should not thus coöperate. If, of course, the trustees are every now and then going to overrule the university in the securing of a teacher or to overrule a physician in his treatment of patients, the situation becomes intolerable and impossible. Instances have occurred, for example, in which the board of women managers of a children's hospital has forbidden the use of lumbar puncture. It is not strange that these things have happened, because neither party to the arrangement has had definite ideas as to the limits of its province. Now, however, that there is no further doubt as to just what the trustees ought to do, on the one hand, and as to just what the university ought to do, on the other, it would appear an auspicious time for extending the experiment. The list of teaching hospitals as above given is so far not large. It may, however, to some extent be lengthened by

[1] At present, clinics at Wesley Hospital are not limited to Northwestern University students.

adding schools with hospitals not as yet adequate in size, of which type the University of Virginia furnishes the most satisfactory example. Long contentedly a didactic school, this institution has just undertaken to develop a modern clinical department. The new and excellent University Hospital, with eighty ward beds, is still under size. But a speedy development may be somewhat confidently anticipated. Its problem is that which Michigan has already shown how to solve; meanwhile it is perfectly clear that the justification of such a school lies in the fact that its situation makes possible the most intimate relations between the clinic and the scientific laboratories, and a discipline in medical technique so thorough and so vigorous that a few gaps in the student's experience may prove relatively insignificant. There is every indication that the University of Virginia thoroughly appreciates both points.

By no means every hospital owned by a medical school is, however, to be reckoned a teaching asset. The details require to be closely scanned. In many cases they are private institutions, in process of being paid for out of their own profits and out of the fees of medical students, who are lured by the advertisement of a school hospital from which they get no good at all. Barnes Medical College (St. Louis) adjoins Centenary Hospital, "which affords clinical facilities surpassed by none and equalled by few;" but except for part of one floor, the building is given over to private rooms.[1]

Where control ceases, ideals necessarily change. A medical school with its own hospital may of course be sterile. Unwise appointments may cut off all possibility of productivity; too much consultant prosperity may be fatal to scientific zeal; inbreeding may exhaust fecundity. On the other hand, an occasional clinician may keep his lamp trimmed despite every obstacle, — poor facilities, a precarious term of service, lack of appreciative sympathy. Neither the one nor the other contingency, however, militates against the position that as between the two systems a school hospital is in America essential to the existence of an efficient department of clinical medicine; that in its absence the general plane of instruction settles down to a distinctly lower level.

The best of the schools without a hospital which they can call their own do not lack for abundance or variety of clinical material. Rush, Northwestern, the College of Physicians and Surgeons (Chicago), Columbia, Cornell, and the University and Bellevue Hospital Medical College (New York), Harvard and Tufts (Boston), are not troubled for clinical material; some of them have more of it than they can possibly use, — much more than several of the university hospitals can ever hope to command. But the conditions to which they submit in order to gain access to it at all, though varying somewhat from place to place, are alike fatal to freedom and continuity of pedagogic policy. Our clinical failure concurs with the clinical success of the Germans in proving that freedom is the very life-breath of scientific progress, — freedom on

[1] Similar is the relation between the medical department of Lincoln Memorial University (Knoxville) and its hospital next door ; between the University Medical College and the University Hospital (Kansas City) ; and between the Milwaukee Medical College and Trinity Hospital.

the part of the university to choose its own teachers, finding them where it may; freedom on the part of the teachers to strike out along whatever path they please. An artificial impediment will in general entail barrenness.

The institutions above named are necessarily confined to the local profession for clinical teachers,—a restriction that they would find intolerable in any other department and that they endure under protest in medicine, only because they are not yet financially in position to throw off the yoke. No disrespect to the practising profession in these large cities is implied: they are doubtless as good doctors as can be found anywhere. But they are not teachers; they have neither time for, nor effective interest in, productive teaching. If they were really as much interested in clinical science as in professional prosperity, they could as a body do much to improve hospital conditions on the pedagogical side. As a matter of fact, professional prominence and institutional rivalry keep the college tenure insecure, often chop the hospital services into short terms, compel hospital authorities to abridge teaching privileges in order to avoid friction, and present a solid and opposing front to the importation of outsiders, even though the outsider chance to reside in the same town. Under such conditions it becomes at once impossible to entertain in clinical medicine the ideals set up in the laboratories of pathology, physiology, or chemistry. One pitches one's expectations lower. It becomes a scramble for abundance and variety of "facilities" on the part of the schools; public hospitals split up and overload their services in order to distribute their favors widely; private institutions promote their prosperity by declining exclusive alliances. In Chicago staff positions in the great Cook County Hospital are awarded every six years by competitive examination; and the schools make what terms they can with the winners, who rotate from ward to ward at stated periods. No bedside clinics are allowed; patients are wheeled into teaching-rooms or amphitheaters for demonstration; anyone who purchases a ticket may attend any clinic that he pleases. The student gets an excellent chance to see detached conditions; what he loses is the opportunity to observe individual cases of disease in process of development and to correlate his own laboratory findings with symptoms observed at the bedside. As for the professors, whisked about in rotation, scientific study is out of the question. At Bellevue Hospital (New York), Columbia, Cornell, and New York University have each a "division," within which, however, they are not supreme; the medical board, composed of the entire visiting staff of all three schools and the fourth division,—the outsiders,—limits the freedom of the several parties in interest; final authority is lodged with a lay board, who have, for example, recently overruled Columbia in its own division. At Boston neither Harvard nor Tufts has the initiative in filling staff positions in the hospitals used in teaching. Appointments are made by seniority; it is well-nigh impossible for the school to break the line. In Boston as in New York, the large hospitals tend to have their own pathological departments, the permanence of whose relation to the corresponding department of the medical schools is decidedly uncertain. Money and educational opportunity are thus both wasted. As a rule, services rotate every three or four months; the hospitals sometimes provide clinical laboratory space in which students work.[1] All these institutions possess supplementary facilities. In general, however, supplementary clinical opportunities are of fragmentary and precarious character; the medical school has as such no uniform constitution, nor is a single department an organized entity; clinical clerks may be employed by one teacher for three months, only to be spurned by his successor in the service at the close of his brief term. Fresh pathological material may be procured by giving a faculty appointment to a coroner's physician, while the professor of pathology scours the city in vain for admission to a dead-room; instead of compact departments pulling as a whole towards a definite goal, a half-dozen professors of medicine and surgery stand on an equal footing, each compelled to conform to conditions imposed by the hospital on the staff of which he is a transient sojourner, or holding the whip-handle over his own school, because the school cannot antagonize the clinical professor without imperiling its clinical opportunities correspondingly. The normal relation of school and teacher is inverted. The question is not, "Who is a good teacher?" but rather, "Who controls a hospital service?" In a large city, the curtain rises on a dozen hospitals, each already provided with a staff, and several medical schools, each requiring a faculty of men who can bring as their dower "clinical facilities." There is a lively competition: at once, every holder of a hospital service finds himself a potential professor of medicine, surgery, or whatnot. When the scramble is over, the counted spoils appear in the catalogue in the form of a list of the hospitals "open to students of this school." The hospital appointments are therefore valuable "plums." They give the holders the call in the matter of school rank; and school positions are still in most places of substantial commercial value. It happens, in consequence, that the schools under discussion are put together of two dissimilar pieces: the laboratory branches are of one texture, the clinical branches of another. The laboratory men are imported; their productivity has been increased by crossing the breed. The clinical men are local[2] and, with some notable exceptions, contentedly non-productive. There is little intercourse across the line in either direction. The redeeming feature of these schools is, then, simply the amount and variety of clinical material that their students see.

The plane drops once more as we leave behind these large schools and approach the next class. Conditions now become rapidly worse through aggravation. Hospital management becomes increasingly unsympathetic or unintelligent, thus keeping the schools on the anxious bench. In truth, not much can be expected. "Amongst the

[1] In a few services a continuous term prevails for the time being, — sometimes by arrangement among the teachers themselves, sometimes by way of personal compliment to an individual. Welcome as such improvements are, they are far from curing the trouble.

[2] One can in a few lines give a complete list of schools that can and do go outside the local profession to procure clinical teachers : Johns Hopkins, University of Michigan, University of Virginia, Yale, Tulane (in medicine), University of Pennsylvania, and Washington University. These institutions have imported perhaps a score or two of clinical teachers ; there are almost 4000 more clinical professors in the United States and Canada who are practising local doctors.

hospital superintendents I know of, there are, besides a very few physicians, an ex-newspaper reporter, a ward boss, a china factory hand, various clerks, and a still more varied assortment of clergymen. . . . In order that domestic complaints may be removed, a committee of ladies is sometimes appointed, . . . their only claim to knowledge being that of the 'born housekeeper' supposed to be inherent in every woman. The organization and management of institution households, however, hav-ing little in common with that of a few maids and no sick people, the management of details by visiting committees is often but an added discomfort."[1]

Such institutions are mere boarding-houses for the sick. Physicians call there as they call at a private house, seeing twenty patients in the former instance, a single patient in the latter. It is the difference between wholesale and retail,—no other; scientifically the "calls" are on the same level. The visiting staff of physicians is ap-pointed through favor, pull, or bargain, and the schools make the best of it. A small clique occasionally controls the situation. Conspicuous fitness cannot be the sole or main consideration. A school rich in facilities to-day may be beggarly to-morrow. The medical department of Toledo University has just lost its main clinical sup-port as one outcome of a local political overturning. The University of Minnesota has been fortunately hastened in the resolution to build its own hospital because a local upset reduced its former privileges. The Woman's Medical College of Phila-delphia adjoins a hospital of which its faculty was once the staff; now there is no commerce between them. The Hering Medical College at Chicago (homeopathic) is in even closer proximity to a homeopathic hospital: a bridge connects them; but the barred doorway bears the legend, " No students admitted." Medical politics are de-cisive at Albany; to keep control in the hands of the dominant clique of the Albany Medical School (the medical department of Union University), the size of the fac-ulty was recently increased, all the new members being adherents of the side in power. The City Hospital at St. Louis, the County Hospital at Denver, are frankly described as being "in politics."[2] Staff appointments made for personal or political reasons may of course be revoked for reasons that are no better. The uncertainty of any one connection constitutes a good reason for getting hold of as many as possible. Columbia, for example, used to be supreme at Roosevelt Hospital, opposite its lab-oratories; it is being gradually edged out,—a deplorable condition for all concerned; but it has recompensed itself abundantly elsewhere. The medical department of the George Washington University protects itself by providing that " every clinical teacher shall cease to be such teacher should his facilities for giving clinical instruc-tion cease before the end of his term of service."[3] If a school drops an indifferent teacher, it may be worse off than if it retained him; for he keeps, and the school loses, the "clinical facilities" that he represents. St. Louis University, in purchasing

[1] Banfield, loc. cit., pp. 42, 43 (abridged). Occasionally, feeling is cordial, as at Topeka, for example.
[2] The same is admitted at Halifax, N. S.
[3] Ordinance to Reorganize the Department of Medicine, section 3.

its present medical department, contracted to keep the clinical professors in their chairs for a term of years. When the term expires, they are free to drop them,—at the cost, however, of cutting down their clinics in the same ratio. In a few places things are held together somewhat more compactly by an arrangement that gives the school faculty the hospital services during term time. Such is the case at Mobile, Birmingham, and Chattanooga. But in general a hospital staff is composed of heterogeneous elements, appointed for reasons that cannot be classified. Representatives of no school and representatives of all schools, serving now through the year, again for a few weeks, now in one ward only, now rotated through several, make up a situation unfavorable to every interest involved. In New York the ancient ecclesiastical evil of plural benefices crops out unexpectedly: one individual may hold several appointments in hospitals so far removed from each other that he cannot possibly do even his perfunctory duty by them; instead of surrendering superfluous perquisites, he sub-lets them at will, according as fancy or personal interest may determine: the staff appointments appended to his name are so many scalps hung about his belt! There is no such thing as hospital policy: the wards have as little wholeness, as little intimacy of relation with each other, as the private homes in which these same physicians treat their personal patients; only a local accident puts one roof over them.

Teaching is obviously but an incident in the routine of these institutions. Not infrequently amphitheaters have been included in their construction; but they usually lack a clinical laboratory in which students may work, not a few lack it altogether. The failure to provide clinical laboratory space thus keeps instruction to the level of passive demonstration. The student has presumably spent two years in mastering certain medical sciences. A large part of this laboratory discipline was designed to enable him to gather a greater variety of facts than the bedside examination will disclose. Blood, sputum, urine, etc., all contain important evidence which the laboratory years equip the student to utilize. He has been taught to do certain things. But at the critical moment, when doing them will count, he may get no chance, in the first place, because at many hospitals, among them those mainly relied on by the University of Nebraska (Omaha), Denver and Gross (Denver), the Hahnemann Medical College (Philadelphia), and most southern schools, there is no clinical laboratory at all. At Denver "there is no equipment to make a culture, and the internes are rarely equal to it, anyway." At Omaha, the clinical microscopist of the university faculty was unable even to get material from the County Hospital; when he wanted gastric juice for demonstration, he had to manufacture it himself. In the second place, where a clinical laboratory is provided, "students" are as a rule not admitted. The work is done by a resident pathologist who has no connection with any of the several "schools" that are permitted to demonstrate cases in the amphitheater or in the wards; or by internes, equally detached and too frequently of very doubtful competency by reason of just the educational limitations we are deploring. To the clinical laboratories connected with the municipal hospitals of St. Louis, Chicago, Minneapolis, students have no access, though in these hospitals, rich in material, the students of St. Louis University, Rush and the College of Physicians and Surgeons (Chicago), the University of Minnesota, respectively, ought to be getting the best part of their clinical training. Not infrequently it is alleged that the students do "carry material for examination back to the college:" the students of the Creighton School (Omaha) and of the Los Angeles schools would thus have to transfer specimens of urine, feces, and gastric contents on the street cars across town,—distances of several miles. At Southwestern University (Dallas, Texas), a section of four students has an assigned patient at the City Hospital, perhaps a mile and a half distant, where there is no clinical laboratory ; to work up material, they must carry it to the college building, —where there is no clinical laboratory, either. Educationally, an "academic" laboratory discipline that thus hangs loose, that cannot be brought to bear on specific clinical cases, must be largely wasted. There is no merit in making a blood-count unless the student has been disciplined to connect the blood-count with all other symptoms of the patient whose blood is counted. As it is, he beholds a patient, sees things pointed out, may even listen to his heart-beat; away off in the college laboratory, he has previously examined some one's urine, counted some one's blood, tested, perhaps, an artificially prepared gastric juice. But there is no connection; the discipline splits in the middle. Scientific habits of practice are not established in that way. Nor are loose habits, thus contracted, cured by an internship. Pupils are more apt to disappoint than to astonish their teachers; they do not generally better their instruction. In consequence hospital records made by internes graduated by these schools are scant and unsystematic. Defective methods at the University of Buffalo were extenuated on the plea that as internes they learn better ; but the meager records of the Buffalo General Hospital disprove the claim. Whoever is responsible, poorly kept records are very apt to denote inferior bedside instruction. The situation is this : there lies the patient ; teacher, interne, and students surround the bed. The case is up for discussion. A question arises that requires for its settlement now a detail of the patient's previous history, now a point covered by the original physical examination, now something brought out by microscopic examination at some time in the course of the disease. If complete, accurate, and systematic records hang at the bedside, there is an inducement to ask questions; doubtful matters can be cleared up as fast as they are suggested. That, then, is the place for the records,—full records, at that. In few instances are the records full; in still fewer are they, full or meager, in easy reach. At the University of Kansas, at Lane Hospital (Cooper Medical College, San Francisco), there is no uniform method of making or keeping records: "some men do better than others;" "it depends on the man." At the Protestant Hospital, Columbus, Starling-Ohio graduates are internes, the records are nurses' charts ; at Trinity Hospital (Milwaukee), attached to the Milwaukee Medical College, the same is true.[1]

[1] Similar instances can be cited from all other sections of the country : the records are nurses' charts at the hospital of the College of Physicians and Surgeons, Little Rock, and at the City Hospital—

The clinical facilities of the ordinary medical school are put together of scraps, the general character of which have now been described. They offer a medical clinic here, an obstetrical clinic there, a skin clinic somewhere else. Faculties numerically out of all proportion to the number of students are assembled in order to piece out the quilt: Fordham University has 72 instructors for 42 students; the New York Medical College for Women has 45 instructors for 24 students; the Toledo Medical College, 48 instructors for 32 students; the Oakland College of Medicine and Surgery, 42 instructors for 17 students. As the hospitals are scattered, time is wasted in going to and fro. All told, our 150 medical schools have resulted, among other things, in some 4000 professorial titles.[1]

Imagine the engineers that would be produced if students were sent to a series of shops to see things done,—as far as they could be seen without interfering with the workmen! In no two of these hospitals is exactly the same kind of teaching privilege granted; and the privileges granted are highly precarious: the hours are arbitrarily limited, and number of beds is usually too small. Nowhere do they approach the ideal which the school might readily institute in its own hospital. They fall short, however, in varying degrees. In St. Louis the situation is lamentable. The City Hospital has a medical and surgical staff who "do no teaching," and a teaching staff who "do no doctoring." Each of the half-dozen schools in the town has one afternoon; the instructor must go out to the hospital the day before to select two cases for demonstration,—an amount of trouble which the better men are reluctant to take. The instruction consists in pointing out features and suggesting what ought to be done: in surgery, it may have been done already; in medicine, there is no telling. In either case, the entire process remains purely hypothetical. These opportunities are not infrequently treated as they deserve: at the St. Louis College of Physicians and Surgeons it was stated: "This is hospital day; lots of them don't go." In the County Hospital at Los Angeles, the main reliance of two university departments of clinical medicine,—one of them (the University of California) requiring for admission three years of college work,—students are not permitted to handle sur-

---

used by two schools—at Memphis; at Ensworth Hospital, one line in a ledger contains all the facts on record; at Topeka, the same is true; it is added that "laboratory reports are not kept, and physical examinations could not be found;" the histories, made up by internes at the Kansas City Hospital, are so irregular that "the visiting staff don't even read them." They are imperfect at the University of Texas (Galveston); defective and careless at the Maine General Hospital (Portland).

[1] See Table in Appendix, for a complete list. The disproportion in point of number between laboratory and clinical chairs is instructive. For example:

NUMBER OF FULL PROFESSORS IN

Institution	Anatomy	Pathology	Physiology	Medicine	Surgery (not including gynecology)
Cornell	2	2	1	5	9
Columbia	2	2	1	8	5
St. Louis	1	1	2	5	6
Denver and Gross	1	1	1	5	5
University of Louisville	1	1	1	4	8
Contrast with these					
Johns Hopkins	1	1	1	2	1

gical patients, and teachers "shall not conduct bedside clinics when possible to re-
move patients from the ward;"[1] on these terms 100 beds are available, for six hours
weekly in surgery, and perhaps for a few more in medicine. At Creighton, students
"witness the operation," and are admitted to about 90 beds. In Denver, students
"are not much at the bedside; they just look on;" the hours are from 8.30 to
10 a.m., daily,—the early hour having been fixed, it is alleged, to prevent the attendance of the state university boys at Boulder. There are "ward classes" at Memphis—
as many as fifty students in a group at once!

Where things are patched up in the way described, it is of course impossible that
proportions and relations should be observed. We have urged that the backbone of
clinical training must be internal medicine. But it is precisely here that the schools
are in general weakest. The sum total of accessible beds may amount to a hundred:
not infrequently less than one-fifth of them will contain medical cases. The "additional facilities" of the larger schools are mainly surgical in character; and in general, the less a school has to offer in the way of clinical facilities, the more heavily
is surgery overweighted. Its pedagogical value is relatively slight; for operations are
performed in large amphitheaters in which the surgeon and his assistants surround
the patient, to whom they give their whole mind, in practical disregard of the
students, who loll in their seats without an inkling of what is happening below. Most
of the students see only the patient's feet and the surgeon's head. Only in rare cases,
previously mentioned, in which the student helps to form the machine, do designated individuals take turns and become part of the operation,—making the examination, watching the procedure at close range, and "cleaning up" afterwards.
Inadequacy in general is thus aggravated by increasing predominance of surgical
over medical clinics. Clinical teaching thus tends more and more to concentrate
in the amphitheater. The laboratory side sinks further and further into the background; the bedside work becomes more and more contracted. The whole thing is
demonstrative—and at steadily increasing remoteness. At the University of Vermont juniors and seniors have most of their medical and surgical clinics together,
averaging in medicine about three hours weekly one year and four hours weekly the
next; and the work is mostly in the amphitheater. Dartmouth Medical School has
access to 24 beds, eighty per cent of the patients occupying which are surgical cases.
Bowdoin—to complete the list of the smaller New England schools—uses the
Maine General Hospital, Portland, where surgery greatly predominates. Tufts has an
imposing array of clinical facilities; but its medical clinic is limited to the Boston Dispensary and one service in the City Hospital. Kansas Medical College relies almost
wholly on three hospitals, in which it gets a total of nine or ten hours' instruction
weekly: in two of the three hospitals all the work is surgery; in the remaining, two-
thirds of it. In the university hospital at Rosedale (University of Kansas), there were
last year 240 patients, 190 of them surgical; six free beds are this year reserved for

[1] *Rules and Regulations, Los Angeles County Hospital,* section 4, rule 12.

medicine. Of course, the school has privileges elsewhere; but this small hospital is all that it controls, though two years of college work are required for admission. The Starling-Ohio Medical College (Columbus) uses several hospitals: in one 150 beds are open, "mostly surgical;" in another 40 beds, "mostly surgery." The Detroit College of Medicine has access to two hospitals; one of them, with 100 teaching beds, is fortunate in a fairly equal division between medicine and surgery; the other describes its work as nine-tenths surgical. The clinical instruction of Epworth University (Oklahoma City) is given in a hospital within which 30 to 40 beds are available, two-thirds to three-quarters of the cases being surgical. Drake University uses 30 beds during a weekly total of twelve or fifteen hours in two hospitals, in neither of which is the student essentially other than a passive witness. The Chicago College of Medicine and Surgery—being the medical department of Valparaiso University—has a hospital of 75 beds, about one-fourth usable for teaching; the Bennett Medical College (Chicago) has a hospital of 40 beds, 20 claimed as free; at Chattanooga, the city hospital contained, all told, in the course of the year 1908 something over 500 patients; at Augusta, about 300. Temple University (Philadelphia) has a hospital with 20 free beds; the Woman's Medical College (Philadelphia), 27; the New York Eclectic Medical College sends parties limited to three students to the Sydenham hospital twice weekly. The Physio-Medical College of Chicago got along last year with 167 patients; Western University (London, Ontario) has access to an average of less than 30 beds a year. At Trinity Hospital (Milwaukee), with 75 beds, mostly pay, — a part of Milwaukee Medical College,—nine-tenths of the cases or more are surgical.

We have, however, by no means even yet exhausted the subject of arbitrary clinical limitations. As a rule, only the general medical and surgical wards are open at all. Few of the hospitals possess an isolating ward, and not all of these permit students to see infectious diseases. The instruction in that important branch is therefore usually didactic. This holds true of some schools that ask two years of college work for entrance, Yale and the University of Kansas among them. It is true, too, of the New York Medical College for Women, the University Medical College (Kansas City), the Starling-Ohio (Columbus), the University of Tennessee, Baylor University and Southwestern University (Dallas), Louisville, Little Rock, Memphis, etc. At Albany it was stated that the hospital has a pavilion for infectious diseases, which the school might use: "it does n't, because the students are afraid." But the very worst showing is made in the matter of obstetrics. Didactic lectures are utterly worthless. The manikin is of value only to a limited degree. For the rest, the student requires discipline and experience. The safety and comfort of both patients — mother and child — depend on the trained care and dexterity of the physician. The practice is a fine art which cannot be picked up in the exigencies of out-patient work, poorly supervised at that. Principles, methods, technique, can be learned and skill acquired only in an adequately equipped maternity hospital; only after that is the student fit to be trusted with the responsibilities of the out-patient department. Difficulties and limitations in such matters sit lightly on most of our medical schools. The hospitals of Atlanta and Los Angeles exclude students from the obstetrical ward; at Burlington there is no obstetrical ward, but the "students see more or less;" at Denver a "small amount" of material is claimed; at Birmingham it is "very scarce;" at Chattanooga there are "about ten cases a year," to which students are "summoned," how or by whom is far from clear. At the Hahnemann Medical College (Chicago) students "look on at internes who do the work;" a committee of the Missouri state board reports of the College of Physicians and Surgeons of St. Louis that it could find only incomplete records of 21 cases for a senior class of 57; at Augusta, Georgia, the cases "always come at night when you can't get students;" at Charlotte 15 cases were available from September 15 to February 4; the medical department of Lincoln Memorial University (Knoxville) has no out-patient department, but alleges "a few deliveries before the class;" Vanderbilt relies on out-patient work mostly. There is a senior class of almost 150 at the American School of Osteopathy (Kirksville, Missouri). In two months they had eight clinical cases in obstetrics. Perhaps most lamentable of all, the Woman's Medical College of Baltimore concedes its opportunities to be "inadequate." At Toledo, Louisville, the University of Tennessee, Kansas City, the University of Kansas, Albany, and Yale, obstetrics is practically altogether out-patient work; that is to say, the student gets about the same training as a mid-wife. At Willamette (Salem, Oregon) he probably does not get even that: for "obstetrics depends on private practice and is very precarious. The student sees a delivery when the doctor is willing to take him."

Not a few of the schools mentioned have elevated their entrance requirements until they already demand one or two years of college work for entrance, or expect to do so presently.[1] Meanwhile their clinical facilities remain what they were. Doubtless some of them will make haste to improve,—Yale, for example. Others will probably recede from their announced elevation,—as several have already done. Assuredly, students who improve their preparation will demand that the schools improve their facilities correspondingly. In the laboratory years this has generally taken place: he will be a dull fellow who does not quickly feel and resent the inferiority of the clinical end. In all fairness, the betterment of the facilities, the change of spirit and ideal, ought to have preceded as the warrant for the higher entrance standard. For the two-year college standard proclaims a university department. It still remains to be demonstrated that towns like Omaha, Washington, San Francisco, Topeka, Milwaukee, can recruit university faculties from the local profession. A university connection or a two-year college entrance requirement do not, of themselves, transform a medical school faculty. They merely impose upon it an additional strain.

The strain to which high entrance standards and good laboratory teaching at

[1] Kansas Medical College, Dartmouth, Yale, Creighton, Denver and Gross, Hahnemann (Chicago), Starling-Ohio, Milwaukee Medical, Wisconsin College of Physicians and Surgeons, etc.

once subject the clinical end is distinctly apparent in the remote half of the divided school. We have already[1] considered the perplexities of the laboratory end without contact with clinics. They appeared not insoluble. Whether two clinical years given by themselves with practising physicians as teachers can ever form a substantial texture is highly problematical. The latter half of a divided school is given by the University of California at San Francisco,[2] by the University of Nebraska at Omaha,[3] by the University of Kansas in a suburb of Kansas City,[4] by Bowdoin College at Portland.[5] The American Medical Missionary College carries division still further. It is divided between Battle Creek and Chicago; but no single year is entirely given in either place. Every class is shifted in the course of the year from one town to the other. Nor does the division end here; for at Chicago, the clinical instruction is divided so that different pieces are given at widely separated places. These pieces do not touch each other, and none of them ever touches the laboratory work given in Battle Creek. Indeed, none of the detached clinical departments is doing well. The vitality of the clinic depends on the closeness of its commerce with the laboratory branches; otherwise the clinical end is not rooted. Thus far none of these has achieved either executive or scientific intimacy. A certain degree of executive unity may perhaps be secured through a dean freely circulating between the two parts, though if he is attached as professor to one end of the department, the other is apt to resent intrusion. Scientific unity seems in any case unattainable. The clinical men at Omaha or San Francisco simply cannot be at home in the laboratories of Lincoln or Berkeley. Laboratories must be duplicated at the clinical site if the clinicians are to be in touch with them: in which case the divided type of school tends to turn into the whole remote type illustrated by the medical departments of the universities of Texas at Galveston, Indiana at Indianapolis, and of Cornell at New York. The truth is that an efficient medical school is a compact whole, in which geographic unity of laboratories and hospital is essential to scientific and educational integrity. The wilted condition of the clinical ends of the divided schools is a warning that Michigan, now contemplating the removal to Detroit of the final year in medicine, may well weigh. Even separation of the two parts within one city is a disadvantage.[6] Division seems justifiable only as a temporary expedient to get clinical material, pending a choice between concentration of the entire school at one point or the other, or outright abandonment of clinical instruction in favor of a two-year school.[7]

[1] Page 74.

[2] First half given at Berkeley. The latter half will be duplicated at Los Angeles. Leland Stanford Junior will shortly give the latter half of its medical course at San Francisco, too; its first half is given at Palo Alto.

[3] First half given at Lincoln.

[4] First half given at Lawrence.

[5] First half given at Brunswick.

[6] As at Rush (University of Chicago).

[7] Several of the southern state universities and the University of Colorado are in this position.

Meanwhile we are not without schools that have practically no hospital connection at all. The Mississippi Medical College (Meridian) has absolutely no hospital facilities or privileges of any sort whatsoever. The Georgia College of Eclectic Medicine and Surgery (Atlanta), the California Eclectic Medical College (Los Angeles), are in the same plight. Others are hardly better: for example, the three Chicago night schools, one of which, the National Medical University, had two lonely patients on the top floor of the school-building, though claiming the usual relations with a private pay institution. Thrice happy for the nonce is the Hippocratean College of Medicine (St. Louis), a night school; it crosses no clinical bridges till it reaches them: as it is only three years old, it need not bother about hospital connections until next year! The Lincoln (Nebraska) Medical College deplores the fact that "there are no poor in Lincoln; hence students have no regular hours at any hospital, but depend on cases as they turn up." The Hahnemann Medical College of Chicago has two surgeons on the Cook County Hospital staff and a hospital of 60 beds; but the lay superintendent "does n't believe in admitting students to the wards, so that there is no regular way for them to see common acute diseases." The College of Physicians and Surgeons, Denver, had access to a hospital of 28 beds, "certain ones free." The medical school at Little Rock that trades on the name of the University of Arkansas, with which it is not even affiliated, is connected by a bridge with a city hospital that has a capacity of from twenty-five to thirty-five patients, some of whom are occasionally transported across into the amphitheater for operation or exhibition. The clinics of the medical department of Willamette University (Salem, Oregon) are somewhat intangible: whether medical clinics are held, and where, "depends on the cases." Not infrequently, schools advertise varied hospital connections that prove on investigation to be baseless or surreptitious. The Philadelphia College of Osteopathy claims "the freedom of every important surgical clinic in the great medical colleges and hospitals" of that city. Its hospital list is almost a page long; at the top stand the University and Jefferson Hospitals, to which its students can gain access only by concealing their identity. Rights or privileges they have none. The College of Physicians and Surgeons of Boston announces that "equal opportunities and privileges are available in the hospitals and institutions" of that city, — a flagrant misstatement; for the students of that institution can on payment of fee attend only certain public clinics of little value.

It is unnecessary to describe dispensary conditions in equal detail: naturally they parallel the hospital situation. The same clinicians are responsible for both; in general, the dispensaries would be likely, therefore, to reflect the same degree of intelligence and conscientiousness. A teaching dispensary needs ample space, equipment for making the necessary diagnostic examinations and for taking simple therapeutic or surgical measures on the spot, a well organized staff, and a thorough record system, in the keeping of which students serve as clerks. Voluminous attendance is an advantage, because it permits selection in the first place, repeated illustration of important conditions in the second. It may be set down as fundamental that a good dispensary will not run itself; that nothing in the way of equipment will be used that is not actually there. Economy of time is of such importance to both teachers and students that makeshift inevitably means neglect. The well conducted dispensaries are the well equipped and well organized dispensaries. The moment that equipment and organization fail, omission begins; no general rule prescribes where it will stop.

Vanderbilt Clinic—the dispensary attached to the College of Physicians and Surgeons, New York (Columbia University)—represents in respect to facilities the school dispensary at its best. Teaching and treatment rooms, ample in size and equipment from the standpoints of both students and patients, are provided; a clinical laboratory, with working space for every student on duty, is part of the building; close correlation of physical examination and laboratory tests is feasible. An admirably kept card index facilitates the keeping and use of data; there was an attendance in 1908 of almost 50,000 patients, making over 160,000 visits. The Johns Hopkins Dispensary and the Lakeside Dispensary, operated by Western Reserve, are equally efficient. Less sumptuously housed, but adequate in all essential respects, are the dispensaries of Cornell, New York University, the three Philadelphia schools, and those open in Boston to Harvard and Tufts. The Polhemus Clinic controlled by the Long Island College Hospital, the Homeopathic Medical Dispensary controlled by the Boston University School of Medicine, must be included in the number of excellently housed, equipped, and organized institutions of this kind.[1] Yale has an excellent building, which the application of a few thousand dollars yearly will readily convert into an effective teaching adjunct.[2]

The first break comes in the care with which an abundant attendance is handled. It would seem probable that, where the records are careless and incomplete, the treatment of patients is likely to be hurried. The compilation and arrangement of data slow the pace. They conduce to, and usually indicate, thoroughness and deliberation,— of fundamental importance if the student is to acquire a cautious habit. Lack of system and superficiality tend to run together. Mere mass of material, swiftly handled, may be useful to experienced practitioners in affording a variety of cases among which occasionally something rare and interesting may turn up; but a student who is in such a dispensary initiated into the routine of practice will be fortunate ever to form methodical and thorough working habits. The Los Angeles clinical branch of the University of California possesses a thoroughly admirable dispensary building. Some of the rooms are well, some ill equipped; the records are brief and non-significant; no report is compiled; and the clinical laboratory, indispensable to intelligent conduct of an out-patient department concerned to mould the student's

---

[1] A few institutions possess small, moderately well equipped dispensaries, the conduct of which indicates conscientious desire to do the best possible under the circumstances. Creditable examples are the dispensary of Drake University (Des Moines) and the South End Dispensary used by the Albany Medical School.

[2] Denver and Gross also has an excellent dispensary building.

habits and to do well by its patients, is both defective and disorderly: the surgical instrument case contained a tack-hammer, candle-ends, and other equally incongruous miscellaneous objects among its instruments. In the medical department of the University of Cincinnati, there is a card index alphabetically arranged; but the results of the physical examination are not given, nor is there any note of the treatment advised. The Starling-Ohio Medical College (Columbus) has a clean dispensary, with adequate attendance, but no records in a proper sense at all; Halifax Medical College requires attendance at a city dispensary that possesses little equipment for treatment, still less for teaching; besides, the college has no voice in its conduct. The students of Syracuse University also attend a city dispensary, but the head clinical professors know nothing about what they get, or fail to get, there. Utterly destructive of good habits of observation or treatment must be a dispensary like the North End Dispensary, Kansas City, attended by the students of the state university; equipment and records are alike defective and confused. But there are others much worse. Dispensary suites are found at the Barnes Medical College and the College of Physicians and Surgeons (St. Louis). The former claims an annual attendance of 10,000 cases. Several rooms are provided, those devoted to branches like gynecology and surgery being especially filthy. The equipment for internal medicine consists of a small dirty room and a few miscellaneous bottles of proprietary drugs scattered on the shelves of a bookcase. The dispensary of the College of Physicians and Surgeons is of the same general character: the gynecological room, for example, is without a window, water, or instruments; all is dark and dingy; there are no records of cases; evasive answers are made to all questions. The fact is that a dispensary, costing little to keep and nothing to run beyond the expense of a drug room, cannot answer for teaching. Nor can youthful volunteers be usually relied on to form an efficient staff. The expenditure on the score of dispensary must be greatly increased if the material that presents itself is to be effectively handled in the training of students.

These schools shade off imperceptibly into those that make no pretense to a dispensary at all, passing on the way institutions like Birmingham Medical College, with a department both small and poor; Augusta, without case records, not even prescriptions put up in the pharmacy being numbered; Portland (Oregon), claiming two to seven a day; the Jenner (Chicago), claiming two to ten nightly; the Physio-Medical (Chicago), with perhaps 250 all of last year; the Eclectic (New York), using "what comes to the college;" Charlotte, with loose unnumbered cards, mostly unintelligible, the prescription files showing an average of four or five a day. At the Detroit Homeopathic College one finds prescriptions written on scraps of paper, envelope backs, etc., with neither numbers nor names; at the Cleveland Homeopathic Medical College "medical cards are kept in pigeonholes that are cleaned out every spring." The Kansas City Eclectic school is hopeful, if not ambitious: its dispensary attendance averages now "about three daily;" they hope to be able "to work it up to six." The medical department of Bowdoin College uses a dispensary at Portland that has an attendance of eight or ten a day : there are no case records, not even a prescription file, no clinical laboratory, and not so much as a microscope on the premises. The University of Alabama (Mobile) is the only small southern school with decent dispensary quarters: an attractive wing has been recently built for the purpose by the state.

There remains still the goodly number of schools that possess absolutely no dispensary provision at all. With some of them we are already familiar as destitute of hospital facilities. Without dispensary teaching of any kind, their students enter the homes of the poor,— to officiate at childbirth, to care for wage-workers on whose well-being depends the independence of the family. Meridian, the Georgia Eclectic, Willamette, the Lincoln Eclectic, the Hospital Medical College (Atlanta), the American Medical College[1] (St. Louis), the Chattanooga Medical College, Western University (London, Ontario), are representative schools of this description. It is painful to include in essentially the same class the Medical College of the State of South Carolina, at Charleston, which in lieu of a school dispensary refers to the out-patient work of the Roper Hospital, with which its students have nothing at all to do. The two Dallas schools—both long without a dispensary—are now starting one; Ensworth Medical College at St. Joseph, Missouri,—a city of 130,000,—has practically no dispensary at all; Epworth University (Oklahoma City) is in the same plight. Not a few of these institutions might develop a fair dispensary service if their opportunities were intelligently cultivated. For example, the University of Buffalo, in a city of 400,000, has a wretched dispensary with a daily attendance of from twelve to fifteen, if one can judge by sampling ; for tabulated records there are none. Such notes as exist are brief and irregular. The poor do better to suffer in silence rather than to trust to the haphazard student medication that such institutions now supply.

Astonishing to relate, the conditions that have been portrayed are defended. It is alleged in extenuation that "our graduates pass state board examinations, get hospital appointments, succeed in practice." It is quite true: what of it? The argument if valid would commit every school above the lowest to deliberate deterioration of its facilities. Bowdoin makes light of a wretched dispensary on the grounds above cited; Dartmouth men succeed by the same tests without any dispensary at all; ergo, Bowdoin may safely forego dispensary teaching altogether. Is it not obvious that both are mistaken? that they take hold of the situation at the wrong end? Medical education is nowadays a definite problem, the factors to which, the end of which, may be specifically stated. We know exactly what it drives at; we can determine to a nicety the means necessary to reach the goal thus set up. It will shortly be demonstrated that the number of doctors needed can in most sections be supplied without material departure from the conditions agreed on. Why, then, should they be abandoned? In order that local doctors may continue to develop their professional

[1] At this school one is naïvely told that they have "a dispensary room, and almost every day some one comes."

business? In order that "historic" schools may continue to produce a slightly ameliorated type of didactically trained physician?

As a matter of fact, many of the schools mentioned in the course of this recital are probably without redeeming features of any kind. Their general squalor consorts well with their clinical poverty: the class-rooms are bare, save for chairs, a desk, and an occasional blackboard; the windows streaked with dust and soot. In wretched amphitheaters students wait in vain for "professors," tardy or absent, amusing the interval with ribald jest and song. The teaching is an uninstructive rehearsal of text-book or quiz-compend: one encounters surgery taught without patient, instrument, model, or drawing; recitations in obstetrics without a manikin in sight,—often without one in the building. Third and fourth year men are frequently huddled together in the same classes. At the Memphis Hospital Medical College the students of all four years attend the same classes in many of the subjects taught.

So much for the worst. It may be, however, that in the case of some schools with weak hospitals and no dispensaries, the didactic instruction is vigorous, clean cut, in its way effective. Such is the claim made at Dartmouth and at Bowdoin. Let us concede its justice: what of it? Logically, the position of these institutions would be stronger if they stuck to didactic instruction altogether. The moment that they offer a course in clinical microscopy, they are committed to an entirely different scale of values. For that they require patients whom they can observe closely and continuously in order that laboratory data and bedside data may be put together as the basis of a specific judgment. In other words, teaching must henceforth be concrete, not abstract; clinical, not didactic. Good didactic instruction may indeed to some extent accompany clinical teaching. We are not especially concerned to determine its actual extent.[1] Let it earn the school an extra credit, if you please. But its excellence is no substitute for missing, defective, or badly balanced clinical opportunities.

---

[1] The subjoined comparative schedule indicates the distribution between clinical and didactic work in schools of various grades. This table is not alone conclusive; for schools with weak clinical resources are not infrequently without illustrative material, so that a clinical lecture may perforce turn into a didactic lecture. Moreover, clinical instruction of the amphitheater type may, if the students are few and the conditions good, be as useful as a bedside demonstration; where, however, the students are many and the conditions poor, it may be no better than a didactic exposition.

COMPARATIVE SCHEDULE, THIRD AND FOURTH YEARS

Third Year

Western Reserve University

Subject	Did.	Lab.	Clin.
anatomy			
Applied anatomy	96		
athology and Preventive Medicine			
Gross pathological anatomy		32	
Autopsy technique		10	
Hygiene and preventive medicine	40		
harmacology, Materia Medica & Therapeutics			
Pharmacology	84	20	
Therapeutics	32		
Advanced prescription writing		6	
edicine			
Physical diagnosis			68
Medicine and clinical medicine	64		96
Clinical microscopy	35	105	
Medical dispensary			24
urgery			
History taking	12		
Surgical diagnosis	20		
Fractures and dislocations	18		
Genito-urinary surgery	12		
Principles of surgery	64		
Clinical surgery			64
Surgical pathology		60	
Surgery dispensary			36
Eye, ear, nose, & throat	32		24
stetrics & Gynecology			
Obstetrics	64		
Gynecology	32		12

New York University

Subject	Did.	Lab.	Clin.
Pathology			
Demonstrations		64	
Applied pathology	32	64	
Bacteriology		64	
Pharmacology			
Lectures	16		
Therapeutics			
Lectures and recitations	96		
Medicine			
Lectures and recitations	192		
Section work: hospital, dispensary, and bedside			96
Clinics			96
Diseases of children	64		
Surgery			
Lectures and recitations	192		
Section work: hospital, dispensary, and bedside			96
Clinics			96
Operative surgery		32	
Obstetrics			
Lectures and recitations	96		
Manikin work	8	3 wks.	
Lying-in hospital			
Gynecology			
Recitations and demonstrations	32		

Medico-Chirurgical College

Subject	Did.	Lab.	Clin.
Anatomy			
Applied anatomy	48		
Path. & Bacteriology			
Pathology	96		
Bacteriology	32		
Surgical pathology	32		
Autopsies		1	
Therapeutics			
Lectures and recitations	128		
Therapeutic clinics			32
Prescription dispensing	16		
Medicine			
Med. & clinical med.	64	64	64
Pathological physical diagnosis			1
Children's diseases	32		32
Nervous and mental diseases	32		32
History taking		1	
Surgery			
Lectures and recitations	192		
Clinics			128
Operative surgery & bandaging	50		
Orthopaedic surgery			32
Obstetrics and Gynecology			
Obstetrics	96		1
Gynecology	32		32
Specialties			
Ophthalmology			32
Laryngology			16
Otology			16
Dermatology			32
Medical Jurisprudence & Toxicology[2]	32		

[1] Section work; exact number of hours not given.
[2] Part of this work is laboratory.

University of Alabama

Subject	Did.	Lab.	Clin.
Anatomy			
Anatomy of the eye, ear, nose, and throat	14		
Pathology			
Lectures, recitations, and laboratory	28	112	
Therapeutics			
Lectures and recitations	56		
Electro-therapeutics[1]		56	
Medicine			
Lectures and clinics	56		112
Physical diagnosis	28		
Clinical diagnosis		56	
Surgery			
Lectures and clinics[3]	38		112
Obstetrics			
Lectures and recitations[3]	112		

[1] On class schedule as "Electricity."
[2] Clinics are the same for 3d and 4th year classes.
[3] Class schedule shows only one recitation per week.

Fourth Year

Western Reserve University

Subject	Did.	Clin.
thology & Preventive Med.		
ygiene	24	
eventive medicine	20	
edical jurisprudence	20	
dicine		
edicine and clinical med.	96	96
ysical diagnosis		50
ard clinics		40
dside work		32
spensary medicine		50
inical microscopy	1	
seases of children	32	50
seases of nervous system	32	23
rmatology and syphilis	64	27
edical ethics, economics, and Roentgenology	1	
rery		
rgical diagnosis	12	
citations	20	
nical surgery		192
spensary surgery		50
ard work, clinical microscopy, and assignment to cases		64
hthalmology	32	
e dispensary		50
r, nose, and throat		50
trics and Gynecology		
stetrics	64	1
nikin work	1	
ical gynecology		64
pensary gynecology		50
ber of hours varies.		

New York University

Subject	Did.	Clin.
Pathology		
Conference	32	
Pathologic chemistry	6	
Autopsies		8
Therapeutics		
Conferences	32	
Hygiene	32	
Special subjects	30	
Medicine		
Recitations & clinics	60	96
Section work		72
Neurology	32	12
Diseases of children	48	20
Mental diseases	16	
Dermatology	32	16
Surgery		
Recitations & clinics	92	96
Section work		72
Genito-urinary surgery	32	24
Orthopaedic surgery	32	4
Obstetrics and Gynecology		
Obstetrics	34	
Gynecology		52
Specialties		
Ophthalmology	32	16
Otology	16	16
Laryngology	16	20

Medico-Chirurgical College

Subject	Did.	Clin.
Pathology		
Autopsies	1	
Therapeutics		
Applied therapeutics		2
Medicine		
Theory and practice	192	
Clinical medicine		96
Medical dispensary		2
Diseases of children		32
Pediatrics dispensary		2
Nervous and mental diseases	16	48
Dermatology	16	32
Dispensary dermatology		2
Surgery		
Lectures and recitations	192	
Clinics		2
Genito-urinary surgery	16	2
Orthopaedic surgery		2
Ophthalmology		2
Laryngology		2
Otology		2
Obstetrics and Gynecology		
Obstetrics	64	
Clinical obstetrics and manikin work		2
Gynecology	64	32
Gynecology ward clinics		2

[1] When material is available.
[2] Section work; number of hours not given.

University of Alabama

Subject	Did.	Clin.
Medicine		
Medical clinics[1]		112
Nervous and mental diseases	42	
Tropical medicine	56	
State medicine	28	
Dispensary, all subjects[2]		28
Dermatology	28	
Surgery		
Lectures and recitations	70	
Clinics[1]		112
Operative surgery	84	
Genito-urinary surgery	28	
Hospital section[2]		70
Obstetrics and Gynecology		
Obstetrics lectures	56	
Gynecology lectures	56	
Other Subjects		
Hygiene and medical jurisprudence	28	
Ear & nose diseases	56	
Eye and throat diseases	84	
Ophthalmology		28

[1] Clinics open to 3d & 4th year classes.
[2] Clinics only for 4th year...

CHAPTER VIII

THE FINANCIAL ASPECTS OF MEDICAL EDUCATION

An examination of the financial aspects of the American medical school will completely account for the conditions that have been described.[1] It is universally conceded that medical education cannot be conducted on proper lines at a profit, — or even at cost; but it does not follow that it has therefore ceased to "pay." It is commonly represented that medical schools are benevolent enterprises, to which selfish financial considerations are nowadays quite alien. Such is not even generally the case. Our best medical schools are indeed far from self-supporting; they absorb the income of large endowments or burden seriously the general resources of their respective universities. But these institutions constitute but a small fraction of the medical schools of the country. The others pay in one or more of several ways, if "paying" is understood to mean that the fees do more than meet the expense of running the school. This use of terms is entirely justifiable; for if fees alone are inadequate to meet the running expenses of an up-to-date medical school, then the difference between actual expenditure on instruction, with its essential incidentals, and the total fee income of the school is profit, whatever the use to which it is applied. In the worst cases this sum is great and goes into the pockets of the teachers; in many others, it may not be large in any single year, though its total over a stretch of years may be quite sufficient to have altered materially the complexion of the institution. In these schools an annual balance to the good is obtained for distribution by slighting general equipment, by overworking laboratory teachers, by wholly omitting certain branches, by leaving certain departments relatively undeveloped, or by resisting any decided elevation of standards. In one or more of these ways, for example, not to go outside the Empire State, the Albany Medical School is enabled to pay some $500 a year apiece to otherwise well-to-do clinicians; the University of Buffalo to distribute "nominal sums" of $1000 to a number of professors in large regular practice; the Long Island College Hospital to apportion a substantial sum out of the fee income in tithes among the faculty; and the University and Bellevue Hospital Medical College to pay out of fees salaries to some of the most successful practitioners in New York city, while the laboratory branches still lack anything like uniform development. More favorable, but still by no means beyond the reach of legitimate criticism, is the case of schools that, admitting the impossibility of providing satisfactory instruction at cost, nevertheless save from current use a not inconsiderable amount to be applied to paying for buildings or plant instead of dividends. Every such saving is necessarily at the expense of instruction; that is to say, if every dollar taken in were consumed in current teaching, unfortunate makeshifts would still have to be employed. With every dollar less than total fee income

[1] See appendix for table showing income of medical schools.

used in providing teaching, the quality of instruction is still further impaired. As the country becomes able and willing to support at a loss the number of schools needed, the ethical justification of other schools that must pay a profit—even though that profit go into buildings and equipment—becomes decidedly dubious.

Most of the existing medical school plants have been provided in this manner; quite commonly those who have participated in the operation fail to reflect on its significance. For if a good medical education costs more than the student pays in fees, then, even though an adequate plant has been provided in advance, his instruction must at some essential points be curtailed if additional income is not available. If, however, fees must provide either initial plant or plant extension, it is clear that proper teaching must be still further refused during the years when fees are employed to accumulate equipment. Historically that is the explanation of our extensive medical school plants in New York, Philadelphia, Baltimore, Louisville, Chicago: instruction far below what was at the moment scientifically feasible was given to the current student body, in order that their fees might be used to provide a better basis for a body of students that would come along in the future. Didactic lectures were given in 1890, to pay for a building in which laboratory instruction could be given in 1900. As conditions improved, one laboratory was put into operation, while a fee surplus was accumulated to install a second. Before the day of medical school support by endowment or taxation, such procedure compared very favorably indeed with the more common practice of doing nothing for the student of to-day and as little as possible for the student of to-morrow. The point now to aim at is the development of the requisite number of properly supported institutions and the speedy demise of all others.

In varying degrees, contented acceptance of these conditions goes along with the survival, however insidiously, of the notion that medical education, whatever else it may be, is something of a business, too. It is questionable whether this notion can ever be uprooted, so long as several competing schools in the same or in adjacent towns solicit patronage that can never again be sufficient in volume to satisfy them all. The essence of a business transaction consists in spending less in producing an article than is paid for it over the counter, how much less depending now on the proximity and competitive eagerness of other dealers, now on the wariness and number of the customers. It matters not that in this instance the article is education, the counter the registrar's latticed window, the profit going in extreme cases in large sums into a doctor's pocket, in the best cases in smaller sums into bricks and microscopes. If, in other words, medical education is a social function, it is not a proper object for either institutional or individual exploitation. Society ought to provide means for its support according to the best light obtainable; and the law should make it impossible for any person or institution to engage in it on any other than the best terms that society is in position to enforce. Great departures from this principle were at one time inevitable: the country was bound to have doctors; it had to take them as it could get them. They need never have been so badly trained as most of them were. But on that point it is useless to dwell. Important for us it is to ascertain whether in this year of grace, 1910, it is still necessary to put up with schools that are seriously defective; and if so, to what extent, and how much longer.

What does it really cost to carry on a medical school that construes its duty in social terms? Initial investment may be put to one side. That, the college income cannot furnish; fees cannot provide buildings and equipment in the first place, or pay for them subsequently in instalments. The medical school must start with an adequate plant, laboratory and clinical, debt free. The value of these plants may vary within very wide limits; size, style, the ratio of teaching to research, all bear on the problem of initial cost. In a measure it is a question of taste, how much one will expend on buildings and equipment. Essential, however, to every venture are class-rooms with the essential teaching paraphernalia, class laboratories in each of the sciences with individual equipment, private quarters with requisite appurtenances for each member of the teaching staff. These facilities cannot be dispensed with because the numbers to be handled are small. The several items may be scaled down, but they do not disappear. Fee income, confessedly inadequate to keep such a plant running, cannot be called on to provide it. The plant, therefore, is taken for granted before we even begin to consider what it costs to teach medicine.

For the sake of simplicity we shall continue the demarcation between laboratory and clinical branches. At present the cost of maintaining the hospital is not usually a school encumbrance. Whether or not it ought to be must be decided as the case arises. Western Reserve is in position to avoid the expense; the University of Michigan must carry it. In general, the school obligation on this point has been shirked. The intolerable compromises described in the preceding chapter are employed in consequence. Nothing will perhaps go further towards destroying superfluous schools or preventing new ones than correct ideas as to necessary hospital conditions. It is quite impossible that most schools should either possess their own hospitals or effect a satisfactory relation with hospitals belonging to other people. At the moment, possession rather than diplomacy seems in most places to furnish the only satisfactory solution, —and possession necessitates an immense increase of the school budget. Meanwhile, this point will not be obscured by provisional separation of the two budgets; for this manner of presentation an additional reason is found in the fact that, to a varying extent, the hospital may be made to carry itself without derogating from its pedagogical purpose.

A schematic outline of the laboratory years calls for at least five departments, (1) anatomy, (2) physiology and pharmacology, (3) chemistry, (4) pathology, (5) bacteriology and hygiene, subject, within limits, to rearrangement. The ultimate cost of the entire school will not be greatly affected by such redistribution. In their internal economy the departments will follow the same general lines. There will be a professor, devoting himself wholly to teaching and research, and in position to do both;

assistants varying in number with the size of the classes and the extent to which the institution is minded to encourage original activity; a departmental helper attached to each department; preferably, too, a technician and a mechanic, who will, however, in the end more than save their cost.

The budget of a department thus organized in a medical school of, say, 250 students, favorably situated, would assign $3000 to $5000 a year to its head, $2000 to $2500 to a first assistant, $1000 to $2000 to additional assistants, $750 to a helper, and $2500 to $5000 to maintenance, including books, new apparatus, material, animals, etc. The total, ranging from $9250 to $15,250, still omits a proportionate share of the general overhead expense of administering the institution. A university department in one of the fundamental medical sciences, none too elaborately provided, cannot, then, on the average be effectively maintained for less than $10,000 to $15,000 per annum. At the moment, of course, the departments are not all equally expensive. Anatomy and pathology cost more than pharmacology and bacteriology. But the average is not thus seriously disturbed; for the former will extend above the line as much as the latter can be reduced below it. All of them, as they are developed, tend to cost more. Where the sum named has not yet been reached, the tendency towards it is unmistakable. It is, of course, true that fairly good instruction is at times furnished more cheaply. In the small two-year schools situated in small towns, the professors receive less, sometimes much less, than the sums stated; and the expense of maintenance does not at times exceed a few hundred dollars per annum. But these departments cannot continue on this makeshift basis: they are now manned by young men, who, finding themselves doomed to routine and sterility, begin fighting at once to get away. The teacher who is content under such circumstances will soon be out of date; and the instruction, however conscientious, will be decidedly limited in range. To live, these departments must be much more liberally supported; and in the small two-year schools where this has been the case—notably at Cornell and Wisconsin—the departmental budgets correspond pretty closely to our present estimate. The organization of a department of, say, physiology on the minimum basis of efficiency, for 25 students or less, would require, after providing the initial plant, $3000 for the professor, $1000 for his assistant, $750 expense on the score of material for class use, $250 to keep some little research going, $300 for books and periodicals, $600 for a janitor,—a total of $5900 for the routine teaching of a few students under undesirable limitations. As it is clear that there is no justification just now for the existence of medical schools that are incapable of greatly bettering the type, it follows that schools unable or indisposed to spend the requisite sums lack a valid reason for being. We may then assume that the five departments of a properly organized medical school, capable of handling 125 students, in its first two years can hardly be properly sustained on a total budget of less than from $50,000 to $75,000 annually. If, now, the student pays $150 a year for tuition, there will be an annual deficit ranging from $31,250 to $56,250 a year. Not all the medical schools that are alive to their responsibility are, as we shall see, at this moment able to provide on this scale for each of the fundamental departments; but they are in no doubt that these departments need such support; and they are straining every effort to procure it for them.[1]

On the clinical side, the problem is more complicated. We have seen that the relation of the medical school to its hospital must be of the same kind as its relation to its laboratories. But laboratories exist only for school purposes; the hospital dis-

[1] A comparison of the estimates above given with corresponding budgets in German universities is highly suggestive. Despite the fact that the cost of apparatus, supplies, etc., is much lower in Germany than here, the sums spent in various universities on laboratory maintenance are as follows:

KÖNIGSBERG (170 *medical students*)		BRESLAU (189 *medical students*)	
Anatomy	16,349 marks	Anatomy	26,618 marks
Pathology	9,860 "	Pathology	14,932 "
BERLIN (1107 *medical students*)		GÖTTINGEN (189 *medical students*)	
Anatomy	57,436 marks	Anatomy	19,850 marks
Physiology	89,766 "	Physiology	9,606 "

(From *Etat des Ministeriums der Unterrichts- und Medizinal Angelegenheiten*, 1909, Beilage 6.)

Still more significant is the ratio between expenditure for salaries and that for laboratory maintenance, and the steady encroachment of the latter: out of every 100 marks spent in German universities, there went in

1868	45.95 marks	to	salaries	37.07 marks	to	laboratories
1878	41.94 "	"	"	40.46 "	"	"
1888	36.00 "	"	"	47.18 "	"	"
1902	29.46 "	"	"	53.77 "	"	"
1906	27.93 "	"	"	55.45 "	"	"

(From *Preussische Statistik*, 204: *Statistik der preussischen Landes Universitäten*, 1906, p. 7.)

Finally, the actual sums spent on salaries and laboratories respectively tell the same significant story:
Total expenditure in Prussian universities in

1868	1,786,108 marks	for	salaries	1,440,955 marks	for	laboratories
1878	2,959,187 "	"	"	2,959,103 "	"	"
1888	3,305,125 "	"	"	4,331,649 "	"	"
1898	3,499,785 "	"	"	6,094,316 "	"	"
1906	4,308,980 "	"	"	8,554,581 "	"	"

(*Ibid.*, p. 14.)
That is, in 38 years, total salaries have increased 141 per cent, total laboratory expense, 490 per cent. In the same period, the total attendance of medical students in the same universities has risen 113 per cent (from 2771 in winter semester, 1868, to 5903, winter semester, 1906).

Paulsen (*German Universities*, translated by Thilly, p. 219, note) quotes from the Rector's Address of Adolph Wagner in 1896:
"Expenditures for salaries and institutes in the University of Berlin show the following growth:

Year	Salaries		Institutes	
1811	116,550 marks (71.8 per cent)		39,294 marks (24.0 per cent)	
1834	193,650 " (64.6 " ")		78,434 " (26.2 " ")	
1880	321,000 " (52.8 " ")		267,000 " (40.1 " ")	
1896–7	865,000 " (30.9 " ")		1,461,000 " (52.9 " ")	"

All the seminaries in the mental sciences (there are 18) cost 17,650 marks annually; the 15 natural-scientific institutes and collections cost 379,798 marks; the 10 medical-scientific institutes 190,054 marks; the 10 clinical institutes, 617,691 marks.
The publications of the Prussian government mentioned above are models, which we would do well to adopt. They enable us to follow in minute detail the educational developments of the last seventy-five years, with their social implications. The American student of similar problems deals with chaos. It is difficult to obtain definite and complete statements from any one institution; and quite impossible to compare data from several institutions without exhaustive inquiry by way of ascertaining whether they cover the same ground. The German statistics prove clearly, however, the point at issue, i. e., the rapidly increasing cost of properly organized medical education.

charging simultaneously a philanthropic office may, as we have seen, be provided for independently of school funds and yet be as intimately a part of the educational organization as if teaching were its main purpose. The school will invariably have to equip and maintain its laboratories; the hospital may be separately financed without burden to the medical school. Further, the initial cost of the hospital establishment may vary within large limits: a plain, but serviceable structure, capable of accommodating 200 patients, with proper teaching facilities, may be erected for a few hundred thousand dollars; or it may cost millions. The cost of maintenance also fluctuates considerably according to situation and scale of support. In the city of New York, it is roughly estimated that it takes $1000 to maintain one bed for one year; a 200 bed hospital may thus readily involve an annual expenditure of $150,000 and upwards. This sum may be reduced by profits derived from pay patients, or by small contributions from charity patients. The extent to which the provision of proper clinical opportunities falls upon the medical school varies, then, from place to place. It is therefore not included in the schematic school budget we are preparing; but it is important to emphasize clearly that where independent endowment or state support does not furnish the medical school with a hospital in which it is thoroughly at home, the burden falls at once upon the school. The substitutes, makeshifts, and compromises now so widely employed in the United States do not relieve the medical schools of their responsibility.

From the standpoint of the medical school, it is perhaps immaterial how its hospital is supported. But it would be unfair not to point out briefly in passing that certain larger considerations give great importance to the source of hospital support. The hospital in the United States is not necessarily privately managed because privately supported, or publicly managed because publicly supported: it may be privately managed, even though in large measure publicly supported. The teaching hospitals connected with the Philadelphia schools and with the proprietary schools of Baltimore are of this description. In respect to management they are private concerns; but they have received large lump subsidies from the state for both buildings and support. It is not the sole objection to this policy that it strengthens proprietary medical schools, though that is surely a legitimate criticism. More serious is the general demoralization that log-rolling always entails. Schools and hospitals, competing in all other matters, join hands in assaulting the state treasury; for coöperative action increases the total largess to be divided. The state or city can indeed legitimately aid medical education by completely handing over to high-grade medical schools the ward service in hospitals financially managed by the proper state or municipal authorities. The public interest would be promoted, not injured, if, for example, Cornell, Columbia, and New York University were each left in unfettered possession of its division at Bellevue (New York); there is no possible source of demoralization there. The Pennsylvania plan, however, tends to transfer the making of appropriations and the accounting for the same from the hands of state officials to private parties whose common interest it is to increase appropriations and to reduce oversight.[1] The size of the appropriation is determined to greater or less degree by the violence of the onset. There is no fixed relation between the charity work done and the amount asked or secured.[2] In pursuance of that policy the state of Pennsylvania last year granted out of the public treasury to private and semi-private hospitals $4,404,500.

However the hospital and dispensary are supported, the teaching budget of the clinical years is necessarily a charge upon the funds of the medical school. The professor of medicine in the medical school will be physician-in-chief to the hospital; surgeon, obstetrician, pediatrist, will likewise occupy the same dual relation. The university hospital will be their laboratory; their salaries will protect them against the distractions of successful practice, be that practice general or consultant,—for a thriving consultation business may prove just as fatal to scientific productivity as any other form of immersion in routine. The clinical departments must embody the same ideals as pathology or physiology in respect to teaching and research; they require, then, the same organization and support. The laboratory service must be extended for them. For the investigator in internal medicine needs not only a clinic, but a laboratory, in whose activities the bedside problem and the fundamental sciences are brought together. The professors of pathology, physiology, physiological chemistry, work on broad lines. The clinician applies what he obtains from them to problems that are narrower in compass. Neither the clinical laboratories, where routine examinations are carried on, nor the fundamental scientific laboratories, serve precisely the needs of the investigating clinician, though the latter are in the most intimate coöperation with him.

What may be called the theory of virtual endowment deserves a word at this point. Let us suppose that ten practitioners give their professorial services gratis. Undoubtedly their ethical position is better than that of practitioner teachers who draw dividends. They contend, however, that their services constitute an endowment. Paid teachers would get, say, $3000 each. The $30,000 saved represents five per cent on $600,000. It is argued that the school is just where it would be if it had an endowment of something more than a half-million. Sanguine calculators of this type occasionally run the virtual endowments up to two or three millions. But virtual endowment is a poor substitute for good bonds. The volunteer teacher may begin well; but as between teaching and practice, the former must always get the worst of it. Slipshod dispensaries, imperfect hospital records, general clinical barrenness, tell the tale.

[1] Experts are of one mind as to the viciousness of this policy. See, for example, *Report on Subsidies*, National Conference of Charities and Corrections, held at Washington, D.C., May 9-15, 1901.

[2] The amounts secured vary from 12 cents to $2 a day for free patients, according to the efficacy of the hospital "pull." In New York city "pull" is eliminated: the hospital is paid a fixed sum for service rendered. Nevertheless, even this method of procedure may have unfortunate educational consequences,—for it enabled the Brooklyn Post-Graduate Medical School to start.

The modern medical establishment that spends $50,000 or $75,000 upon its fundamental laboratories will, if it is to be equally productive in clinical medicine, spend an equal sum on teaching and investigation during the latter two years,—quite apart from the current maintenance of hospital and dispensary. That is to say, $100,000 to $150,000 will be required at the start to pay the minimum cost of a four-year school of medicine accommodating 250 students and consistently organized along sound lines on both laboratory and clinical sides. The outlay will increase, not decrease, as the school grows, not in number, but in scope and power. The proposed budget may look formidable just now, when compared with the scant provision that has been generally made for medical education in this country under men many of whom have had no real appreciation of what good medical training is, or costs; but as public sentiment and educational intelligence develop, the suggested scale will appear not only modest, but insufficient.

The fees received from such a student body would amount to some $40,000; so that it may be fairly estimated that in such an institution fees will at the utmost pay little more than one-third of the expense, provided that proper hospital and dispensary facilities are already supported by endowment or otherwise. A comforting notion is prevalent that "in time" this proportion will rise, and that losses in attendance due to elevation of standards will eventually be "made up." There is no warrant for this belief. Institutions which have always, or long, operated on a high standard, and thus command an established public, find that expense tends to increase more rapidly than fee income. They persistently seek additional funds that may enable them to push ahead. The number of high standard schools supported will tend to be in some definite relation to the public need; there will be no such disproportion between number and need on a high, as there has been on the low, basis. In other words, the total enrolment will shrink; it will tend to concentrate in fewer schools. Under these circumstances schools which have long enjoyed a comparatively low-grade patronage must cut loose from their past, and begin to cultivate a new clientele. They will probably make slow headway in recovering from the initial shock. Most of them must expire or "merge" before their independent salvation can possibly be worked out. Our conclusion is that established schools, secure of their public on a sound basis, may count on fees to the extent of one-third to one-half of the expenditure required to conduct a good school of modern medicine; and that as the department becomes more homogeneously developed, the fees will tend to do even less.

It is interesting to compare this hypothetical budget as a whole, and by separate departments, with the actual outlay of our best schools. The Johns Hopkins most nearly represents desirable conditions; for there a teaching hospital belonging to the medical school is supported by adequate and separate endowment, so that clinical facilities impose no burden on the funds of the medical school proper. Moreover, there from the first clinical teachers have been salaried and, in a measure, withdrawn from general practice. The actual cost of conducting the Johns Hopkins Medical School, with 297 students, is something over $100,000 a year, not including, however, the salaries of clinical professors, which are in this case paid out of the hospital funds. Including these, the total outlay would considerably exceed our estimate. Tuition fees are about one-half of this amount. The Harvard budget runs higher, $251,389, much more than double the income in fees from its 285 students; Michigan, with 389 students, spends $83,000 on its department·of medicine and surgery, and $70,000 more on the university hospital; Columbia, with 312 students, requires $239,072 for the College of Physicians and Surgeons, including the Sloane Maternity Hospital and the Vanderbilt Clinic; Cornell (207 students) expends $209,888 at New York and $32,840 more at Ithaca, and gets back $24,410 in fees. The Toronto (592 students) medical budget is about $85,000, as against $64,500 received in fees; McGill (328 students), $77,000, as against $43,750 received in fees; the University of Minnesota, $71,336, as against $16,546 received in fees. More modest establishments, working towards the same ideals, make a similar exhibit: eighteen years ago the total budget of the Yale Medical School was $10,000;[1] it is now $43,311,—three times the amount received in tuition fees and confessedly inadequate to the aspirations and capacity of the medical faculty. Cornell spends at Ithaca, on a two-year course, $32,840, not including the cost of heating, lighting, administration, etc.

Few of these institutions have developed all departments equally. Even the laboratory branches are not as yet all of the same type. Relatively few even of the best schools are able to cultivate pharmacology to any considerable extent; the same is true of preventive medicine. On the clinical side, makeshifts of which we cannot be too impatient are all but universal. In general, even where intelligent ideals prevail, resources do not suffice for an all-round organization. Wherever a department has been acceptably cared for, the expenditure is apt to exceed our schematic estimate:[2] Johns Hopkins now spends $16,750 a year on anatomy, $14,171 on pathology (not counting $4791 spent on the clinical laboratory), $13,246 on physiology and physiological chemistry. Columbia spends $29,259 on anatomy, $18,400 on pathology,[3] $17,838 on physiology. Cornell (New York) spends $37,000 on pathology,[4] histology, and bacteriology, $15,895 on anatomy, $14,940 on physiology. These appropriations are not extravagant. On the contrary, they are closely approached—sometimes exceeded—wherever modern methods are effectively employed: at Ithaca, Cornell (18 students) spends $9500 on anatomy and $13,500 on physiology and pharmacology; New York University (408 students) spends $15,000 on pathology; Washington

[1] Graham Lusk: "Medical Education," *Journal Amer. Med. Assn.*, vol. lii. p. 1230.

[2] The budgets that follow are not exactly comparable, for the lines are not always drawn in exactly the same way. Nevertheless they represent nearly enough the same thing to illustrate the point under discussion. Unfortunately college accounting does not as yet enable us to say how much goes into ordinary undergraduate teaching, how much into research, etc.

[3] Including clinical pathology, $26,800.

[4] Excluding clinical pathology.

University, St. Louis (178 students), spends $9640 for anatomy, $8550 for physiology and pharmacology; the University of Wisconsin (49 students) spends $10,000 for anatomy and $8100 for physiology. Anatomy costs the University of Michigan $14,300 a year, and the University of Iowa $13,525. Champions of cheapness allege that large sums are needed only for research, where medicine is taught to college graduates who afterwards practise in large cities; but Michigan and Iowa spend these sums in behalf of high school boys who after graduation from the medical school return to the simple surroundings amidst which they grew up. New York University operates also with high school boys, and is mainly a teaching school. Where clinical medicine is on the proper basis, the same result emerges: at Tulane, for example (489 students), the department, recently reorganized on modern lines, requires $9100 for its support. The University of Michigan uses $7830 in medicine, $9405 in surgery. Every one of the important subjects must of course very soon be provided on an adequate scale; for in every acceptable medical school, though large individual variations must occur, the movement to treat the main clinical divisions similarly will not stop. A simple process of multiplication will then give the minimum cost of maintaining a medical establishment in which all the essential subjects are adequately, even though not homogeneously, developed. Endowment or taxation alone can meet this burden,—and endowment and taxation are feasible only if medical education is carried on not only in, but by the university. For of course a medical school supported by fees is just as fettered inside, as it would be outside, the university. Its ideals may be higher; its fee income may be more independently expended. But in no case are the fees adequate to support all the essential departments on a substantial basis. As a rule, these schools "feature" one or two branches; the others pine. The best developed departments show what all ought to be: pathology at New York University, anatomy at Jefferson Medical College, are really strong departments; they belong to institutions dependent on fees; but to provide them, other departments must be denied anything like equal opportunity to expand.

Of course it is not to be supposed that the most expensive teaching is the best; that a department that costs $20,000 is necessarily twice as good as one that spends $10,000; it may be both scientifically and pedagogically inferior. It remains true, however, that in general the equipment and conduct of laboratories are costly; that professorial salaries are rising; that a productive teacher needs competent assistants, expensive apparatus, material, etc., and a certain margin, in case an unforeseen turn necessitate an unusual outlay. The scientist financially hampered so as to be incapable of following out surprises may miss the most valuable result of his tedious labors.

Important is it to observe that the expense does not diminish *pari passu* with the attendance. The formation of two-year schools has recently proceeded apace, many of them feebly equipped and poorly sustained; their initial plant costs little; their total budgets are but a few thousand dollars.[1] A few dollars are expended for books; animals are provided in a gingerly manner; pathological material is small in amount, and comes as a gratuity from distant schools whose needs have been previously supplied; apparatus barely suffices for routine work; no helpers relieve the single departmental teacher of menial drudgery. These schools are of course scientifically sterile; as such, they must rapidly become antiquated, for they are situated in out-of-the-way places and their staff has but little intercourse with active centers. It seems hardly justifiable to start such ventures merely to meet institutional competition. The two-year school can doubtless make good where, as in Wisconsin, liberal support overcomes at many points the defects due to isolation; the heavy charges incurred, however, ought to be seriously pondered by those whose less ample means forbid anything like so adequate an appropriation.

It is now clear that medicine cannot be, and is not, properly taught on the basis of receipts. We have at this date 30-odd schools, all university departments, whose annual budgets call for sums considerably in advance of their receipts from fees. As these institutions will in number and facilities undoubtedly soon be equal to the task of producing physicians enough to supply the need, the coil is tightening around schools not yet in position to devote even all their fees to instruction. Well known institutions can still be cited, whose instruction as offered costs the school less than the fees paid in,—a balance being available for buildings, improvements, or for debt originally incurred for plant. Large receipts mean in most instances[2] low standards,—standards below the four-year high school basis. In order to secure a balance, economies must be effected, as has been already pointed out, at the expense of teaching, by inadequate equipment, uneven development, lack of full-time professors, reliance upon necessarily incompetent student assistants, absence of helpers, employment of volunteers in the dispensary, etc. Tufts College Medical School, with an income of $59,093, is paying off in annual instalments a debt incurred for the building it now occupies; Jefferson Medical College, with receipts of $102,995, must incidentally accumulate a fund to retire a large mortgage. The medical department of Northwestern University must apply its surplus to the discharge of debts incurred for buildings and plant. Vanderbilt University, having invested $83,000 in a medical department, compels the department out of its fees (about $25,000 a year) to pay all its own running expenses, something on the original purchase price, and six per cent interest on the unpaid balance. The University of Maryland, the College of Physicians and Surgeons of Baltimore, the Starling-Ohio (Columbus), pursue substantially the same policy.

[1] The minimum outlay, ordinary working efficiency being considered, for a department of physiology is given on page 129. It is questionable whether just now an institution is justified in undertaking the work if it is unable to do more than this minimum. Only a decided probability of increased resources in the future warrants the step.

[2] Rush (Chicago) is the only exception. No other high standard school contains over 300 students; most of them have a comparatively small enrolment.

Of our 155 medical schools, 120-odd depend on fees alone. Of these, there are better and worse: the former using the fees as far as they go to provide either several laboratory branches decently, or two or three well; the latter devoting but a part, often a small part, of the fee income to pedagogical use, distributing the rest among the teachers, who are in such cases always practising physicians.

The ethics of the case are clear. Let us grant that in the hope of ultimately getting to a sounder basis, it may have been justifiable for the more prosperous fee-supported schools, whose total income is large enough to do something, to fight for survival. Surely they were, and are, morally bound meanwhile to furnish the best medical teaching procurable with such income as they enjoy. Their practitioner teachers were all the time profiting indirectly by their school connection; and this would suffice, if their motives were really as altruistic as is commonly alleged. Meanwhile, laboratories can be kept decent and laboratory teaching can as a rule be thorough only if full-time instructors are employed. These teachers have no income but their salaries. The medical school must therefore devote its fees primarily to paying them and to giving them the necessary facilities. Though the fee-supported school do this unreservedly, it will none the less omit part of its duty, because fees cannot support a complete set of laboratories efficiently organized. The school is therefore not justified in cutting out one or more of its possible laboratories in order to pay its clinical teachers. It must not only use its fees to pay for the right kind of laboratory instruction, but it must organize as many such laboratories as fees will support before paying anything to the clinical teachers, who profit indirectly nevertheless. A school may not be justified in existing even on this basis; that is, if the demand for doctors can be met by institutions that can do better for their students, there is no need to put up with even so altruistic a compromise. Surely an institution that is not willing to do so much as this has absolutely no defense unless a section is so hard run for doctors that it must take them on any terms upon which they can be procured. Such is not the case at this writing in any part of the United States or Canada. The younger men utilized in the dispensary ought probably to be treated on the same basis. For the dispensary is usually turned over to young men still struggling for a livelihood. A small annual stipend would go far to get from them the best service they are capable of rendering. To these two purposes the fee-supported school is in conscience bound to apply its income. As far as fees reach, orderly, even though modest, scientific departments and a well conducted dispensary service should be provided and paid for.

A few schools have squarely met their responsibility in this matter, and with results that prove them deserving of additional support. The medical department of Syracuse University has a total fee income of $28,861, which is spent on the scientific branches; the plant is not elaborate, but it is effective, attractive, and conscientiously managed. Within less than a year, the medical department of the University of Pittsburgh has come under complete university control. Prior to that time it was a highly prosperous concern to its managers; nowhere in the country were worse conditions found. Now, as then, the school has only its fees for support; but they have this year gone into laboratories instead of into professorial pockets: with a result that is hardly less than a transformation. Full-time professors of pathology, physiology, and other branches have brought order out of chaos. The entire atmosphere of the institution has been clarified: students may be found actually studying, in the room in which under other conditions last year "four dozen wooden chairs were broken up" in boisterous horse-play. The medical department of Boston University, with a total income of $12,762, makes a decent and attractive showing in a simple way in its laboratories of bacteriology, pathology, physiology, etc. Highly creditable is the record of Meharry Medical College, the colored school at Nashville; for there the teachers, though practising physicians, are poor men: of the total income of $23,946, the salary list gets only $9665. A violent contrast is afforded by Shaw University (Raleigh, N. C.), another school for colored men, whose teachers are, however, white physicians: its income from fees is $2846; a few contributions increase the total income (not counting the board of students) to $4721; the teachers just referred to draw out $4737. In consequence the school has practically no outfit.

In the majority of the larger schools dependent on fees, an opposite policy is pursued. The laboratories are slighted or starved; the dispensary is neglected in order that dividends or salaries, running sometimes as high as $1000, may be paid to precisely those faculty members who need it least. The Albany Medical School—nominally affiliated with Union College—has a fee income of $20,276. Associated with it is the Bender Laboratory, where practically all its laboratory teaching except chemistry and anatomy is carried on. The school appropriates niggardly sums to provide for the teaching of pathology and bacteriology by the overworked and underhelped chief of the Bender Laboratory; the laboratory has struggled hard, and not unsuccessfully, to be productive at the same time; but it has accomplished, whether in teaching or in research, but a fraction of what it would have achieved, had not a large part of the college receipts been distributed in sums approximating $500 each to fifteen members of the school faculty. At Buffalo similar conditions exist. The dispensary is utterly neglected; some laboratory subjects are unprovided, others are slighted, in order that a "nominal" salary of $1000 may be paid in real money to some of the leading practitioners in the town. This institution collects $4608 in laboratory fees and spends $1105 in carrying the laboratories on. Brooklyn fairly repeats Albany. There the Hoagland Laboratory relieves the Long Island College Hospital of certain subjects; the rest are omitted, for the fees that might furnish them are distributed among well-to-do clinical teachers. Bowdoin, with a total available income of $15,230, appropriates $200 for the maintenance of the bacteriological laboratory, $50 for the physiological laboratory, $200 for chemistry, and $200 for books, as against $12,225 for salaries to men, not one of whom gives his whole time to medical education. At Halifax, the fee income is some $5000 a year and the government makes an appropriation of $1200,—a total of $6200. The faculty apportions this sum as follows: three-fourths of the fees are divided among the teachers; one-fourth of the fees plus the government subsidy must carry all other expense,— heat, light, janitor service, laboratory maintenance: the disgraceful condition of the premises follows as a matter of course. The Hahnemann of Philadelphia, with estimated receipts of $18,500, distributes $11,000 among teaching practitioners and spends perhaps $1500 on equipment and $500 for laboratory material. Advertising and commencement exercises—the latter only another form of advertising—often cost these institutions more than their laboratories. One large eastern institution expends $4700 on publicity, as against $3500 on its laboratories; another—a New York school, this—$1500 on publicity, $1100 on laboratories; another, $2100 on advertising, $1160 on laboratories; another—this time in the south—$1000 on advertising, $500 on laboratories, "including repairs."[1]

The conclusion, then, is irresistible that these schools, far from being the benevolent enterprises that they are alleged to be, still "pay," both directly and indirectly; nor can a genuine altruistic motive be made out for any medical school which does not consistently devote its entire income to providing decent facilities and adequate instruction in the laboratories, where the teachers, if competent, must rely wholly on their salaries. Clinical teachers ought undoubtedly be paid, but not out of fees at the expense of laboratories and laboratory men. Institutions that supplement their fee income out of special endowments or out of their general funds very properly go ahead to pay their clinical teachers; otherwise the practitioner teacher must be subordinated. That these schools have been persistently used for pecuniary advantage is clear when an inventory of their belongings is contrasted with the annual income that has in some cases been earned for many years. They have little or nothing to show in the way of equipment. The medical department of the University of Arkansas is thirty years old; its annual receipts are now $14,100;[2] except for a small recent investment, it is practically bare. The medical department of Georgetown University (Washington, D.C.) has been in operation almost sixty years; its annual income is now estimated at $11,000. Its plant can represent only a small fraction of its receipts during its lifetime. The Medical College of Georgia is seventy years old; it has accumulated no plant worthy the name. The medical department of the University of Oregon, started in 1887, with a present fee income of $8000 and state aid of $1000 a year, has only one small laboratory that represents any investment at all. The medical department of the University of Chattanooga—twenty-one years old— with an income now of $4290, of which the dean draws $1800, would not, if sold under

[1] Additional examples to prove that the schools are operated for the profit of their faculties may be given if necessary: University of Alabama, fee income $19,788, salaries $14,000; University of Vermont, fee income, $22,730, salaries and dividends, $17,489 (laboratories, supplies, etc., $1941, publicity, $1289).
[2] Estimated.

the hammer, bring $500. The St. Louis College of Physicians and Surgeons, with an estimated income of $16,035, cannot afford the simplest equipment for its squalid dispensary and its hopeless laboratories. The osteopaths bid fair to repeat the worst offenses of the medical practitioners: their schools are fairly booming. The receipts of the Kirksville institution probably reach $89,600 a year. The instruction furnished is exceedingly cheap in quality. All in all, there are annually paid in the United States and Canada about $3,000,000 in medical student fees. An equal sum has been paid annually for years. It is obvious that only a small part of the total fee income of our medical schools has been devoted to upbuilding and equipping the schools, though just the reverse is pretended. Undoubtedly, the disfavor with which educational benefactors have regarded medical education is justified by the mercenary record reflected in these figures. But it is highly important that henceforth distinctions be made.

There are in the United States and Canada 56[1] schools whose total annual available resources are below $10,000 each,—so small a sum that the endeavor to do anything substantial with it is of course absurdly futile; a fact which is usually made an excuse for doing nothing at all, not even washing the windows, sweeping the floor, or providing a disinfectant for the dissecting-room. There is not a shred of justification for their continuance: for even if there were need of several thousand doctors annually, the wretched contribution made by these poverty-stricken schools could well be spared. Among them may be mentioned the California Eclectic (Los Angeles), estimated income $1060; Pulte Medical College (Cincinnati), estimated income $1325; Toledo Medical College, with $3240; Willamette University, with $3580; and Southwestern Homeopathic College, with $1100.

Responsibility for the conditions described does not rest on medical men alone; colleges and universities have not infrequently become accessory after the fact. We have repeatedly urged that the proper place for a medical school is within a university; but there is no saving grace in the mere name. Three services may be specified as comprised in the duty of a university which makes itself responsible for a medical school: the definition and enforcement of entrance standards, the upholding of scientific ideals, and responsibility for adequate support. We have mentioned universities that fail in the first or the second or in both; and as a rule these are the institutions that fail likewise in the third. Of the 155 medical schools of the continent, 82 are university departments, actual or so-called. With few exceptions the connection of these universities with medical education began at a time when no one took obligations in the matter seriously. Some of those that entered the field thus lightly have made amends. Others, awakening late to a sense of their obligations, are confronted by an apparently hopeless situation. Their total annual income would not alone suffice for a good medical school,—and it must carry the burden of the entire

[1] There are thirteen more whose fee income is likewise below $10,000 apiece, but they are university departments whose budgets, greatly in excess of fees, are carried by the respective universities.

institution. Their medical departments will, unless discontinued, prove sources of weakness and reproach, until their income is augmented far beyond their immediate expectations. As a matter of fact, few university administrators yet grasp clearly the fundamental principles of modern medical education. Twenty-seven colleges and universities of the United States and Canada have nominal or affiliated medical departments which they do not control and which they do not help to support. The state universities of Arkansas, Georgia, Illinois, and Oregon are in this position. Among endowed institutions that lend their names to proprietary medical schools, for which they can hope to do nothing and which they cannot possibly control as long as they do nothing, are the University of Denver, Washburn College, Cotner University, Epworth, Baylor, Western, and Dalhousie Universities. Some of these institutions are very poor. Among those that are capable of leading respectable lives as colleges, but are little less than absurd as universities, may be mentioned Union University, in New York state, which is the appellation given to the superficial combination of Union College and the Albany Law and Medical Schools. The chancellor of the University of Denver, — a Methodist institution, — affiliated with the Denver and Gross Medical College, finds a strange reason for self-congratulation in the connection. "The University of Denver," he says in a recent report, "has always had a form of organization that is peculiar to itself. From the beginning the professional schools have had autonomous life. The church has never expended one penny for equipment or for buildings or for maintenance of the professional schools. ... It has made a notable extension of its influence in very many ways through the professional schools of the university without the expenditure of a penny for any purpose whatsoever." A highly diverting illustration of the seriousness with which these ties are regarded has been recently furnished at Los Angeles; there a local school, affiliated with the University of Southern California, saw a chance of improving its lot by contracting an alliance with the University of California. A divorce was speedily agreed on, and the University of California, protected by contract, however, against any expenditure for two years, promptly became sponsor for a second clinical school. The University of Southern California, however, enjoyed only a brief widowhood. Into the vacant place, the Los Angeles College of Physicians and Surgeons promptly stepped. The University of Southern California was thus again made whole by the addition of a medical department which, enjoying an estimated total fee income of $4075, will ask nothing for support and still less for supervision.

The strength of the argument advanced in this chapter is not dependent on the absolute accuracy of the figures cited. Actual income may vary from our estimates a few thousand dollars up or down; we may have failed to consider this offset or that. It has been, as a matter of fact, utterly impossible to get figures that represent exactly the same items in all, or even in many, institutions. An improvement in institutional book-keeping would have to be effected in order to make accurate comparison possible. None the less, the picture is on the whole fair and reliable. Medicine is expensive to teach. It can in no event be taught out of fees. Reputable institutions with no other outlook should combine with better favored schools or stop outright. Legal enactment should terminate the career of the others. Abundant benefaction should strengthen up to our need the relatively small number of schools required to deal effectively with the subject. No greater error can be made than to suppose that endowment and university ideals are necessary only to medical schools with high entrance standards. Vanderbilt and Tulane, trying to make intelligent physicians out of high school boys in the south, need the same means and ideals as Harvard and Johns Hopkins, working with college material in another section. Indeed, the more defective the material or the more unfavorable the environment, the greater must be the resources and the higher must be the purposes of those who have undertaken to look after this vital social function.

CHAPTER IX

RECONSTRUCTION

THE necessity of a reconstruction that will at once reduce the number and improve the output of medical schools may now be taken as demonstrated. A considerable sloughing off has already occurred. It would have gone further but for the action of colleges and universities which have by affiliation obstructed nature's own effort at readjustment. Affiliation is now in the air. Medical schools that have either ceased to prosper, or that have become sensitive to the imputation of proprietary status or commercial motive, seek to secure their future or to escape their past by contracting an academic alliance. The present chapter undertakes to work out a schematic reconstruction which may suggest a feasible course for the future. It is not supposed that violent measures will at once be taken to reconstitute the situation on the basis here worked out. A solution so entirely suggested by impersonal considerations may indeed never be reached. But legislators and educators alike may be assisted by a theoretical solution to which, as specific problems arise, they may refer.

This solution deals only with the present and the near future,—a generation, at most. In the course of the next thirty years needs will develop of which we here take no account. As we cannot foretell them, we shall not endeavor to meet them. Certain it is that they will be most effectively handled if they crop up freely in an unencumbered field. It is therefore highly undesirable that superfluous schools now existing should be perpetuated in order that a subsequent generation may find a means of producing its doctors provided in advance. The cost of prolonging life through this intervening period will be worse than wasted; and an adequate provision at that moment will be embarrassed by inheritance and tradition. Let the new foundations of that distant epoch enjoy the advantage of the Johns Hopkins, starting without handicap at the level of the best knowledge of its day.

The principles upon which reconstruction would proceed have been established in the course of this report: (1) a medical school is properly a university department; it is most favorably located in a large city, where the problem of procuring clinical material, at once abundant and various, practically solves itself. Hence those universities that have been located in cities can most advantageously develop medical schools. (2) Unfortunately, however, our universities have not always been so placed. They began in many instances as colleges or something less. Here a supposed solicitude for youth suggested an out-of-the-way location; elsewhere political bargaining brought about the same result. The state universities of the south and west, most likely to enjoy sufficient incomes, are often unfortunately located: witness the University of Alabama at Tuscaloosa, of Georgia at Athens, of Mississippi at Oxford, of Missouri at Columbia, of Arkansas at Fayetteville, of Kansas at Lawrence, of South Dakota at Vermilion; and that experience has taught us nothing is proved by the recent location of the State University of Oklahoma at Norman. Some of these institutions are freed from the necessity of undertaking to teach medicine by an endowed institution better situated; in other sections the only universities fitted by their large support and their assured scientific ideals to maintain schools of medicine are handicapped by inferiority of location. We are not thereby justified in surrendering the university principle. Experience, our own or that of Germany, proves, as we have already pointed out, that the difficulty is not insuperable. At relatively greater expense, it is still feasible to develop a medical school in such an environment: there is no magnet like reputation; nothing travels faster than the fame of a great healer; distance is an obstacle readily overcome by those who seek health. The poor as well as the rich find their way to shrines and healing springs. The faculty of medicine in these schools may even turn the defect of situation to good account; for, freed from distraction, the medical schools at Iowa City and Ann Arbor may the more readily cultivate clinical science. An alternative may indeed be tried in the shape of a remote department. The problem in that case is to make university control real, to impregnate the distant school with genuine university spirit. The difficulty of the task may well deter those whose resources are scanty or who are under no necessity of engaging in medical teaching. As we need many universities and but few medical schools, a long-distance connection is justified only where there is no local university qualified to assume responsibility. A third solution—division—may, if the position taken in previous chapters is sound, be disregarded in the final disposition.[1]

(3) We shall assign only one school to a single town. As a matter of fact, no American city now contains more than one well supported university,[2]—and if we find it unnecessary or impolitic to duplicate local university plants, it is still less necessary to duplicate medical schools. The needless expense, the inevitable shrinkage of the student body, the difficulty of recruiting more than one faculty, the disturbance due to competition for hospital services, argue against local duplication. It is sometimes contended that competition is stimulating: Tufts claims to have waked up Harvard; the second Little Rock school did undoubtedly move the first to spend several hundred dollars on desks and apparatus. But competition may also be demoralizing; the necessity of finding students constitutes medical schools which ought to elevate standards the main obstacles to their elevation: witness the attitude of several institutions in Boston, New York, Philadelphia, Baltimore, and Chicago. Moreover, local competition is a stimulus far inferior to the general scientific competition to which all well equipped, well conducted, and rightly inspired university departments throughout the civilized world are parties. The English have experimented with both forms,—a single school in the large provincial towns, a dozen or more in London,—and their experience inclines them to reduce as far as possible

[1] We shall omit the half-school because it may be considered to divide with the whole school the work of the first two years; it does not greatly affect the clinical output, with which this chapter is mainly concerned.

[2] Chicago is almost an exception, as Northwestern University is situated at Evanston, a suburb.

the number of the London schools. Amalgamation has already taken place in certain American towns: the several schools of Cincinnati, of Indianapolis, and of Louisville have all recently "merged." This step is easy enough in towns where there is either no university or only one university. Where there are several, as in Chicago, Boston, and New York, the problem is more difficult. Approached in a broad spirit it may, however, prove not insoluble; coöperation may be arranged where several institutions all possess substantial resources; universities of limited means can retire without loss of prestige,—on the contrary, the respect in which they are held must be heightened by any action dictated by conscientious refusal to continue a work that they are in no position to do well.

(4) A reconstruction of medical education cannot ignore the patent fact that students tend to study medicine in their own states, certainly in their own sections. In general, therefore, arrangements ought to be made, as far as conditions heretofore mentioned permit, to provide the requisite facilities within each of the characteristic state groups. There is the added advantage that local conditions are thus heeded and that the general profession is at a variety of points penetrated by educative influences. New Orleans, for example, would cultivate tropical medicine; Pittsburgh, the occupational diseases common in its environment. In respect to output, we may once more fairly take existing conditions into account. We are not called on to provide schools enough to keep up the present ratio. As we should in any case hardly be embarrassed for almost a generation in the matter of supply, we shall do well to produce no doctors who do not represent an improvement upon the present average.

The principles above stated have been entirely disregarded in America. Medical schools have been established regardless of need, regardless of the proximity of competent universities, regardless of favoring local conditions. An expression of surprise at finding an irrelevant and superfluous school usually elicits the reply that the town, being a "gateway" or a "center," must of course harbor a "medical college." It is not always easy to distinguish "gateway" and "center:" a center appears to be a town possessing, or within easy reach of, say 50,000 persons; a gateway is a town with at least two railway stations. The same place may be both,—in which event the argument is presumably irrefragable. Augusta, Georgia, Charlotte, North Carolina, and Topeka, Kansas, are "centers," and as such are logical abodes of medical instruction. Little Rock, St. Joseph, Memphis, Toledo, Buffalo, are "gateways." The argument, so dear to local pride, can best be refuted by being pursued to its logical conclusion. For there are still forty-eight towns in the United States with over 50,000 population each, and no medical schools: we are threatened with forty-eight new schools at once, if the contention is correct. The truth is that the fundamental, though of course not sole, consideration is the university, provided its resources are adequate; and we have fortunately enough strong universities, properly distributed, to satisfy every present need without serious sacrifice of sound principle. The German Empire contains eighty-four cities whose population exceeds 50,000 each. Of its twenty-two medical schools, only eleven are to be found in them: that is, it possesses seventy-three gateways and centers without universities or medical schools. The remaining eleven schools are located in towns of less than 50,000 inhabitants, a university town of 30,000 being a fitter abode for medical study than a non-university town of half a million, in the judgment of those who have best succeeded with it.

That the existing system came about without reference to what the country needed or what was best for it may be easily demonstrated. Between 1904 and 1909 the country gained certainly upwards of 5,000,000 in population; during the same period the number of medical students actually decreased from 28,142 to 22,145, i.e., over 20 per cent. The average annual production of doctors from 1900 to 1909 was 5222; but last June the number dropped to 4442. Finally, the total number of medical colleges which reached its maximum— 166[1]— in 1904 has in the five years since decreased about 10 per cent. Our problem is to calculate how far tendencies already observable may be carried without harm.

We have calculated that the south requires for the next generation 490 new doctors annually, the rest of the country, 1500. We must then provide machinery for the training of about 2000 graduates in medicine yearly. Reckoning fatalities of all kinds at ten per cent per annum, graduating classes of 2000 imply approximately junior classes of 2200, sophomore classes of 2440, freshman classes aggregating 2700,— something over 9000 students of medicine. Thirty medical schools, with an average enrolment of 300 and average graduation classes of less than 70, will be easily equal to the task. As many of these could double both enrolment and output without danger, a provision planned to meet present needs is equally sufficient for our growth for years to come. It will be time to devise more schools when the productive limit of those now suggested shall come in sight.

For the purpose here in mind, the country may be conceived as divided into several sections, within each of which, with due regard to what it now contains, medical schools enough to satisfy its needs must be provided.[2] Pending the fuller development of the states west of the Mississippi, the section east will have to relieve them of part of their responsibility. The provisional nature of our suggestions is thus obvious; for as the west increases in population, as its universities grow in number and strength, the balance will right itself: additional schools will be created in the west and south rather than in the north and east. It would of course be unfortunate to over-emphasize the importance of state lines. We shall do well to take advantage of every unmistakably favorable opportunity so long as we keep within the public need; and to encourage the freest possible circulation of students throughout the entire country.

[1] Not including osteopathic schools.
[2] This chapter now recapitulates and summarizes the more detailed accounts contained in Part II, in which the schools of each state are described and the general state situation discussed.

(1) New England represents a fairly homogeneous region, comprising six states, the population of which is increasingly urban. Its population increased, 1908-9, somewhat less than 75,000, requiring, on the basis of one doctor to every increase of 1500 in population, 50 new doctors. About 150 physicians died. Seventy-five men would replace one-half of these. In all, 125 new doctors would be needed. To produce this number two schools, one of moderate size and one smaller, readily suffice. Fortunately they can be developed without sacrificing any of our criteria. The medical schools of Harvard and Yale are university departments, situated in the midst of ample clinical material, with considerable financial backing now and every prospect of more. It is unwise to divide the Boston field; it is unnecessary to prolong the life of the clinical departments of Dartmouth, Bowdoin, and Vermont. They are not likely soon to possess the financial resources needed to develop adequate clinics in their present location; and the time has passed when even excellent didactic instruction can be regarded as compensating for defective opportunities in obstetrics, contagious diseases, and general medicine. The historic position of the schools in question counts little as against changed ideals. Dartmouth and Vermont can, however, offer the work of the first two years with the clinical coloring made feasible by the proximity of a hospital, as is the case with the University of Missouri at Columbia; with that they ought to be content for the time being.

(2) The middle Atlantic states comprise for our purpose New York, New Jersey, Pennsylvania, Delaware, Maryland, and the District of Columbia. Their population grows at the rate of 300,000 annually, for whom 200 doctors can care; 230 more would fill one-half the vacancies arising through death: a total of 430 needed. Available universities are situated in New York city, Syracuse, Philadelphia, Pittsburgh, Baltimore. The situation is in every respect ideal; the universities located at New York, Philadelphia, and Baltimore are strong and prosperous; those of Syracuse and Pittsburgh, though less developed, give good promise. Without sacrifice of a ' single detail, these five university towns can not only support medical schools for the section, but also to no small extent relieve less favored spots. The schools of Albany, Buffalo, Brooklyn, Washington,[1] would, on this plan, disappear,—certainly until academic institutions of proper caliber had been developed. Whether even in the event of their creation they should for some years endeavor to cultivate medicine is quite doubtful. Appreciation of what is involved in the undertaking might well give them pause. Meanwhile, within the university towns already named there would be much to do: better state laws are needed in order to exterminate the worst schools; merger or liquidation must bring together many of those that still survive. The section under consideration ought indeed to lead the Union; but the independent schools of New York and Pennsylvania are powerful enough to prove a stubborn obstacle to any progressive movement, however clearly in the public interest.

[1] Except Howard University which, patronized by the government, is admirably located for the medical education of the negro.

(3) Greater unevenness must be tolerated in the south;[1] proprietary schools or nominal university departments will doubtless survive longer there than in other parts of the country because of the financial weakness of both endowed and tax-supported institutions. All the more important, therefore, for universities to deal with the subject in a large spirit, avoiding both overlapping and duplication. An institution may well be glad to be absolved from responsibilities that some other is better fitted to meet. Tulane and Vanderbilt, for example, are excellently situated in respect to medical education; the former has already a considerable endowment applicable to medicine. The state universities of Louisiana and Tennessee may therefore resign medicine to these endowed institutions, grateful for the opportunity to cultivate other fields. Every added superfluous school weakens the whole by wasting money and scattering the eligible student body. None of the southern state universities, indeed, is wisely placed: Texas has no alternative but a remote department, such as it now supports at Galveston; Georgia will one day develop a university medical school at Atlanta; Alabama, at Birmingham,—the university being close by, at Tuscaloosa. The University of Virginia is repeating Ann Arbor at Charlottesville; whether it would do better to operate a remote department at Richmond or Norfolk, the future will determine. Six schools are thus provided:[2] they are sufficient to the needs of the section just now. The resources available even for their support are as yet painfully inadequate: three of the six are still dependent upon fees for both plant and maintenance. It is doubtful whether the other universities of the south should generally offer even the instruction of the first two years. The scale upon which these two-year departments can be now organized by them is below the minimum of continuous efficiency; they can contribute nothing to science, and their quota of physicians can be better trained in one of the six schools suggested. Concentration in the interest of effectiveness, team work between all institutions working in the cause of southern development, economy as a means of improving the lot of the teacher—these measures, advisable everywhere, are especially urgent in the south.

(4) In the north central tier—Ohio, Indiana, Michigan, Wisconsin, Illinois—population increased 239,685 the last year: 160 doctors would care for the increase; 190 more would replace one-half of those that died: a total of 350. Large cities with resident universities available for medical education are Cincinnati, Columbus, Cleveland, and Chicago. Ann Arbor has demonstrated the ability successfully to combat the disadvantages of a small town. The University of Wisconsin can unquestionably do the same, with a slighter handicap, at Madison whenever it chooses to complete its work there. Indiana University has undertaken the problem of a distant connection at Indianapolis. Four cities thus fulfil all our criteria, two more develop the small town type, one more is an experiment with the remote university department.

[1] The south includes eleven states, viz., Virginia, Kentucky, North Carolina, South Carolina, Florida, Georgia, Tennessee, Mississippi, Louisiana, Arkansas, Texas.
[2] A seventh, Meharry, at Nashville, must be included for the medical education of the negro.

Surely the territory in question can be supplied by these seven medical centers. Chicago alone is likely to draw a considerable number of students from a wider area. It has long been a populous medical center. Nevertheless the number of high-grade students it just now contains is not large. If the practice of medicine in this area rested on a two-year college basis, as it well might, there would to-day be perhaps 600 students of medicine in that city. Coöperative effort between the two universities there and the state university at Urbana would readily provide for them.

(5) The middle west comprises eight states, Minnesota, Iowa, Missouri, Oklahoma, Kansas, Nebraska, South Dakota, North Dakota, with a gain in population last year of 216,036, requiring 140 more physicians, plus 160 to replace half the deaths: a total of 300. To supply them, urban universities capable of conducting medical departments of proper type are situated in Minneapolis and St. Louis; and both deserve strong, well supported schools. For Minneapolis must largely carry the weight of the Dakotas and Montana; St. Louis must assist Texas and have an eye to Arkansas, Oklahoma, and the southwest. The University of Nebraska, now dispersing its energies through a divided school, can be added to this list; for it will quite certainly either concentrate the department on its own site (Lincoln, population 48,232), or bring the two pieces together at Omaha, only an hour's distance away. The University of Kansas will doubtless combine its divided department at Kansas City. The State University of Iowa emulates Ann Arbor at Iowa City. These five schools must produce 297 doctors annually. Their capacity would go much farther. Oklahoma[1] and the Dakotas might well for a time postpone the entire question, supporting the work of the first two years, which they have already undertaken, on a much more liberal basis than they have yet reached. With the exception of St. Louis, all these proposed schools belong to state universities, and even at St. Louis the coöperation of the state university may prove feasible. A close relation may thus be secured between agencies concerned with public health and those devoted to medical education. The public health laboratory may become virtually part of the medical school,—a highly stimulating relation for both parties. The school will profit by contact with concrete problems; the public health laboratory will inevitably push beyond routine, prosecuting in a scientific spirit the practical tasks referred to it from all portions of the state. The direct connection of the state with a medical school that it wholly or even partly maintains will also solve the vexed question of standards: for the educational standard which the state fixes for its own sons will be made the practice standard as well. Private corporations, whether within or without its borders, will no longer be permitted to deluge the community with an inferior product.

(6) Seven thinly settled and on the whole slowly growing states and territories form the farther west: New Mexico, Colorado, Wyoming, Montana, Idaho, Utah, Arizona. Their increase in population was last year about 45,000. They contain now

[1] Should it be possible for the State University of Oklahoma, by engaging in clinical work at Oklahoma City, to get and to retain a monopoly of the field, the step would doubtless be advisable even now.

one doctor for every 563 persons. In view of local conditions, let us reckon one additional doctor for every additional 750 persons: 60 will be required. And, further, let us make up the death-roll man for man: 60 more would be needed—altogether 120. There are at the moment in this region only two available sites, Salt Lake City and Denver. At the former the University of Utah is situated; the latter could be occupied by the University of Colorado, located at Boulder, practically a suburb. The outlying portions of this vast territory will long continue to procure their doctors by immigration or by sending their sons to Minneapolis, Madison, Ann Arbor, Chicago, or St. Louis.

(7) The three states on the Pacific coast, California, Oregon, Washington, are somewhat self-contained. They increased last year by 53,454 persons, requiring 36 more physicians; 50 more would repair one-half the losses by death: a total of 86. Available sites, filling the essential requirements, are Berkeley and Seattle. The former, with the adjoining towns of Alameda and Oakland, controls a population of 250,000 or more; the medical department of the University of California concentrated there would enjoy ideal conditions. At present the clinical ends of two divided schools share San Francisco, and the outlook for medical education of high quality is rendered dubious by the division. With unique wisdom the University of Washington and the physicians of Seattle[1] have thus far refrained from starting a medical school in that state. They have held, and rightly, that in the present highly overcrowded condition of the profession on the coast, there is no need for an additional ordinary school; and the resources of the university are not yet adequate to a really creditable establishment. The field will therefore be kept clear until the university is in position to occupy it to advantage.

(8) In Canada the existing ratio of physicians to population is 1:1030. The estimated increase of population last year was 239,516, requiring 160 new physicians; losses by death are estimated at 90. As the country is thinly settled and doctors much less abundant than in the United States, let us suppose these replaced man for man: 250 more doctors would be annually required. The task of supplying them could be for the moment safely left to the Universities of Toronto and Manitoba, to McGill and to Laval at Quebec. Halifax, Western (London), and Laval at Montreal have no present function. At some future time doubtless Dalhousie University at Halifax will need to create a medical department. The future of Queen's depends on its ability to develop halfway between Toronto and Montreal, despite comparative

---

[1] *Copy of Extract of Minutes*
Of the King County Medical Society (State of Washington), June 20, 1904.
Committee. On motion a committee consisting of F. H. Coe, P. W. Willis, and R. W. Schoenle was appointed to draw up suitable resolutions regarding the establishment of any medical preparatory course in the University of Washington, condemning the same and directed to the regents of the institution.

Committee. A committee, consisting of H. M. Read, L. R. Dawson, J. E. Harris, N. D. Pontius, C. A. Smith, and I. A. Parry, was also appointed with directions to visit Dr. Kane personally and urge the importance of our position upon the same subject.

inaccessibility, the Ann Arbor type of school. As for the rest, the great northwestern territory will, as it develops, create whatever additional facilities it may require.

In so far as the United States is concerned, the foregoing sketch calls for 31 medical schools[1] with a present annual output of about 2000 physicians, i. e., an average graduating class of about 70 each. They are capable of producing 3500. All are university departments, busy in advancing knowledge as well as in training doctors. Nineteen are situated in large cities with the universities of which they are organic parts; four are in small towns with their universities; eight are located in large towns always close by the parent institutions. Divided and far distant departments are altogether avoided.

Twenty states[2] are left without a complete school. Most of these are unlikely to be favorably circumstanced for the next half century, so far as we can now judge. Several may, however, find the undertaking feasible within a decade or two. The University of Arkansas might be moved from Fayetteville to Little Rock; Oklahoma, if its rapid growth is maintained, may from Norman govern a medical school at Oklahoma City; Oregon may take full responsibility for Portland. Unfortunately, of the three additional schools thus created, only one, that at Little Rock, would represent conditions at their best. There is therefore no reason to hasten the others; for their problem may, if left open, be more advantageously solved.

To bring about the proposed reconstruction, some 120 schools have been apparently wiped off the map. As a matter of fact, our procedure is far less radical than would thus appear. Of the 120 schools that disappear, 37 are already negligible, for they contain less than 50 students apiece; 13 more contain between 50 and 75 students each, and 16 more between 75 and 100. That is, of the 120 schools, 66 are so small that their student bodies can, in so far as they are worthy, be swept into strong institutions without seriously stretching their present enrolment. Of the 30 institutions that remain, several will survive through merger. For example, the Cleveland College of Physicians and Surgeons could be consolidated with Western Reserve; the amalgamation of Jefferson Medical College and the University of Pennsylvania would make one fair-sized school on an enforced two-year college standard; Tufts and Harvard, Vanderbilt and the University of Tennessee, Creighton and the University of Nebraska, would, if joined, form institutions of moderate size, capable of considerable expansion before reaching the limit of efficiency.

In order that these mergers may be effective, not only institutional, but personal ambition must be sacrificed. It is an advantage when two schools come together; but the advantage is gravely qualified if the new faculty is the arithmetical sum of both former faculties. The mergers at Cincinnati, Indianapolis, Louisville, Nashville,

---

[1] The accompanying maps contrast the existing with the suggested number and distribution. Meharry and Howard are included.

[2] They are Maine, New Hampshire, Vermont, West Virginia, North Carolina, South Carolina, Florida, Mississippi, Kentucky, Arkansas, Oklahoma, North Dakota, South Dakota, Montana, Wyoming, Idaho, New Mexico, Arizona, Nevada, Oregon. One school will not long content the state of Texas.

I. MAP SHOWING THE ACTUAL NUMBER, LOCATION, AND DISTRIBUTION OF MEDICAL SCHOOLS

● Complete School.   + Half-School.   *Note.* When two parts of a divided school are in close proximity to each other they are represented by one dot.

II. MAP SHOWING THE SUGGESTED NUMBER, LOCATION, AND DISTRIBUTION OF MEDICAL SCHOOLS

● Complete School.   + Half-School.

have been arranged in this way. The fundamental principles of faculty organization are thus sacrificed. Unless combination is to destroy organization, titles must be shaved when schools unite. There must be one professor of medicine, one professor of surgery, etc., to whom others are properly subordinated. What with superabundant professorial appointments, due now to desire to annex another hospital, and again to annexation of another school, faculties have become unmanageably large, viewed either as teaching, research, or administrative bodies.

Reduction of our 155 medical schools to 31 would deprive of a medical school no section that is now capable of maintaining one. It would threaten no scarcity of physicians until the country's development actually required more than 3500 physicians annually, that is to say, for a generation or two, at least. Meanwhile, the outline proposed involves no artificial standardization: it concedes a different standard to the south as long as local needs require; it concedes the small town university type where it is clearly of advantage to adhere to it; it varies the general ratio in thinly settled regions; and, finally, it provides a system capable without overstraining of producing twice as many doctors as we suppose the country now to need. In other words, we may be wholly mistaken in our figures without in the least impairing the feasibility of the kind of renovation that has been outlined; and every institution arranged for can be expected to make some useful contribution to knowledge and progress.

The right of the state to deal with the entire subject in its own interest can assuredly not be gainsaid. The physician is a social instrument. If there were no disease, there would be no doctors. And as disease has consequences that immediately go beyond the individual specifically affected, society is bound to protect itself against unnecessary spread of loss or danger. It matters not that the making of doctors has been to some extent left to private institutions. The state already makes certain regulations; it can by the same right make others. Practically the medical school is a public service corporation. It is chartered by the state; it utilizes public hospitals on the ground of the social nature of its service. The medical school cannot then escape social criticism and regulation. It was left to itself while society knew no better. But civilization consists in the legal registration of gains won by science and experience; and science and experience have together established the terms upon which medicine can be most useful. "In the old days," says Metchnikoff,[1] "anyone was allowed to practise medicine, because there was no medical science and nothing was exact. Even at the present time among less civilized people, any old woman is allowed to be a midwife. Among more civilized races, differentiation has taken place and childbirths are attended by women of special training who are midwives by diploma. In case of nations still more civilized, the trained midwives are directed by obstetric physicians who have specialized in the conducting of labor. This high degree of differentiation has arisen with and has itself aided the progress of obstetrical science." Legislation

[1] *The Nature of Man* (translated by Chalmers), p. 300.

which should procure for all the advantage of such conditions as is now possible would speedily bring about a reconstruction quite as extensive as that described.

Such control in the social interest inevitably encounters the objection that individualism is thereby impaired. So it is, at that level; so it is intended. The community through such regulation undertakes to abridge the freedom of particular individuals to exploit certain conditions for their personal benefit. But its aim is thereby to secure for all others more freedom at a higher level. Society forbids a company of physicians to pour out upon the community a horde of ill trained physicians. Their liberty is indeed clipped. As a result, however, more competent doctors being trained under the auspices of the state itself, the public health is improved; the physical well-being of the wage-worker is heightened; and a restriction put upon the liberty, so-called, of a dozen doctors increases the effectual liberty of all other citizens. Has democracy, then, really suffered a set-back? Reorganization along rational lines involves the strengthening, not the weakening, of democratic principle, because it tends to provide the conditions upon which well-being and effectual liberty depend.

CHAPTER X

THE MEDICAL SECTS

In the reconstruction just sketched, no allusion has been made to medical sectarianism. We have considered the making of doctors and the increase of knowledge; allopathy, homeopathy, osteopathy, have cut no figure in the discussion. Is it essential that we should now conclude a treaty of peace, by which the reduced number of medical schools shall be so pro-rated as to recognize dissenters on an equitable basis?

The proposition raises at once the question as to whether in this era of scientific medicine, sectarian medicine is logically defensible; as to whether, while it exists, separate standards, fixed by the conditions under which it can survive, are justifiable. Prior to the placing of medicine on a scientific basis, sectarianism was, of course, inevitable. Every one started with some sort of preconceived notion; and from a logical point of view, one preconception is as good as another. Allopathy was just as sectarian as homeopathy. Indeed, homeopathy was the inevitable retort to allopathy. If one man "believes" in dissimilars, contrary suggestion is certain to provide another who will stake his life on similars; the champion of big doses will be confronted by the champion of little ones. But now that allopathy has surrendered to modern medicine, is not homeopathy borne on the same current into the same harbor?

The modern point of view may be restated as follows: medicine is a discipline, in which the effort is made to use knowledge procured in various ways in order to effect certain practical ends. With abstract general propositions it has nothing to do. It harbors no preconceptions as to diseases or their cure. Instead of starting with a finished and supposedly adequate dogma or principle, it has progressively become less cocksure and more modest. It distrusts general propositions, *a priori* explanations, grandiose and comforting generalizations. It needs theories only as convenient summaries in which a number of ascertained facts may be used tentatively to define a course of action. It makes no effort to use its discoveries to substantiate a principle formulated before the facts were even suspected. For it has learned from the previous history of human thought that men possessed of vague preconceived ideas are strongly disposed to force facts to fit, defend, or explain them. And this tendency both interferes with the free search for truth and limits the good which can be extracted from such truth as is in its despite attained.

Modern medicine has therefore as little sympathy for allopathy as for homeopathy. It simply denies outright the relevancy or value of either doctrine. It wants not dogma, but facts. It countenances no presupposition that is not common to it with all the natural sciences, with all logical thinking.

The sectarian, on the other hand, begins with his mind made up. He possesses in advance a general formula, which the particular instance is going to illustrate, verify, reaffirm, even though he may not know just how. One may be sure that facts so read will make good what is expected of them; that only that will be seen which will sustain its expected function; that every aspect noted will be dutifully loyal to the revelation in whose favor the observer is predisposed: the human mind is so constituted.

It is precisely the function of scientific method—in social life, politics, engineering, medicine—to get rid of such hindrances to clear thought and effective action. For it, comprehensive summaries are situate in the future, not in the past; we shall attain them, if at all, at the end of great travail; they are not lightly to be assumed prior to the beginning. Science believes slowly; in the absence of crucial demonstration its mien is humble, its hold is light. "One should not teach dogmas; on the contrary, every utterance must be put to the proof. One should not train disciples but form observers: one must teach and work in the spirit of natural science."[1]

Scientific medicine therefore brushes aside all historic dogma. It gets down to details immediately. No man is asked in whose name he comes—whether that of Hahnemann, Rush, or of some more recent prophet. But all are required to undergo rigorous cross-examination. Whatsoever makes good is accepted, becomes in so far part, and organic part, of the permanent structure. To plead in advance a principle couched in pseudo-scientific language or of extra-scientific character is to violate scientific quality. There is no need, just as there is no logical justification, for the invocation of names or creeds, for the segregation from the larger body of established truth of any particular set of truths or supposed truths as especially precious. Such segregation may easily invest error with the sanctity of truth; it will certainly result in conferring disproportionate importance upon the fact or procedure marked out as of pivotal significance. The tendency to build a system out of a few partially apprehended facts, deductive inference filling in the rest, has not indeed been limited to medicine, but it has nowhere else had more calamitous consequences.

The logical position of medical sectarians to-day is self-contradictory. They have practically accepted the curriculum as it has been worked out on the scientific basis. They teach pathology, bacteriology, clinical microscopy. They are thereby committed to the scientific method; for they aim to train the student to ascertain and interpret facts in the accepted scientific manner. He may even learn his sciences in the same laboratory as the non-sectarian. But scientific method cannot be limited to the first half of medical education. The same method, the same attitude of mind, must consistently permeate the entire process. The sectarian therefore in effect contradicts himself when, having pursued or having agreed to pursue the normal scientific curriculum with his student for two years, he at the beginning of the third year produces a novel principle and requires that thenceforth the student effect a compromise between science and revelation.

[1] Johannes Orth : *Berliner Klinische Wochenschrift*, vol. xliii. p. 818.

Once granted the possibility of medical dogma, there can be no limit to the number of dissenting sects. As a matter of fact, only three or four are entitled to serious notice in an educational discussion. The chiropractics, the mechano-therapists, and several others are not medical sectarians, though exceedingly desirous of masquerading as such; they are unconscionable quacks, whose printed advertisements are tissues of exaggeration, pretense, and misrepresentation of the most unqualifiedly mercenary character. The public prosecutor and the grand jury are the proper agencies for dealing with them.

Sectarians, in the logical sense above discussed, are (1) the homeopathists, (2) the eclectics, (3) the physiomedicals, (4) the osteopaths. All of them accept in theory, at least, the same fundamental basis. They admit that anatomy, pathology, bacteriology, physiology, must form the foundation of a medical education, to use the words broadly so as to include all varieties of therapeutic procedure. They offer no alternative to pathology or physiology; there is, they concede, only one proper science of the structure of the human body, of the abnormal growths that afflict it. So far, they make no issue as against scientific medicine. Much is involved in agreement up to this point. The standards of admission to the medical school, the facilities which the schools must furnish in order effectively to teach the fundamental branches, are the same for all alike. A student of homeopathy or of osteopathy needs to be just as intelligent and mature as a student of scientific medicine; and he is no easier to teach; for during the first and second years, at least, he is supposed to be doing precisely the same things.

At the beginning of the clinical years, the sectarian interposes his special principle. But educationally, the conditions he needs thenceforth do not materially differ from those needed by consistently scientific medicine. Once more, whatever the arbitrary peculiarity of the treatment to be followed, the student cannot be trained to recognize clinical conditions, to distinguish between different clinical conditions, or to follow out a line of treatment, except in the ways previously described in dealing with scientific medicine. He must see patients and must follow their progress, so as to discover what results take place in consequence of the specific measures employed. A sectarian institution, being a school in which students are trained to do particular things, needs the same resources and facilities on the clinical side as a school of scientific medicine.

Sectarian institutions do not exist in Canada; in the United States there are 32 of them, of which 15 are homeopathic, 8 eclectic, 1 physiomedical, and 8 osteopathic. Without attempting to indicate the peculiar tenets of each, we shall briefly review them as schools, seeking to ascertain how far they are in position effectively to teach, quite regardless of the individual doctrine each sect may desire to promote.

None of the fifteen homeopathic schools [1] requires more than a high school educa-

[1] Hahnemann (San Francisco), Hahnemann and Hering (Chicago), state universities of Iowa and Michigan, Southwestern Homeopathic (Louisville), Boston University, Detroit Homeopathic, Kan-

tion for entrance; only five[1] require so much. The remaining eleven get less,—how much less depending on their geographical locations rather than on the school's own definition. The Louisville, Kansas City, and Baltimore schools cannot be said to have admission standards in any strict sense at all; Pulte at Cincinnati is bound to be careful in dealing with Ohio candidates: outsiders are responsible for themselves. The minimum at Boston University, to judge from the examinations which, in default of acceptable credentials, the candidate must pass, covers less than two years of a good high school course.

On the laboratory side, though the homeopaths admit the soundness of the scientific position, they have taken no active part in its development. Nowhere in homeopathic institutions, with the exception of one or two departments at Boston University, is there any evidence of progressive scientific work. Even "drug proving" is rarely witnessed. The fundamental assumption of the sect is sacred; and scientific activity cannot proceed where any such interdict is responsible for the spirit of the institution. The homeopathic departments at Iowa and Michigan are in this respect only half-schools,—clinical halves. For their students get their scientific instruction in pathology, anatomy, etc., in the only laboratories which the university devotes to those subjects, under men none of whom sympathizes with homeopathy. Their disadvantage is increased by the fact that the instruction is adapted to students who have had one or two years of college work. The general argument in favor of higher standards is here reinforced by the consideration that the homeopathic students should certainly qualify themselves for the only grade of scientific instruction that the two universities offer.

Of complete homeopathic schools, Boston University, the New York Homeopathic College, and the Hahnemann of Philadelphia alone possess the equipment necessary for the effective routine teaching of the fundamental branches. None of them can employ full-time teachers to any considerable extent. But they possess fairly well-equipped laboratories in anatomy, pathology, bacteriology, and physiology,[2] a museum showing care and intelligence, and a decent library. Boston University deserves especial commendation for what it has accomplished with its small annual income.

Of the remaining homeopathic schools, four are weak and uneven: the Hahnemann of San Francisco and the Hahnemann of Chicago have small, but not altogether inadequate, equipment for the teaching of chemistry, elementary pathology and bacteriology; the Cleveland school offers an active course in experimental physiology. Beyond ordinary dissection and elementary chemistry, they offer little else. There is, for example, no experimental physiology in the San Francisco Hahnemann: "the instructor does n't believe in it;" the Chicago Hahnemann contains a small outfit and

sas City (Kansas) Hahnemann, New York Medical College for Women, New York Homeopathic, Pulte (Cincinnati), Cleveland Homeopathic, Hahnemann (Philadelphia), Atlantic Medical (Baltimore).
[1] State universities of Iowa and Michigan, Detroit Homeopathic, and the two New York schools.
[2] The Philadelphia Hahnemann is defective in experimental physiology.

a few animals for that subject; the Cleveland equipment for pathology and bacteriology is meager. The New York Homeopathic College for Women is well intentioned, but its means have permitted it to do but little in any direction.

Six schools remain—all utterly hopeless: Hering (Chicago), because it is without plant or resources; the other five,[1] because in addition to having nothing, their condition indicates the total unfitness of their managers for any sort of educational responsibility. The buildings are filthy and neglected. At Louisville no branch is properly equipped; in one room, the outfit is limited to a dirty and tattered manikin; in another, a single guinea pig awaits his fate in a cage. At Detroit the dean and secretary "have their offices downtown;" the so-called laboratories are in utter confusion. At Kansas City similar disorder prevails. At the Atlantic Medical appearances are equally bad; to make matters worse, the school has lately omitted the word "homeopathic" from its title so as to gather in students dropped from other Baltimore schools.

In respect to hospital facilities, the University of Michigan, Boston University, and the New York Homeopathic alone command an adequate supply of material, under proper control, though modern teaching methods are not thoroughly utilized even by them. The Iowa school controls a small, but inadequate, hospital. All the others are seriously handicapped by either lack of material or lack of control, and in most instances by both. The Hahnemann of San Francisco relies mainly on 30 beds supported by the city and county in a private hospital; the Detroit school is cordially welcome at the Grace Hospital, but less than 60 beds are available, and they are mostly surgical; the Woman's Homeopathic of New York[2] controls a hospital of 35 available beds, mostly surgical; the Southwestern (Louisville) and the Cleveland school get one-fifth of the patients that enter the city hospitals of their respective towns, but these hospitals are not equipped or organized with a view to teaching. The Kansas City school holds clinics one day a week at the City Hospital; Pulte (Cincinnati) and the Atlantic (Baltimore) have, as nearly as one can gather, nothing definite at all. Several of the schools appear to be unnecessarily handicapped. The Chicago Hahnemann adjoins a hospital with 60 ward beds. But as the superintendent " does n't believe in admitting students to wards," there is little or nothing beyond amphitheater teaching. A bridge connects Hering (Chicago) with a homeopathic hospital, but "students are not admitted." The Cleveland school is next door to a hospital with which it was once intimate; their relations have been ruptured. An excellent hospital is connected with the building occupied by the Philadelphia Hahnemann, but there is no ward work.

The dispensary situation is rather worse. Iowa and Ann Arbor have little opportunity. Of the others, Boston University alone has a really model dispensary, comparing favorably in equipment, organization, and conduct with the best institutions

---

[1] Southwestern (Louisville), Pulte (Cincinnati), Atlantic (Baltimore), and the Detroit and Kansas City schools.

[2] This school has scattered supplementary facilities, as is the way of New York schools.

of the kind in the country. The New York Homeopathic, the Chicago Hahnemann, and the Philadelphia Hahnemann command material enough. The others lack material, equipment, or care; in some instances,— Atlantic Medical, Pulte, Detroit, Kansas City,—they lack everything that a dispensary should possess.

Financially, the two state university departments and the New York Homeopathic school are the only homeopathic schools whose strength is greater than their fee income. All the others are dependent on tuition. Their outlook for higher entrance standards or improved teaching is, therefore, distinctly unpromising. Only a few of them command tuition fees enough to do anything at all: the Chicago Hahnemann, Boston University, and the Philadelphia Hahnemann, with annual fees ranging between $12,000 and $18,000.[1] Nine of them are hopelessly poor: the San Francisco Hahnemann, Hering (Chicago), the Detroit Homeopathic, and the Atlantic Medical operate on less than $4000[1] a year; the Southwestern (Louisville) and Pulte (Cincinnati) on less than $1500.[1]

In the year 1900 there were twenty-two homeopathic colleges in the United States; to-day there are fifteen; the total student enrolment has within the same period been cut almost in half, decreasing from 1909 to 1009;[2] the graduating classes have fallen from 413 to 246. As the country is still poorly supplied with homeopathic physicians, these figures are ominous; for the rise of legal standard must inevitably affect homeopathic practitioners. In the financial weakness of their schools, the further shrinkage of the student body will inhibit first the expansion, then the keeping up, of the sect.

Logically, no other outcome is possible. The ebbing vitality of homeopathic schools is a striking demonstration of the incompatibility of science and dogma. One may begin with science and work through the entire medical curriculum consistently, exposing everything to the same sort of test; or one may begin with a dogmatic assertion and resolutely refuse to entertain anything at variance with it. But one cannot do both. One cannot simultaneously assert science and dogma; one cannot travel half the road under the former banner, in the hope of taking up the latter, too, at the middle of the march. Science, once embraced, will conquer the whole. Homeopathy has two options: one to withdraw into the isolation in which alone any peculiar tenet can maintain itself; the other to put that tenet into the melting-pot. Historically it undoubtedly played an important part in discrediting empirical allopathy. But laboratories of physiology and pharmacology are now doing that work far more effectively than homeopathy; and they are at the same time performing a constructive task for which homeopathy, as such, is unfitted. It will be clear, then, why, when outlining a system of schools for the training of physicians on scientific lines, no specific provision is made for homeopathy. For everything of proved value in

[1] Estimated.

[2] Journal of the American Institute of Homeopathy, vol. i., 1909, no. 11, p. 537. The Journal of the American Medical Association, Aug. 14, 1909 (pp. 556, 557), gives figures somewhat lower: 869 instead of 1009; 909 instead of 246. The discrepancy does not alter our interpretation.

homeopathy belongs of right to scientific medicine and is at this moment incorporate in it; nothing else has any footing at all, whether it be of allopathic or homeopathic lineage. "A new school of practitioners has arisen," says Dr. Osler, "which cares nothing for homeopathy and less for so-called allopathy. It seeks to study, rationally and scientifically, the action of drugs, old and new."[1]

There are eight eclectic schools.[2] One of them — that in New York City — requires the Regents' Medical Student Certificate, i. e., a four-year high school education, for admission; the Cincinnati school must require an equal preliminary education of students expecting to practise in Ohio, others taking the matter into their own hands. Just how the instruction is thus accommodated to various levels is not clear. The remaining six schools have either nominal requirements or none at all.

None of the schools has anything remotely resembling the laboratory equipment which all claim in their catalogues. The Cincinnati institution possesses a new and attractive building, thus far meagerly fitted out; the New York school has a clean building with a chemical laboratory in which elementary chemistry can be and apparently is taught properly. It has little else: a small room for the microscopic subjects, but no adequate equipment for teaching them; a few thousand books, mostly old; a few models, a lantern, etc., — and this is most satisfactorily equipped of all the eclectic institutions. The Hospital School at Atlanta, starting on four weeks' notice, had time to get students, but not to get means of teaching them. The private laboratory of the instructor in pathology and bacteriology was meanwhile at their service: other equipment there was, at the time of the visit, none.

The remaining five eclectic schools are without exception filthy and almost bare. They have at best grimy little laboratories for elementary chemistry, a few microscopes, some bottles containing discolored and unlabeled pathological material, an incubator out of commission, and a horrid dissecting-room,—when dissecting is in progress. The St. Louis school was the proud possessor of some new physiological apparatus, the state board having recently issued an edict requiring its purchase; but there was no place to use it and no sign of its use. The Kansas City institution had likewise made a recent investment to the same extent, having just taken on the faculty the "laboratory man" of the local homeopathic and osteopathic schools. The other Atlanta, the Los Angeles, and the Lincoln schools have even less. The Lincoln institution alleges that its scientific training is given at Cotner University, where the only material available for medical instruction consists of a chemical laboratory, some microscopes, and a small collection of stuffed birds.

Of the eight schools under discussion, none has decent clinical opportunities. The New York school can send three students twice weekly to the Sydenham Hospital; the Cincinnati school is affiliated with the Seton Hospital, with 24 available beds,

---

[1] Loc. cit., p. 268.
[2] One each at Los Angeles, Kansas City (Kansas), St. Louis, Lincoln (Nebraska), Cincinnati, New York City, and two at Atlanta.

80 to 90 per cent surgical, and can send its men to look on at the public clinics given in the City Hospital; the St. Louis students have a day a week at the City Hospital and profit occasionally elsewhere through professorial connection. All this is criminally inadequate, yet it is the best that the eclectics offer; for the other five schools have literally nothing at all. One of the Atlanta "colleges" is connected with a private infirmary; the other has not even such a semblance. The Los Angeles school claims "private hospitals only;" the Kansas City school claims to give clinics at the new City Hospital, but the hospital authorities deny it. At Lincoln "there are no regular hours at any hospital; they depend on cases as they turn up."

The dispensaries may be even more briefly described. The Atlanta, Lincoln, and Los Angeles schools have none at all. The Cincinnati school uses poorly the small dispensary at the Seton Hospital. The New York school has three rooms in its own building and access to another dispensary. At St. Louis there is one room and "some one comes almost every day;" at Kansas City, one room likewise, with a present daily attendance of three and a confident aspiration that this number can be swelled to six.

The utter hopelessness of the future of these schools is apparent on a glance at their financial condition. All are dependent on fees. Only three of them — the New York, the Cincinnati, and one Atlanta school — enjoy an income between $5000 and $8500[1] a year; the St. Louis, Lincoln, and second Atlanta schools have something over $3000[1] annually; those at Los Angeles and Kansas City not much above $1000;[1] and these modest sums are not always spent within the schools. Statistics confirm the unfavorable prognosis: the ten schools which the sect possessed in 1901 have now dwindled to eight; a maximum enrolment of 1014 in 1904 has already shrunk to 413; graduates numbered 186 in 1906, 84 in 1909.

So far as sectarian creeds go, there is, of course, no reason why these schools should be elaborately equipped for scientific instruction. They talk of laboratories, not because they appreciate their place or significance, but because it pays them to defer thus far to the spirit of the times. Culpable indeed they are, however, for their utter failure to make good what their own tenets prescribe. The eclectics are drug mad; yet, with the exception of the Cincinnati and New York schools, none of them can do justice to its own creed. For they are not equipped to teach the drugs or the drug therapy which constitutes their sole reason for existence.[2]

The eight osteopathic schools[3] fairly reek with commercialism. Their catalogues are a mass of hysterical exaggerations, alike of the earning and of the curative power of osteopathy. It is impossible to say upon which score the "science" most confidently appeals to the crude boys or disappointed men and women whom it successfully

---

[1] Estimated.

[2] The physio-medical sect can be dismissed in a note. It had three schools in 1907; only one, that in Chicago, is left. The reader will find it described in Part II, under Illinois, no. (11). There were 149 physio-medical students in 1904; there are now 59; there were 90 graduates in that year, 15 in 1909.

[3] One school is found in each of the following cities: Chicago, Des Moines, Kirksville (Missouri), Kansas City (Missouri), Philadelphia, Cambridge (Massachusetts), and two at Los Angeles.

exploits. "In no case has a competent osteopath made a failure in his attempt to build up a paying practice. . . . His remuneration, counted in dollars, will be greatly in excess of what he could reasonably expect in most other lines of professional work."[1] "It is only fair to say that many of our graduates are earning as much in single months as they were formerly able to earn by a full year's work."[2] "The average osteopath has a better practice than ninety out of every hundred medical practitioners."[3] "A lucrative practice is assured to every conscientious and capable practitioner."[4] "The graduate who does not make as much as the total cost of his osteopathic education in his first year of practice is the exception."[5] Standards these concerns have none; the catalogues touch that point very tenderly. At the parent school at Kirksville an applicant will be accepted "if he pass examinations in English, arithmetic, history, and geography;" but if he should fail to meet these lofty scholastic requirements, he may be admitted anyway. In Massachusetts—the most homogeneously educated state in the Union—the Cambridge school diplomatically posits that "a diploma may be accepted or an examination be required if deemed advisable by the directors," —the word "is" being conspicuous by its absence; the Pacific College, "chancing it," finds that "most make good."

Whatever his notions on the subject of treatment, the osteopath needs to be trained to recognize disease and to differentiate one disease from another quite as carefully as any other medical practitioner. Our account of the sect proceeds wholly from this point of view. Whether they use drugs or do not use them, whether some use them while others do not, does not affect this fundamental question. Whatever they do, they must know the body, in health and disease, before they can possibly know whether there is an occasion for osteopathic intervention, and if so, at what point, to what extent, etc. All physicians, summoned to see the sick, are confronted with precisely the same crisis: a body out of order. No matter to what remedial procedure they incline,—medical, surgical, or manipulative,—they must first ascertain what is the trouble. There is only one way to do that. The osteopaths admit it, when they teach physiology, pathology, chemistry, microscopy. Let it be stated, therefore, with all possible emphasis that no one of the eight osteopathic schools is in position to give such training as osteopathy itself demands. The entire course is only three years. In so simple and fundamental a matter as anatomy—assuredly the corner-stone of a "science" that relies wholly on local manipulation—they are fatally defective. At Kirksville the accommodations are entirely unequal to the teaching of its huge student body. Hence the first year is devoted to text-book study of anatomy, part of the second year to dissection; at Kansas City they consider that the student dissects better if he has learned anatomy first: hence

[1] *Catalogue*, Pacific College of Osteopathy, 1909–10, p. 9.
[2] *Catalogue*, Los Angeles College of Osteopathy, 1909–10, p. 9.
[3] *Catalogue*, Central College of Osteopathy, 1908–9, p. 22.
[4] *Catalogue*, Philadelphia College of Osteopathy, 1909–10, p. 48.
[5] *Catalogue*, Massachusetts College of Osteopathy, 1909–10, p. 10.

dissection comes in the latter half of the course, being completed just one-half year before graduation. The supply of material is also scant: the school had had one cadaver early in the fall and was looking ahead to a second the latter part of the winter. The Los Angeles college has a small room with five tables for a student body numbering 250; it solves the difficulty by giving separate squads two hours a week each. At Philadelphia the department of anatomy occupies an outhouse, whence the noisome odor of decaying cadavers permeates the premises. Other subjects fare even worse. A small chemical laboratory is occasionally seen,—at Philadelphia it happens to be in a dark cellar. At Kirksville a fair-sized room is devoted to pathology and bacteriology; the huge classes are divided into bands of 32, each of which gets a six weeks' course, following the directions of a rigid syllabus under a teacher who is himself a student. At Cambridge pathology comes in the last year. A professor in the Kansas City school said of his own institution that it had practically no laboratories at all; the Still College at Des Moines has, in place of laboratories, laboratory signs; the Littlejohn at Chicago, whose catalogue avers that the "physician should be imbued with a knowledge of the healing art in its widest fields, and here is the opportunity,"[1] has lately in rebuilding wrecked all its laboratories but that of chemistry without in the least interfering with its usual pedagogic routine.[2]

Nowhere is there the faintest effort to connect the "laboratory teaching" with "clinical osteopathy;" perhaps because no school has anything approaching the requisite clinical opportunities. Once more, their tenets are not in question. Much difference of opinion prevails among them as to whether they should teach everything or only some things; as to whether they may use drugs in certain conditions or must confine themselves wholly to manipulation for "osteopathic lesions." However this may be, the osteopath cannot learn his technique and when it is applicable, except through experience with ailing individuals. And these, for the most part, he begins to see only when his prosperity begins after receiving his "D.O." degree. The Kirksville school (560 students) has indeed a hospital of 54 beds, of which, however, only 20 are in the wards, and practically all are surgical. Eight obstetrical cases were obtained in April and May of last year. The Des Moines and Kansas City schools have no hospitals at all; the students see no acute cases "unless the doctors can take them along." The Pacific College has a hospital of from twelve to fifteen surgical and obstetrical beds, all pay; "the students have no regular work at the hospital as there are so few acute cases; they don't see as much acute work as they should, but they treat everything." The Littlejohn (Chicago) has also a pay hospital, of 20 beds, mostly surgical. The Philadelphia school, whose "opportunities for practical work" are highly extolled in its catalogue, has an infirmary with three beds, occupied by

---

[1] *Bulletin*, June 15, 1909, p. 7.

[2] This school teaches medicine as well as osteopathy. It offers instruction in materia medica and therapeutics, practice of medicine,—and yet it is a three-year school.

maternity cases if at all; the Cambridge student must travel an hour or more to the Chelsea Hospital, a pay institution of from ten to fifteen rooms.

The mercenary character of osteopathic instruction is nowhere more conspicuously displayed than in the dispensaries, designed in theory to turn a humanitarian impulse to educational account. The osteopathic schools insert a cash nexus: the patients almost always pay. At Kansas City students give treatment to patients who pay three dollars a month; those paying more are treated by the professors. At Kirksville two dollars a treatment is charged. The cases are mostly chronics, an instructor being present at the first treatment; afterwards, only if summoned. At Los Angeles the cheapest obtainable treatment is three dollars for "examination" and one month's treatment before the class; at Des Moines the "professor administers to high-priced patients, the students to others."

The eight osteopathic schools now enroll over 1800 students, who pay some $200,000 annually in fees. The instruction furnished for this sum is inexpensive and worthless. Not a single full-time teacher is found in any of them. The fees find their way directly into the pockets of the school owners, or into school buildings and infirmaries that are equally their property. No effort is anywhere made to utilize prosperity as a means of defining an entrance standard or developing the "science."[1] Granting all that its champions claim, osteopathy is still in its incipiency. If sincere, its votaries would be engaged in critically building it up. They are doing nothing of the kind. Indeed, in none of the sectarian schools does one observe progressive effort even along the lines of its own creed. And very naturally: dogma is sufficient unto itself. It may not search its own assumptions; it does well to adopt from the outside, after forced restatement in its own terms.[2]

In dealing with the medical sectary, society can employ no special device. Certain profound characteristics in one way or another support the medical dissenter: now, the primitive belief in magic crops up in his credulous respect for an impotent drug; again, all other procedure having failed, what is there to lose by flinging one's self upon the mercy of chance? Instincts so profound cannot be abolished by statute. But the limits within which they can play may be so regulated as to forbid alike their commercial and their crudely ignorant exploitation. The law may require that all practitioners of the healing art comply with a rigidly enforced preliminary educational standard; that every school possess the requisite facilities; that every licensed physician demonstrate a practical knowledge of the body and its affections. To these terms no reasonable person can object; the good sense of society can enforce them upon reasonable and unreasonable alike. From medical sects that can live on these conditions, the public will suffer little more harm than it is destined to suffer anyhow from the necessary incompleteness of human knowledge and the necessary defects of human skill.

[1] At the Pacific College of Osteopathy alone were two workers doing some research.
[2] In this fashion homeopathy handles serum-therapy as a case of similars.

CHAPTER XI

THE STATE BOARDS

THE state boards are the instruments through which the reconstruction of medical education will be largely effected. To them the graduate in medicine applies for the license to practise. Their power can be both indirectly and directly exerted. They may after examination reject an applicant,— an indirect method of discrediting the school which has vouched for him by conferring its M.D. degree. A small percentage of failures the doctrine of chance would lead one to expect; an increasing proportion must cast increasingly serious doubt on any institution. A more direct and therefore more salutary method is needed, however, in dealing with schools bad beyond a reasonable doubt. In such instances the board should summarily refuse to entertain the applicant's petition because his medical education rests upon no proper preliminary training or was received under conditions that forbade thorough or conscientious instruction: the full weight of its refusal would fall with crushing effect upon the school which sent him forth. No institution can long survive the day upon which it is thus publicly branded as feeble, unfit, or disreputable. For the purpose, however, of saving the victims whose cruel disappointment will in time destroy these schools, the arm of the state boards should for the present go beyond the rejection of individuals to the actual closing up of notoriously incompetent institutions. The law that protects the public against the unfit doctor should in fairness protect the student against the unfit school.

With the manifold duties and responsibilities of the state boards we cannot here fully deal. Our attention is necessarily confined to their educational function. They examine candidates for license; but admission to examination should be granted only after a fair presumption of intellectual fitness in favor of the applicant has been established by the record of his preliminary education, and a fair presumption of sufficient professional training by his graduation from a recognized or reputable medical school. Neither of these points can for the present be overlooked. So long as the medical school has as such no determinate position in the school system, the public health authorities must be empowered to fix at least the lowest point to which it can safely be permitted to fall; moreover, so long as any group of physicians may in most states incorporate a medical school under general laws that offer no safeguard at all, and license examinations are not yet deliberately constructed to frustrate their activity, summary protective power against mercenary and incompetent faculties must be lodged somewhere. The boards therefore touch at three points the problems with which this report has dealt: for they deal (1) with the preliminary educational requirement, (2) with the facilities of medical schools, (3) with examinations for licensure.

In all these respects, the scope of the state board is of course determined by statute. Let us consider briefly what powers in respect to each are needed if the boards are to be effective in the reconstruction to which we look forward.

(1) However the educational prerequisite be defined, the board must be authorized to insist upon it as an educational, and not as a practice, preliminary. The sole reason for a preliminary requirement of any kind is as a method of restricting the study of medicine to those in whose favor an initial presumption of fitness exists. An ordinary secondary school education may be taken as indicating minimum competency only if it chronologically precede admission to the medical school. As a matter of fact, some state boards legally empowered to enforce the high school basis are often strangely careless as to the significance of dates; so that a requirement whose sole value resides in its priority to medical education is held to be satisfied if fulfilled just prior to graduation or to licensure.

The evaluation of preliminary credentials is a task requiring expert knowledge and experience. Certain boards have striven hard to discharge this function effectively; but they lack an organization competent to deal with it. It may be that as the feasibility of federated action is increased by an approach to uniformity in laws and ideals, a central authority can be constituted by voluntary coöperation of the state boards, maintained by contributions from their several funds, and charged with the business of procuring first-hand information respecting secondary schools and colleges. Such an agency could, by communication with the proper educational organizations engaged in the study and improvement of secondary schools, command reliable data for the evaluation of credentials prior to matriculation. In default thereof, the board of each state, instead of endeavoring to act on such knowledge as it can obtain, should get at once into effective relations with the state university, or with some endowed institution accustomed to pass upon questions of this kind; and the medical schools should be compelled to have a student's application "viséd" by the state board before matriculation is regarded as complete. If neither time nor subject credit could be given by the medical school for any work prior to completed matriculation, an actual four-year high school preliminary requirement would be in force.[1]

(2) The enforcement of even the four-year high school standard will so far clean up the medical field that the state boards will at once be relieved of the duty of dealing with actually disreputable schools. Until that has been accomplished, these boards should be empowered to refuse applications from the graduates of schools scandalously defective in teaching facilities. The power here in question, if extended too far, would involve serious dangers. For boards authorized to decide whether schools are satisfactory may be led to specify the details which determine their judgment. In some quarters they have already shown a tendency to prescribe minutely the contents of a proper medical education. Their motive has been excellent; they have tried to compel poor schools to give a good education. Unfortunately, that is quite impossible: teachers may sign a register showing due attendance upon their classes, just as students may scrupulously attend specified exercises in every essen-

[1] The same process can be employed in the south to enforce whatever standard is there decided on.

tial branch for a fixed number of hours; but the instruction will probably be no whit improved by such police regulation. Meanwhile every competent and earnest instructor is seriously hampered by the vain effort to aid those who are beyond human help. The fact is that an enforced entrance requirement at one end and a proper examination at the other will of themselves limit the survival of schools to those that are financially and educationally competent. Only so long as an entrance requirement cannot be enforced or a proper examination arranged, do the state boards need the power to close schools obviously and notoriously defective.

(3) The examination[1] for licensure is indubitably the lever with which the entire field may be lifted; for the power to examine is the power to destroy. At present, these examinations are not only without stimulating effect; they are actually depressing. There is only one sort of licensing test that is significant, viz., a test that ascertains the practical ability of the student confronting a concrete case to collect all relevant data and to suggest the positive procedure applicable to the conditions disclosed. A written examination may have some incidental value; it does not touch the heart of the matter. It tends, indeed, to do just the reverse. Written examinations are notably apt to follow beaten paths. A collection of state board examinations covering even a brief period of years will contain most of the questions that will be asked hereafter. An effective, but purely mechanical and entirely useless drill may be employed to make examination-proof a student who in the presence of a sick person would be quite helpless. As a matter of fact, prominent publishers put forth "State Board Questions" and "Quiz-compends" with "answers." These manuals, well conned, guarantee the candidate's safety. Do not the several states appear to do almost everything in their power to resist the production of a well trained body of physicians? In the first place, they permit a half-dozen men to start a medical school as lightly as they permit them to open a printing-shop; and they then offer them every inducement to furnish poor training by permitting the graduates to undergo an examination for which they can satisfactorily prepare by an inexpensive drill that has no bearing on the practical ends for which doctors are needed. A proper examination would go far to correct all the defects that this report has sought to point out. For low entrance standards, deficient equipment, bad teaching, lack of clinical material, failure to correlate laboratory and clinic, would be detected and punished by a searching practical examination.

If the written examination were relegated to a subordinate position, the weight of the test would fall upon the applicant's ability to do things; schools incapable for whatever reason of training students in the necessary technique would be rapidly exposed through the annual publication of statistics proclaiming their failure. The state board results, now so frequently misleading, would be a trustworthy index which the more intelligent students would carefully scan; and those schools only would sur-

[1] For an excellent discussion, see Councilman: "Methods and Objects of State Board Examinations," *Journal of American Medical Association*, Aug. 14, 1909, pp. 515-19.

vive whose records entitle them to live. Of such overwhelming importance, indeed, is the character of the license examination that, if thorough practical examinations were instituted, all the other perplexing details we have discussed would become relatively immaterial.

How far we now are from this ideal realized in other countries, hardly aspired to in America, a few facts make plain. In 1906, the worst of the Chicago schools—a school with no entrance requirement, no laboratory teaching, no hospital connections—made before state boards the best record attained by any Chicago school in that year. This school, essentially the same now as then, has only recently been declared "not in good standing" with the state board of Illinois. Everywhere in Canada and the United States wretched institutions refute criticism by pointing to their successful state board records. Halifax and Western University candidates pass in Canada side by side with students from McGill and Toronto, though not in an equal proportion; for even in the written examination, better opportunities tell in the long run. Good didactic teaching at Bowdoin or Dartmouth proves capable of satisfying examinations that should strongly stress clinical experience. One or two of the states have latterly begun to introduce certain practical features into their examinations. These timid beginnings are hopeful signs, as yet, however, hardly extensive enough anywhere materially to affect either the kind of teaching employed or the outcome of the examination. The army and navy have gone a little further towards developing a practical examination than has any state board; and their written tests are probably also more severe; with the result that between the years 1900 and 1909, 46 per cent of graduated doctors applying for the naval medical corps failed; between 1904 and 1909, 81 per cent of the applicants for the Marine Hospital service failed; and out of 1512 candidates for the army medical corps between 1888 and 1909, 72 per cent failed:[1] this, although very few of the applicants examined came from the unmitigatedly bad schools.

To do their duty fully, the state boards require to be properly constituted, organized, and equipped. At present none of them fulfils all these conditions. In consequence it is difficult to know where to lodge responsibility. In some states the law is so weak that a board can be successfully "mandamused" the moment it raises a finger. Elsewhere, a good law is practically negatived by the inactivity, if not worse, of a board that excuses itself by the apathy of the public or by the "pull" of the medical schools. In general the boards have not been strongly constituted. In many states appointments are regarded as political spoils; quite generally teachers are ineligible for appointment. It happens, therefore, that the boards are sometimes weak, and either unwilling to antagonize the schools or legally incapable of so doing; again, well meaning but incompetent; in some cases unquestionably neither weak nor well

---

[1] For the records upon which these statements are based, acknowledgments are due to the Surgeon-General of the Navy, the Surgeon-General of the Marine Hospital Service, and to the Surgeon-General of the Army, respectively.

meaning, but cunning, powerful, and closely aligned with selfish and harmful political interests. In a few instances, that stand out, the boards are vigorous, intelligent, and public spirited,— notably in Colorado, Michigan, and Minnesota.

In the matter of organization they are decidedly defective. The whole weight rests usually upon a single executive officer, the secretary, whose sole staff consists of a stenographer, if that. As long as everything depends on the personality of a single individual, administration will be liable to marked fluctuations. There can be neither security nor continuity. For enlightened public opinion and accepted ideals have not as yet established definite and correct policy. Organization would within limits be independent of individuals; for it embodies a routine that fortifies every gain won, and makes possible the division of labor that is indispensable to system and thoroughness.

A bureau properly organized cannot live on small fees. It requires liberal support; for it must be in position to take trouble to secure information and to defend its rights. The power that validates the diploma with its license must have the strength to protect its issues against either debasement or infringement. The physician, like the lawyer, is an agent of the state. If he proves unworthy, the same board that vouched for him must have power to recall its act; and its function must extend to the prosecution of fraudulent or unwarranted attempts to practise without its official sanction. Any effort to exercise powers of recall or restraint will of course be resisted. The state must therefore provide funds that will enable the board to defend its action in the courts.

A model state board law must therefore guard the following points: the membership of the board must be drawn from the best elements of the profession, including —not, as now, prohibiting—those engaged in teaching; the board must be armed with the authority and machinery to institute practical examinations, to refuse recognition to unfit schools, and to insist upon such preliminary educational standards as the state's own educational system warrants; finally, it must be provided either by appropriation or by greatly increased fees with funds adequate to perform efficiently the functions for which it was created. The additional powers needed in order to deal as effectively with the practice of medicine, lie outside the present discussion.

Far-reaching legislative changes would be required in most states before the state boards could play the part here assigned to them. Yet for it they are clearly destined. As a matter of fact, recent legislation has been self-contradictory. The boards have been strengthened, their powers more satisfactorily defined ; and thereupon the end thus sought has been partially defeated by the creation of sectarian boards with lower standards and looser ideas. Minnesota, for example, obtained an excellent law, consolidated the medical schools of the state, established a high standard, and quarantined against invasion by a low-grade product from without; and then, having fairly secured for the people of the state the best attainable conditions in the matter of protecting the public health, it proceeded partly to undo the good work by establishing a separate osteopathic board with power to license osteopaths — who will treat all diseases, and quite possibly in all sorts of ways — according to standards and methods fundamentally at variance with the main statute already outlined. The creation of separate boards is thus a roundabout method of recommitting the errors that the main currents of scientific thinking and effort are endeavoring to remedy. Our forty-nine states and territories have now eighty-two different boards of medical examiners. The province of the state in this matter is plain. It cannot allow one set of practitioners to exist on easier and lower terms than another. It cannot indeed be a party to scientific or sectarian controversy. But it can and must safeguard the conditions upon which such controversy may be fought to its finish. The mooted points concern only therapeutics; in respect to all else there is complete agreement. If matters in dispute are omitted from the examination, enough is left for all essential purposes. A single board should subject all candidates, of whatever school, to the same tests at every point. The license of the state is a guarantee of knowledge, education, and skill. The layman is in no position to make allowances. The state's M.D. and the state's D.O. offer themselves for essentially the same purposes. The state stands equally as guarantor of both. No citizen can indeed be wholly protected by the state against his own ignorance, fanaticism, or folly. A man who does not "believe" in doctors cannot be forced to call them in or to heed them, any more than a man who does not "believe" in wearing rubbers can be compelled to don them in slushy weather. The state is powerless there. But having undertaken to visé practising physicians for the protection of those who summon them, it must see to it that the licenses to which it gives currency bear a fairly uniform value. Between the graduate of Harvard and the graduate of the Boston College of Physicians and Surgeons, the layman could not judge even if he knew the origin of each; as a matter of fact, he rarely knows so much. But in the act of licensing both for one purpose, the state assures its citizens of their substantial equality. It is shocking to reflect that, what with written examinations and separate boards, the divergencies run all the way from a high degree of competency to utter ignorance and unfitness.

There is no question that in the end the medical sects will disappear. The dissenter cannot live on high entrance and educational standards. Pending his disappearance, the combination board is the least of the evils to which we are liable. The terms upon which these boards are now obtainable throw a strong light on the backward state of public opinion. In New York state, homeopaths, eclectics, and osteopaths, making together but a negligible proportion of the practising physicians of the state, have together a majority on the state examining board.

Under existing conditions, though the state boards might well be constituted on a uniform plan and with the same powers, a certain degree of diversity is unavoidable; but a certain degree of inevitable diversity is no excuse for hopeless confusion. The variations now found both in the laws and in their administration are fairly chaotic. In one state the board can and does fix entrance requirements; in the next it can, but does not; in a third it neither does nor can. Six boards[1] have announced the requirement of one or more years of college work preliminary to medical schooling as the basis of practice in their respective states; but, seventy-six remain to be converted. Their conversion, with the necessary changes in the state laws, must precede the actual elevation of the entire medical profession. For though agreed elevation of standard by individual schools improves their own product and indirectly leavens the mass, it does not stop the making of low-grade doctors. Temporarily it even assists the low-grade school. The ultimate improvement of the entire mass will come from control of all schools through the state boards, and not merely from voluntary action on the part of the more self-respecting institutions. The middle west seems likely—the osteopaths permitting—first to realize this condition; for the states will surely not leave the practice of medicine within their borders open to strangers on terms denied to their own sons.

Whether or not it will be left for the osteopaths to say, depends just now on making the public appreciate the fact that the point at issue is not a matter of business. A clever hue and cry has been raised to give the controversy the appearance of a competition between rival claimants for business patronage. The instinct for fair play, opposition to exclusive or aristocratic privileges, have thus won for the sectarian a chance on his own terms. Unfortunately, this leaves the sick man wholly out of account. Medicine, curative and preventive, has indeed no analogy with business. Like the army, the police, or the social worker, the medical profession is supported for a benign, not a selfish, for a protective, not an exploiting, purpose. The knell of the exploiting doctor has been sounded, just as the day of the freebooter and the soldier of fortune has passed away.

Despite imperfect and discordant laws and inadequate resources, the state board has abundantly justified itself. It is indeed hardly more than quarter of a century old; yet, in summing up the forces that have within that period made for improved conditions, the state boards must be prominently mentioned. Their rôle is likely to be increasingly important. They have developed considerable *esprit de corps*. Their power of combined action on broad lines has distinctly increased even in the last few years. Reciprocity between states whose laws are measurably concordant and whose ideals are taking similar shape tends to demonstrate the fundamental sameness of the problems requiring solution. Out of these first coöperative efforts, a model law will emerge; federated action may become possible. Perhaps the entire country may some day be covered by a national organization engaged in protecting the public health against the formidable combination made by ignorance, incompetency, commercialism, and disease.

---

[1] Minnesota, North Dakota, South Dakota, Connecticut, Colorado, Kansas.

CHAPTER XII

THE POSTGRADUATE SCHOOL

THE postgraduate school as developed in the United States may be characterized as a "compensatory adjustment." It is an effort to mend a machine that was predestined to break down. Inevitably, the more conscientious and intelligent men trained in most of the medical schools herein described must become aware of their unfitness for the responsibilities of medical practice; the postgraduate school was established to do what the medical school had failed to accomplish.

"When I graduated in the spring of 1869," says Dr. John A. Wyeth,[1] "I can never forget the sinking feeling that came over me when I realized how incompetent I was to undertake the care of those in the distress of sickness or accident. A week later, after arriving in my native village in Alabama, I rented a small office and attached my sign to the front door. Within two months, the tacks were withdrawn by the hand which had placed them there and the sign was stowed away in the bottom of my trunk. Two months of hopeless struggle with a Presbyterian conscience had convinced me that I was not fit to practise medicine, and that nothing was left for me but to go out into the world of business to earn money enough to complete my education. I felt the absolute need of clinical experience, and a conviction, which then forced itself upon my mind, that no graduate in medicine was competent to practise until he had had, in addition to his theoretical, a clinical and laboratory training, was the controlling idea in my mind when, in later years the opportunity offered, it fell to my good fortune to establish in this city the New York Polyclinic Medical School and Hospital."

The postgraduate school was thus originally an undergraduate repair shop. Its instruction was necessarily at once elementary and practical. There was no time to go back to fundamentals; it was too late to raise the question of preliminary educational competency. Urgency required that in the shortest possible time the young physician already involved in responsibility should acquire the practical technique which the medical school had failed to impart. The courses were made short, frequently covering less than a month; and they aimed preëminently to teach the young doctor what to "do" in the various emergencies of general practice.

As the general level of medical education has risen, the function of these institutions has been somewhat modified. The general course, aiming to make good deficiencies at large, has tended to give way to special courses adapted to the needs of those inclined to devote themselves more or less exclusively to some particular line of work. Simultaneously, as the facilities of the schools have enlarged, they have become centers to which at intervals men practising in isolated places may return for

[1] *Proceedings of the Nineteenth Annual Meeting of the Association of American Medical Colleges,* pp. 25, 26 (abridged).

brief periods in order to catch up with the times. Once more the training offered is of a practical, not of a fundamental or intensive, kind. It is calculated to "teach the trick"—or, perhaps better, to exhibit an instructor in the act of doing it. For, as nothing is known of individuals in the stream of students who course through the schools, it is impossible to give them an active share in the work that goes on at the bedside or in the operating-room. Their part is mainly passive; they look on at expert diagnosticians or operators. The danger of permitting an unknown student, tarrying for a brief stay, to participate at close range is prohibitive. In surgery the so-called practical courses are not usually worked out in such fashion that cadaver work, animal work, and service as dresser might prepare for actual participation : the school lacks means and facilities ; the students lack the time. In medicine the absence of sufficient material, the lack of proper hospital organization and equipment, the scrappiness of professional service, combine to prevent a systematic, thorough, and intimate discipline.

Of the thirteen postgraduate schools,[1] the best of them reflect the conditions and purposes above described. The Postgraduate and Polyclinic of New York and the Polyclinic of Philadelphia command large dispensary services and considerable hospital clinics, partly in their own hospitals, partly in public and private hospitals in the city. No unkind criticism is intended when the teaching is characterized as too immediately practical to be scientifically stimulating: it has the air of handicraft, rather than science. Comparatively little is done in internal medicine: surgery and the specialties predominate. The courses, being practical and definite, are disconnected ; the faculties are huge and unorganized. In the main, demonstrative instruction is offered to small bodies of physicians, who come and go uninterruptedly through the year. Only one of the three — the Philadelphia school — has a laboratory building, and in that no advanced work is in progress; the two New York schools have laboratory space or equipment adequate only to routine clinical examinations. The teaching is in the main more elementary than the upper class instruction of a good undergraduate school of medicine. It is, of course, also at times more special in character. With the exception of the New York Postgraduate, these schools are without endowment: they live on fees, donations, and hospital receipts.

Two departmental postgraduate schools are conducted by the government at Washington for those accepted for service in the army or navy medical corps. Eligible for these appointments are graduated physicians who have had a year of hospital experience or three years of practice. Excellent practical instruction is furnished by way of supplementing the usual undergraduate course. The needs of the services can

[1] Four are situated in Greater New York : (1) The New York Polyclinic Medical School, (2) New York Postgraduate Medical School, (3) Brooklyn Postgraduate Medical School, (4) Manhattan Eye, Ear, and Throat Postgraduate School ; four in Chicago : (5) Postgraduate Medical School, (6) The Chicago Polyclinic, (7) Illinois Postgraduate Medical School, (8) Chicago Ear, Eye, Nose, and Throat College ; one each in Philadelphia, (9) The Philadelphia Polyclinic ; Kansas City, (10) Postgraduate Medical School ; New Orleans, (11) New Orleans Polyclinic (affiliated with Tulane University) ; and two in Washington, (12) Army Medical School, (13) Navy Medical School. A number of schools offer special courses to graduates, in special summer and regular winter sessions.

be very definitely formulated; the course worked out aims to meet them. The accepted surgeons get in this way a concentrated practical drill in bacteriology, hygiene, and military surgery. The laboratories are excellently equipped, though cramped for space. The army school enjoys the advantage of contact with the great library and museum of the surgeon-general's office. The schools, as yet in their infancy, may not improbably develop into research laboratories dealing with the specific problems that crop up in naval and military service in various quarters of the globe.

Postgraduate, like other schools, vary in character. We have spoken of the best. The others are weak concerns wearing a commercial hue. The Brooklyn Postgraduate School, for instance, entertains less than half a dozen students on the average at a time, in a wretched hospital, really a death-trap, heavily laden with debt, and without laboratory equipment enough to make an ordinary clinical examination; the Kansas City affair had, when visited, no students in its improvised hospital containing 25 ward beds, only 13 of them occupied; it ekes out its opportunities with clinics at the public hospital. Chicago, varied and picturesque in this as in all else pertaining to medical education, supports four postgraduate institutions. None of them has a satisfactory plant. All are stock companies. Only unmistakable scientific activity could dislodge the unpleasant suspicion of commercial motive thus suggested. No such activity is in any of them observable. A cynical candor admits in one place that "it pays the teachers through referred cases;" in another, "it establishes the reputation of a man to teach in a postgraduate school;" in a third, "it pays through advertising teachers." In one a youth was observed working with a microscope. Inquiry elicited the fact that he was the teacher of clinical laboratory technique, lecturing in the absence of the "professor." The following dialogue took place:

"Are you a doctor?"

"No."

"A student of medicine?"

"Yes."

"Where?"

"At the Jenner Night School."

"In what year?"

"The first."

A first-year student of medicine in a night school was thus laboratory instructor and *pro tempore* lecturing professor in clinical microscopy in the Chicago Polyclinic.

Improved medical education will undoubtedly cut the ground from under the independent postgraduate school as we know it. This is not to say that the undergraduate medical curriculum will exhaust the field. On the contrary, the undergraduate school will do only the elementary work; but that it will do, not needing subsequent and more elementary instruction to patch it up. Graduate instruction will be advanced and intensive, — the natural prolongation of the elective courses now coming into vogue. For productive investigation and intensive instruction, the medical school will use its own teaching hospital and laboratories; for the elaboration of really thorough training in specialties resting on a solid undergraduate education, it may use the great municipal hospitals of the larger cities. But advanced instruction along these lines will not thrive in isolation. It will be but the upper story of a university department of medicine. The postgraduate schools of the better type can hasten this evolution by incorporating themselves in accessible universities, taking up university ideals, and submitting to reorganization on university lines.

CHAPTER XIII

THE MEDICAL EDUCATION OF WOMEN

MEDICAL education is now, in the United States and Canada, open to women upon practically the same terms as men. If all institutions do not receive women, so many do, that no woman desiring an education in medicine is under any disability in finding a school to which she may gain admittance. Her choice is free and varied. She will find schools of every grade accessible: the Johns Hopkins, if she has an academic degree; Cornell, if she has three-fourths of one; Rush and the state universities, if she prefers the combined six years' course; Toronto on the basis of a high school education; Meridian, Mississippi, if she has had no definable education at all.

Woman has so apparent a function in certain medical specialties and seemingly so assured a place in general medicine under some obvious limitations that the struggle for wider educational opportunities for the sex was predestined to an early success in medicine. It is singular to observe the use to which the victory has been put. The following tables show recent developments in coeducational and in women's medical schools taken separately:

Year	Number of Coeducational Medical Schools	Number of Women Students	Number of Women Graduates
1904	97	946	198
1905	96	852	165
1906	90	706	200
1907	86	718	172
1908	88	649	139
1909	91	752	129

Year	Women's Medical Schools	Number of Students	Number of Graduates
1904	3	183	56
1905	3	221	54
1906	3	189	33
1907	3	210	39
1908	3	186	46
1909	3	169	33

COMBINED

Year	Number of Schools	Number of Women Students	Number of Women Graduates
1904	100	1129	254
1905	99	1073	219
1906	93	895	233
1907	89	928	211
1908	91	835	185
1909	94	921	162

Now that women are freely admitted to the medical profession, it is clear that they show a decreasing inclination to enter it. More schools in all sections are open to them; fewer attend and fewer graduate. True enough, medical schools generally have shrunk; but as the opportunities of women have increased, not decreased, and within a period during which entrance requirements have, so far as they are concerned, not materially altered, their enrolment should have augmented, if there is any strong demand for women physicians or any strong ungratified desire on the part of women to enter the profession. One or the other of these conditions is lacking,— perhaps both.

Whether it is either wise or necessary to endow separate medical schools for women is a problem on which the figures used throw light. In the first place, eighty per cent of women who have in the last six years studied medicine have attended coeducational institutions. None of the three women's medical colleges now existing can be sufficiently strengthened without an enormous outlay. The motives which elsewhere recommend separation of the sexes would appear to be without force, all possible allowance being made for the special and somewhat trying conditions involved. In the general need of more liberal support for medical schools, it would appear that large sums, as far as specially available for the medical education of women, would accomplish most if used to develop coeducational institutions, in which their benefits would be shared by men without loss to women students; but, it must be added, if separate medical schools and hospitals are not to be developed for women, interne privileges must be granted to women graduates on the same terms as to men.

CHAPTER XIV

THE MEDICAL EDUCATION OF THE NEGRO

The medical care of the negro race will never be wholly left to negro physicians. Nevertheless, if the negro can be brought to feel a sharp responsibility for the physical integrity of his people, the outlook for their mental and moral improvement will be distinctly brightened. The practice of the negro doctor will be limited to his own race, which in its turn will be cared for better by good negro physicians than by poor white ones. But the physical well-being of the negro is not only of moment to the negro himself. Ten million of them live in close contact with sixty million whites. Not only does the negro himself suffer from hookworm and tuberculosis; he communicates them to his white neighbors, precisely as the ignorant and unfortunate white contaminates him. Self-protection not less than humanity offers weighty counsel in this matter; self-interest seconds philanthropy. The negro must be educated not only for his sake, but for ours. He is, as far as human eye can see, a permanent factor in the nation. He has his rights and due and value as an individual; but he has, besides, the tremendous importance that belongs to a potential source of infection and contagion.

The pioneer work in educating the race to know and to practise fundamental hygienic principles must be done largely by the negro doctor and the negro nurse. It is important that they both be sensibly and effectively trained at the level at which their services are now important. The negro is perhaps more easily " taken in " than the white; and as his means of extricating himself from a blunder are limited, it is all the more cruel to abuse his ignorance through any sort of pretense. A well-taught negro sanitarian will be immensely useful; an essentially untrained negro wearing an M.D. degree is dangerous.

Make-believe in the matter of negro medical schools is therefore intolerable. Even good intention helps but little to change their aspect. The negro needs good schools rather than many schools,— schools to which the more promising of the race can be sent to receive a substantial education in which hygiene rather than surgery, for example, is strongly accentuated. If at the same time these men can be imbued with the missionary spirit so that they will look upon the diploma as a commission to serve their people humbly and devotedly, they may play an important part in the sanitation and civilization of the whole nation. Their duty calls them away from large cities to the village and the plantation, upon which light has hardly as yet begun to break.

Of the seven medical schools for negroes in the United States,[1] five are at this moment in no position to make any contribution of value to the solution of the problem

[1] Washington, D.C.: Howard University; New Orleans: Flint Medical College; Raleigh (N.C.): Leonard Medical School; Knoxville: Knoxville Medical College; Memphis: Medical Department of the University of West Tennessee; Nashville: Meharry Medical College; Louisville: National Medical College.

above pointed out; Flint at New Orleans, Leonard at Raleigh, the Knoxville, Memphis, and Louisville schools are ineffectual. They are wasting small sums annually and sending out undisciplined men, whose lack of real training is covered up by the imposing M.D. degree.

Meharry at Nashville and Howard at Washington are worth developing, and until considerably increased benefactions are available, effort will wisely concentrate upon them. The future of Howard is assured; indeed, the new Freedman's Hospital is an asset the like of which is in this country extremely rare. It is greatly to be hoped that the government may display a liberal and progressive spirit in adapting the administration of this institution to the requirements of medical education.

Meharry is the creation of one man, Dr. George W. Hubbard, who, sent to the south at the close of the war on an errand of mercy, has for a half-century devoted himself singly to the elevation of the negro. The slender resources at his command have been carefully husbanded; his pupils have in their turn remembered their obligations to him and to their school. The income of the institution has been utilized to build it up. The school laboratories are highly creditable to the energy and intelligence of Dr. Hubbard and his assistants. The urgent need is for improved clinical facilities — a hospital building and a well equipped dispensary. Efforts now making to acquire them deserve liberal support.

The upbuilding of Howard and Meharry will profit the nation much more than the inadequate maintenance of a larger number of schools. They are, of course, unequal to the need and the opportunity; but nothing will be gained by way of satisfying the need or of rising to the opportunity through the survival of feeble, ill equipped institutions, quite regardless of the spirit which animates the promoters. The subventions of religious and philanthropic societies and of individuals can be made effective only if concentrated. They must become immensely greater before they can be safely dispersed.

PART II

MEDICAL SCHOOLS OF THE UNITED STATES
AND CANADA

ARRANGED ALPHABETICALLY BY STATES AND PROVINCES
AND SEPARATELY CHARACTERIZED

NOTE: *Facts given are as of date when the school was visited, which is specified in each case.*

The estimates of population have, with the few exceptions noted, been kindly made by the Director of the Census, through the courtesy of the Secretary of Commerce and Labor.

MEDICAL SCHOOLS
OF THE UNITED STATES AND CANADA
ALPHABETICALLY ARRANGED BY STATES AND PROVINCES

ALABAMA

Population, 2,112,465. Number of physicians, 2287. Ratio, 1: 924.
Number of medical schools, 2.

BIRMINGHAM: *Population,* 55,945.

BIRMINGHAM MEDICAL COLLEGE. Organized 1894. A stock company, paying annual dividends of 6 per cent.

Entrance requirement: Nominal.

Attendance: 185, of whom 168 are from Alabama.

Teaching staff: 32, 18 being professors, none of them whole-time teachers.

Resources available for maintenance: Fees, amounting to $14,550 (estimated).

Laboratory facilities: The teaching of anatomy, for which there is abundant material, is limited to dissecting on old-fashioned lines; there is the usual chemical laboratory and a small outfit for instruction in bacteriology and pathology; the material used for the latter is purchased in the east, not obtained from autopsies or clinics. No animals are provided for experimental purpose beyond the use of dogs for surgical work. There are no physiological, pharmacological, or clinical laboratories. The building is poorly kept, and there is neither library nor museum.

Clinical facilities: The school adjoins the Hillman Hospital, 98 beds, of which the faculty has charge during term time. Bedside clinics are held, but the students make no blood or urine examinations; obstetrical cases are rare; the hospital is largely given over to surgical patients,—gunshot and other wounds being decidedly abundant.

The dispensary service is as yet unorganized.

Date of visit: January, 1909.

MOBILE: *Population,* 56,385.

MEDICAL DEPARTMENT OF THE UNIVERSITY OF ALABAMA. Established 1859. Now an organic department of the state university, with which, however, its connection is legal only. The two institutions are at opposite ends of the state, so that the medical department is practically a local school.

Entrance requirement: Less than three-year high school education.

Attendance: 204.

Teaching staff: 25, of whom 8 are professors. No one devotes full time to medical instruction.

Resources available for maintenance: The school receives from the state an annual appropriation of $5000, in return for which, however, sixty-seven free scholarships are given, one to each county; the school is therefore in effect wholly dependent on tuition fees, amounting to $17,300, for its support, most of which is paid out in salaries.

Laboratory facilities: The laboratory equipment is practically limited to inorganic chemistry, elementary bacteriology and pathology, and anatomy, taught by dissecting first the goat, then the human cadaver. The school occupies a well kept old-fashioned building, recently remodeled. It possesses a few old books, but no funds with which to add to them; and a small museum, mostly composed of antiquated wax or papier-maché models.

Clinical facilities: For clinical instruction the school has access to the Sisters' Hospital, 100 beds, the faculty being the staff in term time. The senior students make blood and urine examinations in connection with clinical cases.

Connected with the college building is a new, well arranged dispensary, for the conduct of which an appropriation of $50 a month is available.

Date of visit: January, 1909.

General Considerations

THE foregoing account makes it clear that really satisfactory medical education is not now to be had in Alabama. The entrance standards are low; the schools are inadequately equipped; and they are without proper financial resources. To get together their present numbers, standards must be kept low; in consequence, the medical schools do nothing to promote or to share the secondary school development of the state. To that and to any higher movement they are likely to be obstacles. Neither Alabama nor the rest of the south actually needs either school at this time; but as the state has become a patron of medical education, it will hardly retire from the field. Under these circumstances, its policy should aim to bring about a genuine and effective connection between the medical department and the rest of the state university. The task of elevating entrance standards in the medical department and of furnishing a higher quality of scientific training would probably be assisted for the time being by removing the instruction in the first and second years to the university itself at Tuscaloosa; for in no other way can whole-time instructors be now procured. An improvement in the quality of training furnished in the scientific branches will ultimately compel a higher quality of clinical instruction. It is difficult to see how the influence or control of the university can in any event be made effective in Mobile, 232 miles distant, at the opposite end of the state, and in a hospital in whose clinical management there is no continuity. Birmingham is much closer, being only 56 miles distant, and promises to offer a larger supply of clinical material. If, therefore, the state is able to look at the question on its own merits, without regard to the rival claims of competing towns, it should establish a practice requirement that would automatically suppress proprietary instruction. For the present, the university might offer two years' work at Tuscaloosa, reserving to a more propitious time the entire question of organizing under effective university control a complete medical school at Birmingham, which is the nearest feasible location. As the state now contains one physician to every 924 inhabitants, the restriction or suspension of clinical teaching for some years to come involves no danger to the community.

ARKANSAS

Population, 1,476,582. Number of physicians, 2535. Ratio, 1 : 582.
Number of medical schools, 2.

LITTLE ROCK: *Population, 44,931.*

(1) MEDICAL DEPARTMENT, UNIVERSITY OF ARKANSAS. Organized 1879. An independent institution, not even "affiliated" with the state university whose name it bears.

Entrance requirement: Nominal.

Attendance: 179, 81 per cent from Arkansas.

Teaching staff: 35, 18 being professors.

Resources available for maintenance: Fees, amounting to $14,100 (estimated).

Laboratory facilities: After an existence of thirty years without any laboratory facilities except a dissecting-room and a laboratory for inorganic chemistry, a frame building has recently been supplied with a meager equipment for the teaching of pathology and bacteriology. The session was, however, already well started and the new laboratory not yet in operation. No museum, no books, charts, models, etc., are provided.

Clinical facilities: Hardly more than nominal. The school adjoins the City Hospital, with a capacity of 30 beds. From this hospital patients are brought into the amphitheater of the school building. There are no ward visits. The students see no contagious diseases; obstetrical work is precarious; of post-mortems there is no mention.
    There is a small dispensary, of whose attendance no record is procurable.

Date of visit: November, 1909.

(2) COLLEGE OF PHYSICIANS AND SURGEONS. Organized 1906. An independent organization, formed by men not in the older school.

Entrance requirement: Nominal.

Attendance: 81, 59 per cent from Arkansas.

Teaching staff: 34, 25 being professors.

Resources available for maintenance: Fees, amounting to $6450 (estimated).

Laboratory facilities: Separate, recently organized, and very disorderly laboratories for pathology, bacteriology, and chemistry, which with pharmacy work are all in charge of a single teacher, who is also pathologist to the County Hospital, three miles off. He proposes shortly to add physiology. The usual wretched dissecting-room is also provided. None of the necessary illustrative paraphernalia are at hand in the shape of books, charts, museum, etc.

Clinical facilities: The faculty of the school controls an adjoining hospital, from which patients are brought into the amphitheater for demonstration or operation. At operations it is claimed that students assist. No ward rounds are made. Occasional clinics are also held at two distant hospitals (county and penitentiary). Obstetrical and acute medical cases are rare; contagious diseases are not seen. There are no post-mortems. A small daily dispensary attendance is claimed. There is no adequate dispensary equipment.

Date of visit: November, 1909.

General Considerations

BOTH the Arkansas schools are local institutions in a state that has at this date three times as many doctors as it needs; neither has a single redeeming feature. It is incredible that the state university should permit its name to shelter one of them. The general educational interests of the state require that the state university, now inconveniently located at Fayetteville, should be moved to Little Rock. Once there, it could probably get possession of both schools and organize something better than either, which it could improve as its resources increase with the general prosperity of the state.

CALIFORNIA[1]

Population, 1,729,543. Number of physicians (exclusive of osteopaths), 4313. Ratio, 1 : 401.

Number of medical schools, 10.

LOS ANGELES: *Population,* 116,420.

(1) COLLEGE OF PHYSICIANS AND SURGEONS. Established 1903 as an independent

---

[1] The Director of the Census states: "The cities of Los Angeles, Oakland, Berkeley, and San Francisco have had such an exceptionally rapid increase that no estimates of their population have been prepared." The figures given are taken from the census of 1900.

school, it suddenly became, in 1909, nominally the medical department of the University of Southern California, when the former medical department of that institution cut loose in order to become the Los Angeles clinical department of the University of California. The seriousness with which the University of Southern California treats medical education may be gathered from this amusing performance.

Entrance requirement: High school graduation or "equivalent."

Attendance: 32.

Teaching staff: 41, 28 being professors. The teachers are practising physicians; no one gives his entire time to the school.

Resources available for maintenance: Fees, amounting to $4075 (estimated).

Laboratory facilities: The school is ordinary in type. It possesses a small chemical laboratory, a single laboratory in common for pathology, histology, and bacteriology, with meager equipment and supplies, and no animals; a dissecting-room with sufficient anatomical material, and clay for modeling bones; a limited number of wet specimens, and a small number of books in a room that is locked, though opened to students on request. There is no laboratory for physiology or pharmacology. The building is new, attractive, and fairly well kept.

Clinical facilities: A considerable part of one floor is used for a dispensary. The rooms are poorly equipped and cared for; there is no clinical laboratory. The attendance is very small, for the neighborhood is decidedly well-to-do.

The school adjoins a private hospital in which many of the teachers are interested. It is, however, of no teaching use. The catalogue describes it as "not a charity hospital by any means. . . . In fact it is a twentieth century classy hospital." For clinical instruction the students have access to the County Hospital, several miles distant, where the school has the use of 100 beds, holding clinics for senior students two days weekly. In surgery, students witness an operation without taking part in it; in medicine, the students make brief histories, which are, however, no part of the hospital records. Autopsies are done by the internes, who have no connection with the medical school. Students are not admitted to the obstetrical ward. Clinical facilities are thus extremely limited, for the management of the hospital is in no essential respect controlled by educational considerations.

Date of visit: May, 1909.

(2) UNIVERSITY OF CALIFORNIA : CLINICAL DEPARTMENT. Up to March, 1909, this school offered a four-year course as the medical department of the University of Southern California; it has now become a second clinical department of the University of California, and will therefore offer after June, 1910, only the third and fourth years' work. *See* (6).

Clinical facilities: Its present facilities for offering the instruction of the last two years are, for a university department on a two-year college basis, distinctly meager. It enjoys at the County Hospital the same facilities as the local College of Physicians and Surgeons, *i.e.*, access to 100 beds, two or three days weekly being devoted to clinics for the senior class. Additional opportunities, depending on the personal connections of members of the faculty, are usually of slight pedagogic value. The school has an excellent dispensary building, fairly equipped in certain respects, but indifferently conducted, though the attendance is good. It is also in close proximity to a good medical library. The clinical teachers are all local practitioners. The state university will incur no expense on account of this department for two years at least.

Date of visit: May, 1909.

(3) CALIFORNIA MEDICAL COLLEGE. Eclectic. Organized at Oakland in 1879, this school has led a roving and precarious existence in the meanwhile.

Entrance requirement: Nominal.

Attendance: 9, of whom 7 are from California.

Teaching staff: 27, of whom 26 are professors.

Resources available for maintenance: Fees, amounting to $1060 (estimated).

Laboratory facilities: The school occupies a few neglected rooms on the second floor of a fifty-foot frame building. Its so-called equipment is dirty and disorderly beyond description. Its outfit in anatomy consists of a small box of bones and the dried-up filthy fragments of a single cadaver. A few bottles of reagents constitute the chemical laboratory. A cold and rusty incubator, a single microscope, and a few unlabeled wet specimens, etc., form the so-called "equipment" for pathology and bacteriology.

Clinical facilities: There is no dispensary and no access to the County Hospital.

The school is a disgrace to the state whose laws permit its existence.

Date of visit: May, 1909.

(4) LOS ANGELES COLLEGE OF OSTEOPATHY. Emigrated from Iowa in 1905. A stock company.

Entrance requirement: Less than an ordinary grammar school education, with conditions. Many of the students are men and women of advanced years.

Attendance: Began two years ago with 60, now claims "more than 250."

Teaching staff: 19. All the teachers are practitioners.

Resources available for maintenance: Fees, the annual income being about $37,500 from tuitions and a considerable sum from "treatments" (*see below*). As the instruction provided is inexpensive, the stock must be a very profitable investment.

Laboratory facilities: The school occupies a five-story building containing a chemical laboratory, with meager equipment and limited desk space, and a single laboratory for histology, pathology, and bacteriology. The dissecting-room contains five tables, but sufficient material. The rest of the building is mainly devoted to treatment rooms and the business office.

Clinical facilities: There is no free dispensary. Patients who are willing to undergo treatment before a class pay not less than $3 a month; patients who are treated in the presence of a single student pay $5. A hospital is now under construction.

The general aspect is that of a thriving business. An abundance of advertising matter, in which the profits of osteopathy are prominently set forth,[1] is distributed.

Date of visit: May, 1909.

(5) PACIFIC COLLEGE OF OSTEOPATHY. A stock company, established in 1896.

Entrance requirement: Ostensibly high school graduation; but "mature men and women who have been in business are given a chance and usually make good."

Attendance: 85.

Teaching staff: 38, 19 being professors.

Resources available for maintenance: Fees, amounting to $12,750 (estimated).

Laboratory facilities: The school has an ordinary chemical laboratory, a fairly equipped laboratory for pathology, histology, and bacteriology, with a private laboratory for the instructor in these branches adjoining, the usual dissecting-room, and a limited amount of apparatus for experimental work in physiology.

Clinical facilities: A dispensary is carried on at the school, which also owns a hospital for obstetrical and surgical cases. The catalogue fails, however, to state that the students have no regular work in this hospital. They rarely see medical cases; "they don't have as much acute work as they should." Nevertheless, they are drilled to "treat gonorrhea by diet and antiseptics; syphilis with ointments and dietetics, and without mercury; typhoid, pneumonia, etc.," along the same lines.

Date of visit: May, 1909.

OAKLAND: *Population, 73,812.*

(6) COLLEGE OF MEDICINE AND SURGERY. Established 1902 as a stock company, stock partly subscribed by merchants of the town.

---

[1] "People are ready to pay for relief from distress and sickness. It is only fair to say that many of our graduates are earning as much in single months as they were formerly able to earn by a full year's work." (*Catalogue*, p. 9.)

Entrance requirement: "High school or equivalent."

Attendance: 17.

Teaching staff: 32, 13 being professors. There are no full-time teachers.

Resources available for maintenance: The school lives on fees, amounting to $2760 (estimated), and on contributions from the faculty.

Laboratory facilities: It occupies a new, well kept building, has a small laboratory for experimental physiology, small separate laboratories for bacteriology, histology, and pathology, a beautiful, though not extensive, collection of pathological specimens, a laboratory for chemistry, a dissecting-room with provision for modeling, and a small library of slight value. Though there are no full-time teachers, there is evidence of active interest in pathology. Post-mortems are abundant and are intelligently used, through a fortunate connection of the instructor in pathology.

Clinical facilities: In respect to both dispensary and hospital, the clinical facilities are decidedly inadequate.

Date of visit: May, 1909.

SAN FRANCISCO: *Population, 355,919.*

(7) UNIVERSITY OF CALIFORNIA MEDICAL DEPARTMENT. Established as such 1872. An organic department of the university. The first and second years' work is given at Berkeley. *See* (2).

Entrance requirement: Two years of college work, strictly enforced.

Attendance: 36, all but 2 from California.

Teaching staff: 60, of whom 12 are professors. The laboratory courses at Berkeley are given by full-time teachers.

Resources available for maintenance: The department shares the university funds, its budget calling for $33,396. The total receipts from fees are $7004.

Laboratory facilities: The equipment and instruction are of the highest quality. The laboratories, though temporary in structure, are completely fitted up, in charge of high-grade teachers, abundantly provided with assistants and helpers. The sole question to be raised concerns the medical atmosphere, which, in several departments, is not strongly in evidence. In consequence, post-mortem work has not been hitherto cultivated, though abundant opportunities for it exist. The biological point of view prevails. This is not the case with anatomy, the teaching of which—thoroughly scientific in method and spirit—frankly meets the main purpose of the students.

Clinical facilities: Clinical instruction is given in San Francisco. The university hospital, its main reliance, is small but modern. It contains 75 beds, practically all available for instruction.[1] Bedside teaching is carried on; but post-mortem work for the benefit of the students is meager. Some additional clinical work is procured at hospitals maintained by the city and by the United States government. In general, the laboratory and clinical departments are not as yet effectively correlated. The teachers of the third and fourth years are, excepting the dean, practitioners who are not in touch with the laboratory work and ideals as realized at Berkeley. Efforts are, however, making to bridge the gap.

The hospital is unfortunately situated from the standpoint of a dispensary; such material as there is, is not well used from a teaching point of view. The students do not in all departments take an active part in the dispensary work. For example, in some of them they have nothing to do with making up the records, which are separately kept in the several departments. No report, showing the number of the distribution of cases, is obtainable.

Date of visit: May, 1909.

(8) LELAND STANFORD JUNIOR UNIVERSITY SCHOOL OF MEDICINE, ON THE COOPER MEDICAL COLLEGE FOUNDATION. Until 1908, the Cooper Medical College offered a four-year course based on high school graduation. Its property has now been deeded to Stanford University, its buildings being the seat of the clinical department of Stanford University School of Medicine, the instruction of the last five semesters being given in Cooper Hall and Lane Hospital. That of the first three semesters is given at Palo Alto. As its present classes graduate, the Cooper Medical College passes out of existence and its faculty disbands.

Entrance requirement: Three years of college work.

Attendance: 16 in first year (fourth collegiate year). No other year's work has yet been given.

Teaching staff: 21, of whom 16 are professors. Six professors and one assistant professor give their entire time to medical work. The clinical professors thus far chosen have been taken from the former faculty of the Cooper Medical College.

Resources available for maintenance: The department will share in the general income of the university. A special library endowment amounts to about $250,000.

Laboratory facilities: These are provided at Palo Alto on the same scale as other departments there (anatomy, pharmacology, bacteriology, physiology, physiological chemistry). The school has an unusually valuable library of some 85,000 volumes and receives the main current medical periodicals, American and foreign.

Clinical facilities: Clinical work on the part of Stanford University is not yet begun. The university now owns the Lane Hospital of 125 beds, which has hitherto been conducted as a pay institution. Patients paying $10 a week are used for clinical

[1] During four months of 1909, there was a daily average of 44 free patients.

teaching; seventy-odd beds are thus available, part of these being temporarily supported by the city.[1] The hospital is now under temporary control of Cooper Medical College until needed by the university. Its organization at present, from the teaching point of view, is seriously defective. Records are meager; no surgical rounds are made in the wards; obstetrical work exists only in the form of an out-patient department; post-mortems are scarce. No hospital report is obtainable. The catalogue statement that the hospital is a teaching hospital is hardly sustained by the facts.

The dispensary in the college building adjoining had in 1907 an attendance of 20,000, including both old and new cases. But the material, though adequate in amount, was not thoroughly used by the Cooper Medical College.

Date of visit: May, 1909.

(9) COLLEGE OF PHYSICIANS AND SURGEONS. Established 1896. An independent school.

Entrance requirement: "High school education or equivalent."

Attendance: 70.

Teaching staff: 53, 23 being professors. There are no full-time teachers.

Resources available for maintenance: The institution has no resources but fees, amounting to $7715 (estimated).

Laboratory facilities: The school has no laboratories worthy the name.

Clinical facilities: There are no adequate clinical or dispensary facilities.

Date of visit: May, 1909.

(10) HAHNEMANN MEDICAL COLLEGE OF THE PACIFIC. Established 1881. Homeopathic. · An independent school.

Entrance requirement: "High school graduation or equivalent."

Attendance: 23.

Teaching staff: 35, 13 being professors, none of them full-time teachers.

Resources available for maintenance: The institution has practically no resources but fees, amounting to $2685 (estimated).

Laboratory facilities: The school occupies a small, well kept building containing the usual dissecting-room, a laboratory for elementary chemistry, one fairly equipped laboratory in common for histology, bacteriology, and pathology, and a small orderly library.

Clinical facilities: Several neatly kept but inadequately equipped rooms are set aside for a dispensary; the attendance is fair, the records meager. The main clinical reli-

---

[1] During four months of 1909, there was a daily average of 60.

ance now is on a small number of beds paid for by the city in the Hahnemann Hospital, a modern institution close by.[1]

Date of visit: May, 1909.

General Considerations

CONSIDERATION of medical education in California may well start from the fact that, without taking into account the osteopaths—who abound—the state has now one physician to every 401 inhabitants, that is, in round numbers, about four times as many doctors as it needs or can properly support. Such an enormous disproportion can hardly be rectified within less than a generation; it makes radical measures in the interest of sound medical education not only immediately feasible, but urgently necessary.

Legal enactment fixing a sound basis for future practitioners, of whatever school, the grant of authority to the state board to close schools flagrantly defective in either laboratory or clinical facilities, or the institution of practical examinations for license,—any one of these measures would at once wipe out at least seven of the ten existing schools, with distinct advantage to the public health of the state. As none of these schools has the resources indispensable to meet the rising tide in medical education, this outcome is in any case inevitable; legal regulation of the type indicated would merely hasten the day.

Even then the situation of medical education in the state is not altogether clear. The University of California has not yet solved its problem. The sums it now devotes to medical education are relatively small; its clinical facilities in San Francisco are inadequate; it has not effectively organized what it there offers; it has not brought about team work between the two severed branches that constitute the department. If now it has proved difficult to perfect an organization covering two places separated by San Francisco Bay, what reason is there to be confident when the distance involved is five hundred miles? Nor does any practical need compel a step educationally questionable. The attendance in Los Angeles in the last two years on a high school or equivalent basis is less than thirty; it will fall still lower when the two-year college basis is enforced and transplantation from Berkeley to Los Angeles is required at the beginning of the third year. Moreover, the clinical prospects are by no means up to university standard. The dispensary may indeed be adequately developed, but one hundred beds in the general medical and surgical wards of an old-fashioned public hospital, however supplemented by courtesies elsewhere, constitute a fragile support for a university department of medicine. The difficulty of controlling the teaching at Los Angeles by the scientific ideals of the university at Berkeley can hardly be overstated. Finally, with the present needs of the clinical department at San Francisco, it is not likely that the university can divert to Los Angeles the sums necessary to create a satisfactory department there. The move is explained on the

[1] During four months of 1909 there was a daily average of 55 city patients.

ground that peculiar conditions exist in the state; it is, however, not clear why a long narrow state is educationally in any different plight from a short broad one; in either case, needless multiplication of medical schools is economically wasteful and professionally demoralizing.

The university has undertaken to dominate two detached clinical departments, manned by local practitioners. There is nothing in the present status of detached clinical departments of this type to encourage confidence in the outcome. Before too far committing itself to this policy, it is at least worth inquiring into the advisability of concentrating its medical instruction across the bay, where a population of over two hundred thousand affords sufficient clinical material, and where a compact, effective, and organically whole university department of medicine, with a faculty, laboratory and clinical, selected on educational principles, could be readily developed.

These considerations apply in some respects with equal force to the action of Stanford University in taking over the Cooper Medical College at San Francisco. It was well enough to offer the laboratory sciences at Palo Alto, where the resources and ideals of the university insure high-grade instruction; but the entrance of the university into the San Francisco field in all probability portends the division and restriction of whatever opportunities the city may hereafter create. Lane Hospital can be developed into a teaching hospital of adequate size only if very large sums are available for the purpose; its organization and conduct have been in the past pedagogically very defective; and the clinical professors so far appointed have been taken with one exception from the former Cooper faculty. With one university medical school already on the ground, a second—and a divided school at that—is therefore a decidedly questionable undertaking. There is no need of it from the standpoint of the public; it must, if adequately developed, become a serious burden upon the finances of Stanford University. If the experience of other schools and cities is to be heeded, the question arises whether Stanford would not do well to content itself with the work of the first two years at Palo Alto, and to coöperate with the state university in all that pertains to the clinical end.

The situation just presented deserves to be studied carefully by all interested in medical education. What has happened in California is likely to happen elsewhere. Scores of schools are beginning a desperate struggle for existence. Their first impulse is to throw themselves into the lap of some prosperous university. The universities, not as yet themselves realizing that medical education is no longer either profitable or self-supporting, are prone to complete themselves by accepting a medical department as an apparent gift. From the standpoint of the university this blunder will soon prove a serious drain, as increased expenditure on instruction and reduced income from fees reveal the actual state of affairs. From the standpoint of medical education and practice, the tendency in question is still more deplorable. The curse of medical education is the excessive number of schools. The situation can improve only as weaker and superfluous schools are extinguished.

COLORADO

Population, 658,506. Number of physicians, 1690. Ratio, 1: 328.
Number of medical schools, 2.

DENVER: *Population, 158,329.*

(1) DENVER AND GROSS COLLEGE OF MEDICINE. Organized by consolidation 1902. Nominally the medical department of the University of Denver, with which institution it has, however, only a six months' contract; to all intents and purposes, a proprietary school, managed by its own faculty.

Entrance requirement: Less than high school graduation, loosely enforced.

Attendance: 109, over one-half from Colorado.

Teaching staff: 44 professors and 35 of other grade, none of them giving their whole time to teaching.

Resources available for maintenance: The school has no resources but fees, amounting to $12,624 per annum (estimated).

Laboratory facilities: Its equipment consists of a chemical laboratory of the ordinary medical school type, a dissecting-room, containing a few subjects as dry as leather, a physiological laboratory with slight equipment, and the usual pathology and bacteriology laboratories. There is a total absence of scientific activity. The rooms are poorly kept. A few cases of books are found in the college office behind the counter.

Clinical facilities: The college owns a new and exceedingly attractive dispensary building. Separate rooms nicely equipped are occupied by the various specialties. The attendance averages 90 a day; the records are inadequate. There is an outpatient obstetrical service.

For hospital facilities the school depends largely on the County Hospital, the management of which is political. Clinics are held daily from 8.30 to 10, "purely through courtesy." Students from all schools merely "look on;" they are "not much at the bedside." Obstetrical work is limited, post-mortems rare. Hospital staff appointments are secured through "pull;" the college must take into the faculty the men who are already on the hospital staff. Supplementary opportunities are furnished by several local institutions. In several of these, however, the clinics are not regularly scheduled: "announcements appear upon the bulletin board of the college."

Date of visit: April, 1909.

BOULDER: *Population, 9,652.*

(2) UNIVERSITY OF COLORADO SCHOOL OF MEDICINE. Organized 1883. An integral part of the university.

Entrance requirement: A four-year high school education or its equivalent. Credentials are passed on by the dean.

Attendance: 85.

Teaching staff: 45, of whom 25 are professors, 20 of other grade.

Resources available for maintenance: The school is supported out of the total university income of $200,000 per annum. Its fee income is $4043; its budget, $28,000.

Laboratory facilities: The school is in general satisfactorily equipped to do undergraduate teaching in the medical sciences. Full-time men are in charge of pathology, bacteriology, and physiology, though the departments lack trained assistants. Histology and embryology are taught in the department of biology. The chair of anatomy is occupied by a non-resident surgeon. There is a good library, with a subscription list including the best German and English journals. A regular fund is available for the purchase of books and apparatus.

Clinical facilities: The university hospital is entirely inadequate, even though the school is small. It contains 35 beds and averages 16 patients available for teaching. Its management has only recently been modernized. It now contains a clinical laboratory where students work, keeping excellent records of their findings. There are from 12 to 15 obstetrical cases annually in the hospital; these are supplemented by an out-patient service.

The dispensary is slight.

Date of visit: April, 1909.

General Considerations

The state is overcrowded with doctors. It can therefore safely go to a higher standard; indeed, the new law provides that after 1912, all applicants for license must have had, previous to their medical education, a year of college work. As this is a practice, and not an educational, requirement, the Denver school may still continue to train low-grade men for adjacent states;[1] but it is probable that if it continues on a standard below the legal practice minimum, it will be too discredited, and if it arises to the aforesaid minimum, too much reduced, to continue. The state university alone, so far as we can now see, can hope to obtain the financial backing necessary to teach medicine in the proper way regardless of income from fees, and to it a monopoly should quickly fall. Its laboratory facilities are steadily increasing, but adequate clinical resources are not at present assured. It is important, therefore, that as a first step the state university gain access to the clinical facilities at Denver, from which it is now cut off, first, by a constitutional provision forbidding the state university to teach except at Boulder, second, by the fact that the City Hospital is

---

[1] It is, however, equally in the interest of these states that a further low-grade supply should be cut off. Though none of the following states has a medical school, all have too many doctors. The ratios are: Wyoming, 1: 541; Arizona, 1: 697; Idaho, 1: 663; New Mexico, 1: 618.

in the hands of the local school. These conditions, so common in American cities, are plainly against the general interest of the community. It may be that an arrangement can be made by which the Denver and Gross school will be handed over to the university, thus clearing the field of all obstacles to the upbuilding of a creditable school; for as Boulder is practically a suburb of Denver, the difficulties in the way of effective management at Denver are not insuperable. Whether the entire medical school shall be permanently concentrated at Denver or, following the Ann Arbor plan, a liberally supported hospital at Boulder be relied on to overcome the disadvantage of location in the matter of clinical material, need not be decided just now. The important steps to take at this moment comprise (1) passage of the constitutional amendment opening the clinical facilities of Denver to the state university, (2) more liberal state appropriations for the medical school, and (3) the consolidation of the Denver and Boulder schools as the medical department of the state university.[1]

CONNECTICUT

Population, 1,054,366. Number of physicians, 1424. Ratio, 1 : 740.
Number of medical schools, 1.

NEW HAVEN: *Population, 130,027.*

YALE MEDICAL SCHOOL. Organized 1813. An organic part of Yale University.

Entrance requirement: Two years of college work, enforced with such unusual conscientiousness that in passing from the high school to the college standard this year, deficient members of last year's class were refused re-admission. Moreover, the advanced requirement has been actually exacted; out of an entering class of 23, one only is conditioned, — in part of biology. This is probably the lowest percentage of "conditions" that the country affords.

Attendance: 138; 72 per cent from Connecticut.

Teaching staff: 64, 14 being professors. Of these, the teachers in the fundamental branches devote full time to instruction, though they are overworked and without a proper force of assistants; in the clinical branches, the professor of medicine with two assistants is salaried. Small sums are also paid to a few other teachers in the clinical years.

Resources available for maintenance: Fees amounting to $15,325, income from endowment amounting to $10,000, university appropriation of $17,986, making annual budget $43,311.

Laboratory facilities: Well equipped student laboratories for organic chemistry,

[1] As this Report goes to press, announcement is made that a consolidation of the Denver and Gross School with the medical department of the state university has been arranged.

physiology, and pharmacology; the provision for bacteriology, pathology, and anatomy is less satisfactory. In physiology alone is there internal evidence of progressive activity. The instructors in other branches are overworked, being called on to carry the routine work of extensive subjects in all their parts without adequate assistance. Under such circumstances, the work, however conscientious, is bound to be limited.

Clinical facilities: The New Haven Hospital, in which the school controls a small number of beds, is very intelligently employed. The obstetrical and gynecological wards, however, are not used for teaching; nor is there a contagious disease pavilion. Post-mortems are scarce. Clinical laboratories and teaching-rooms have been improvised close by the hospital; students are thereby enabled to do the clinical laboratory work in connection with assigned cases. Provision is also made there for the independent work of the professors of medicine and surgery.

The dispensary occupies a new and excellent building, but lacks systematic organization as a teaching adjunct. The attendance is adequate; but as the staff service is gratis, it varies greatly in quality in various departments.

Date of visit: January, 1910.

General Considerations

As the school now stands, it would, in point of facilities, still have to be classed with the better type of those on the high school basis; for, though it has advanced to a two-year college basis, there has been as yet no corresponding improvement of facilities. In order to deserve the higher grade student body which it invites, a more liberal policy ought to be pursued. The laboratory branches ought to be better manned, so that the instructors may create within them a more active spirit. A university department of medicine cannot largely confine itself to routine instruction,—certainly not after requiring two years of college work for admission to its opportunities. For the same reason the clinical facilities should be extended, probably through a more intimate connection with the present hospital. Its wards should be more generally used; more beds should be made accessible within them; and the missing pavilion for contagious diseases be provided. Enough money ought to be spent on the dispensary to ensure in every department systematic and thorough discipline, in examining patients, keeping records, etc.

To make these improvements, larger permanent endowment is required. As the school is one of a very few in New England so circumstanced as to have a clear duty and opportunity, it behooves the university to make a vigorous campaign in behalf of its medical department.

[For general discussion see " New England," p. 261.]

DISTRICT OF COLUMBIA

Population, 322,212. Number of physicians, 1231. Ratio, 1: 262.

Number of medical schools 3, plus two postgraduate (Army and Navy Medical) schools.

WASHINGTON: *Population, 327,044.*

(1) GEORGE WASHINGTON UNIVERSITY, DEPARTMENT OF MEDICINE. Organized 1825. Now an integral department of the university.

Entrance requirement: Less than a four-year high school course.

Attendance: 117.

Teaching staff: 69 instructors, 25 being professors, none of whom is a full-time teacher; three instructors of other grade devote entire time to the school.

Resources available for maintenance: The school budget calls for $23,779; its income in fees is $21,833; the hospital is self-supporting.

Laboratory facilities: The laboratories of physiology, pathology, chemistry, and anatomy are well equipped; the building is admirably kept, and there is evidence of independent activity on the part of the several instructors. Animals are provided; there is a fair library enjoying a small annual appropriation, and a small but attractive museum. Post-mortems are scarce.

Clinical facilities: The University Hospital and Dispensary, under complete control, adjoins the medical school; 56 beds are available for teaching purposes. The staff has been recently reorganized on modern lines in order to increase the scope of bedside work. Supplementary opportunities are furnished under the usual conditions by several other hospitals.

The dispensary has an annual attendance of something over 1000.

Date of visit: March, 1909.

(2) GEORGETOWN UNIVERSITY SCHOOL OF MEDICINE. Organized 1851. A university department in name only.

Entrance requirement: Less than a four-year high school course.

Attendance: 89.

Teaching staff: 74, of whom 20 are professors; no one gives whole time to the medical school, except the dean, who has the chair of hygiene and is treasurer of both medical and dental schools.

Resources available for maintenance: Fees only, amounting to $11,000 a year.

Laboratory facilities: The equipment consists of a good dissecting-room, a single fairly well stocked laboratory for pathology, bacteriology, and histology, a fair equipment for experimental physiology, and an ordinary chemical laboratory. There is no library accessible to students, no museum, and no pharmacological laboratory.

Clinical facilities: The school has recently built a hospital, in which there are 100 ward beds, not free, but available for clinical use. It is several miles distant. The usual supplementary clinics are held in other places also. A few rooms at the hospital are set aside for a dispensary; the attendance is small.

Date of visit: March, 1909.

(3) HOWARD UNIVERSITY MEDICAL COLLEGE. Organized 1869. An integral part of Howard University.

Entrance requirement: A high school course or its equivalent.

Attendance: 205, most of whom are working their way through. Practically all the students are colored.

Teaching staff: 52, 22 being professors, 30 of other grade.

Resources available for maintenance: The school budget calls for $40,000, of which $26,000 are supplied by student fees, most of the remainder by government appropriation. Though the school has been changed from a night to a day school, the fees raised from $80 to $100, and the admission requirements stiffened, the attendance has nevertheless increased.

Laboratory facilities: The laboratory equipment includes anatomy, pathology, histology, bacteriology, and chemistry. There is no organized museum, though the school possesses a number of specimens, normal and pathological, charts, models, etc.

Clinical facilities: Clinical facilities are provided in the new, thoroughly modern, and adequate government hospital of 278 free beds, with its dispensary, closely identified with the medical school. A pavilion for contagious diseases alone is lacking.

Date of visit: January, 1910.

(4) ARMY MEDICAL SCHOOL. Organized 1822. Offers laboratory courses, covering eight months, to candidates who have passed their preliminary examinations as army surgeons.

Attendance: 57.

Teaching staff: 10 instructors, detached from the army for the purpose.

Laboratory facilities: Excellent teaching and working laboratories in cramped quarters are provided in the building occupied by the great library and museum of the Surgeon-General's office.

Date of visit: January, 1910.

(5) NAVY MEDICAL SCHOOL. Offers laboratory courses, covering six months, to candidates who have passed preliminary examinations as navy surgeons.

Attendance: 20.

Teaching staff: Several instructors, detached from the service for three years or less.

Laboratory facilities: Good teaching and working laboratories are provided in the building formerly used for the naval observatory.

Date of visit: January, 1910.

General Considerations

OF the medical schools in Washington, Howard University has a distinct mission —that of training the negro physician—and an assured future. The government has to some extent been the patron of the institution, and has done its medical department an incalculably great service by the erection of the Freedman's Hospital. Sound policy—educational as well as philanthropic—recommends that this hospital be made a more intimate part of Howard University, so that students may profit to the uttermost by its clinical opportunities. Its usefulness as a hospital in its immediate vicinity will be thereby increased; and its service to the colored race at large will be augmented to the extent to which it is used to educate their future physicians.

The other two schools lack adequate resources as well as assured prospects. They are surrounded by medical schools—those of Richmond, Baltimore, Philadelphia— whose competition they cannot meet. Finally, the District of Columbia has relatively more physicians than any other part of the country. Should the District require, as it ought, a higher basis, or even enforce an actual four-year high school standard, both would suffer seriously. Neither school is now equal to the task of training physicians of modern type.

GEORGIA

Population, 2,557,412. Number of physicians, 2887. Ratio, 1: 886.
Number of medical schools, 5.

ATLANTA: *Population,* 118,243.

(1) ATLANTA COLLEGE OF PHYSICIANS AND SURGEONS. Organized through merger, 1898. An independent school.

Entrance requirement: Nominal.

Attendance: 286, about 63 per cent from Georgia.

Teaching staff: 51, of whom 20 are professors. None of the teachers devotes full time to the school.

Resources available for maintenance: The school has practically no resources but fees, amounting to $28,000.

Laboratory facilities: It is perhaps the best equipped of all the schools of its grade; it has good buildings, containing a good dissecting-room,—dissecting material, however, somewhat scarce,—a fairly equipped laboratory for physiology and physiological chemistry, one of the same character for histology and pathology, and a separate laboratory, well equipped, for bacteriology. Unfortunately, the school has no full-time instructors in these branches, so that, what with practitioner teachers and an inferior student body, the equipment cannot be used at its real value. There is a small library, but no museum.

Clinical facilities: Hospital facilities are furnished by the Grady (free city) Hospital, close by. Except in obstetrics, to which department students are not admitted, the clinical material is fairly abundant; but it cannot be effectively used,[1] and the students are so unappreciative of their opportunities that attendance in the wards is very irregular.

In the school building a large suite of rooms is set aside for a dispensary. The attendance is ample, the methods old-fashioned.

Date of visit: January, 1909.

(2) ATLANTA SCHOOL OF MEDICINE. Organized 1905. An independent school.

Entrance requirement: Nominal.

Attendance: 230; not quite 70 per cent from Georgia.

Teaching staff: 44, of whom 17 are professors, no one devoting whole time to the school.

Resources available for maintenance: Fees and gifts, amounting together to $20,000–$25,000 annually.

Laboratory facilities: Its laboratory equipment is slight, though it possesses some features uncommon in schools of its type,—an excellent projectoscope, an X-ray machine, and a small, useful library. There is no museum.

Clinical facilities: A suite of rooms in fair condition only is provided for a dispensary. Likewise, in the basement of the college, two wards, containing 20 beds, have been arranged; so far as they go, they are fairly well used. For the rest of its clinical instruction the school depends mainly on the Grady Hospital, so far off, however, that the students do not conscientiously attend.

Date of visit: January, 1909.

(3) GEORGIA COLLEGE OF ECLECTIC MEDICINE AND SURGERY. Organized 1877. An independent institution.

[1] The consent of ward patients must be obtained before bedside instruction can be given.

Entrance requirement: Nominal.

Attendance: 66.

Teaching staff: 20, of whom 14 are professors and 6 of other grade.

Resources available for maintenance: Fees, amounting to $5655 (estimated).

Laboratory facilities: The school occupies a building which, in respect to filthy conditions, has few equals, but no superiors, among medical schools. Its anatomy room, containing a single cadaver, is indescribably foul; its chemical "laboratory" is composed of old tables and a few bottles, without water, drain, lockers, or reagents; the pathological and histological "laboratory" contains a few dirty slides and three ordinary microscopes.

Clinical facilities: The school is practically without clinical facilities. Its outfit in obstetrics is limited to a tattered manikin.

Nothing more disgraceful calling itself a medical school can be found anywhere.

Date of visit: February, 1909.

(4) HOSPITAL MEDICAL COLLEGE. Eclectic. Organized 1908. This institution occupies the rear of a private infirmary. Started in 1908 "on four weeks' notice" by seceders from the Georgia College of Eclectic Medicine and Surgery (*see* (3) *above*), it graduated 17 doctors at the close of its first year.

Entrance requirement: Nominal.

Attendance: 48.

Teaching staff: 16, all of whom are professors.

Resources available for maintenance: Fees, amounting to $3950 (estimated).

Laboratory facilities: In the matter of equipment, it is impossible to say what belongs to the school and what to the infirmary. At any rate, there is only one laboratory with any equipment worthy the name,—that of pathology and bacteriology.

Clinical facilities: The clinical facilities comprise the infirmary above mentioned, containing 16 beds. It is, of course, a pay infirmary.

Date of visit: February, 1909.

AUGUSTA: *Population, 45,582.*

(5) MEDICAL COLLEGE OF GEORGIA. Organized in 1828, it has been since 1873 nominally the medical department of the state university; but it is entirely controlled by its own separate board, and "no liability for its debts or expenses shall be incurred by the university."[1] The institution is therefore in effect a proprietary school.

[1] Agreement between Medical College of Georgia and University of Georgia, article 4.

Entrance requirement: Nominal.

Attendance: 99, mostly from Georgia. Twenty-six of these hold free county scholarships, in addition to which number the dean admits as many more as he pleases, generally at the request of congressmen. Eighteen students were admitted free in this way last year. Hence 44 of the 99 students are free.

Teaching staff: 33, of whom 18 are professors.

Resources available for maintenance: The institution has no resources but fees, amounting to $6835.

Laboratory facilities: The school occupies a building which contains an exceedingly foul dissecting-room, a meager equipment for elementary chemistry, a fair equipment for histology and pathology, and practically nothing for bacteriology. There is a small museum and a collection of several thousand books of mainly antiquarian interest.

Clinical facilities: The city hospital adjoining, containing 100 beds,—less than half of them occupied at the time of the inspection,—offers most of the clinical facilities; the Lamar Hospital is also available, but is more than a mile off, though described in the official catalogue of the state university as "located only a short distance from the college." At the city hospital the students get no obstetrical work because "the cases mostly come at night and you can't get the students;" at the Lamar Hospital they get none because "they are too busy." There is no evidence anywhere of clinical laboratory work. It was learned that at the city hospital there had been "two post-mortems in six years."

There is a dispensary at the city hospital, but no records are kept.

Date of visit: February, 1909.

General Considerations

THE situation to be dealt with in this state is so simple that there is no room for difference of opinion as to what ought to be done. That every state in the south is overcrowded with doctors is generally admitted. Florida alone of surrounding states lacks a medical school, and there is an excess of doctors there (ratio 1 : 865). The two eclectic schools, as utterly incapable of training doctors, should be summarily suppressed. The Augusta situation is hopeless. There is no possibility of developing there a medical school controlled by the university. The site is unpropitious, the distance too great. The university ought not much longer permit its name to be exploited by a low-grade institution, whose entrance terms—if the phrase can be used—are far below that of its academic department. It should snap the slender thread; the medical school will not long survive amputation.

Two schools remain at Atlanta, a growing city in close proximity to the university at Athens. It would be easy to consolidate these two institutions to form the medical department of the University of Georgia. The department could immediately adopt the general entrance requirements of the university, to be enforced by the university authorities. The faculty should, of course, be reconstructed and governed without restriction on university lines. The city's growth ensures a fair clinic and probably material aid.

ILLINOIS

Population, 5,717,229. Number of physicians, 9744. Ratio 1: 586.
Number of medical schools, 14, plus 4 postgraduate schools.

CHICAGO: *Population, 2,282,927.*

(1) RUSH MEDICAL COLLEGE. A divided school. Since 1900 the instruction of the first and second years has been given wholly at the University of Chicago, of which it is an integral part; the third and fourth years, given at the Cook County, the Presbyterian, and the Children's Memorial Hospitals and in the laboratory buildings adjoining them, are merely affiliated with the university. Pedagogically, the two branches do not form an organic whole.

Entrance requirement: Two years of college work, strictly enforced, though a considerable part of the entering class is conditioned in part of the scientific requirement.

Attendance: 488.

Teaching staff: 89 professors and 141 of other grade: total 230. The laboratory work is in charge of men devoting their entire time to teaching and research.

Resources available for maintenance: The instruction provided by the university is paid for out of the university funds and costs annually $45,738; the clinical division, carried by student fees and by contributions, costs $36,714: a total cost of $82,452. The total income in fees is $60,485.

Laboratory facilities: The laboratory branches are most liberally provided for on the university grounds; the laboratories are complete in number and equipment, each manned by a full staff, all the members of which are engaged in investigation as well as in teaching. There is considerable difference of opinion among those engaged in teaching the scientific subjects as to how far the presentation should be deliberately medical in aim.

Clinical facilities: Clinical facilities are provided by the Presbyterian Hospital, the staff of which is the faculty of the Rush Medical School, by the Cook County Hospital, and by other connections. The Presbyterian Hospital is an important adjunct, though thus far it is not by any means a genuine teaching hospital. It contains about 150 beds available for instruction. The Cook County Hospital will be discussed in connection with the general state situation. It is sufficient to say here that its abundant material is in a high degree valuable, though serious limitations upon its use exist. Rush holds 21 staff appointments.

Dispensary facilities are entirely adequate.   .   •

Date of visit: April, 1909.

(2) NORTHWESTERN UNIVERSITY MEDICAL DEPARTMENT. Organized 1859, it has borne its present title since 1891. An integral part of the university.

Entrance requirement: One year of college work, hitherto loosely enforced.

Attendance: 522.

Teaching staff: 54 professors and 89 of other grade: 143 in all, ten of whom devote their entire time to the school.

Resources available for maintenance: Except for two professorships, endowed to the extent of $60,700, the department lives on and pays for plant addition out of its fees now amounting to $89,076.

Laboratory facilities: The school has the necessary laboratories, well equipped for routine work; more could be done but that the full-time teachers lack the necessary assistants.

Clinical facilities: These are provided by Mercy Hospital, Wesley Hospital, the Cook County Hospital, and other institutions. The Wesley Hospital, the staff of which comes wholly from the faculty of this school,[1] contains 80 free beds. It is, however, not primarily a teaching hospital, though it might apparently be reorganized as such with much advantage both to itself and to the medical school. The Cook County Hospital will be discussed below; Northwestern holds 12 staff appointments there. In general, material is abundant in amount and variety; the defects of the situation arise from the lack of financial resources and pedagogical control.

Dispensary requirements are amply met.

Dates of visits: April, 1909; December, 1909.

(3) COLLEGE OF PHYSICIANS AND SURGEONS. Organized in 1882; since 1896 nominally the medical department of the University of Illinois, with which, however, only a contractual relation exists.

Entrance requirement: A high school education or its equivalent, the latter hitherto very loosely interpreted, though somewhat stricter action has been enforced this year. The policy of the institution had been to accept students who satisfied the Illinois law as administered by the present state board; the requirement has, therefore, been more or less nominal. Advanced standing has been accorded to students from decidedly inferior schools, some of them among the worst institutions

[1] Students from the American Medical Missionary College attend certain clinics.

in the country. These students were examined, only those who passed being accepted; but the fact that, with the teaching they have had, they can pass is conclusive as to the nature of the examination.

Attendance: 517, about 60 per cent from Illinois.

Teaching staff: 198, of whom 42 are professors, 156 of other grade.

Resources available for maintenance: The institution is practically dependent on its fees, amounting to $80,155 (estimated), and has a large floating debt.

Laboratory facilities: The school has the following laboratories: physiology, well equipped; pharmacology and chemistry, mediocre; anatomy, pathology, and bacteriology, adequate. There are full-time professors of anatomy and physiology, without skilled assistants or helpers. Their work is limited to routine. The school has a large library.

Clinical facilities: For these the school relies on the Cook County Hospital, on the staff of which it holds 11 appointments, and on a number of other institutions to which its students are admitted under the usual limitations. Prominent among these is the so-called "University Hospital," which may be cited as a typical instance of the misleading character of catalogue representations. The title itself is a misnomer; for the hospital is a university hospital not in the sense that large teaching advantages exist for the benefit of the university, but only in the sense that to the existing opportunities, restricted as they are, students from other schools are not admitted at all. The catalogue states that "it contains one hundred beds, and its clinical advantages are used exclusively for the students of this college." Not, however, the "clinical advantages" of the "one hundred beds," for 52 of them are private. Its "clinical advantages" shrink on investigation to three weekly amphitheater clinics of slight pedagogic value and four ward clinics in obstetrics, —each of the latter attended by some 12 or 14 students in a ward containing 13 beds. Supplementary connections give access to large surgical clinics.

The dispensary service is in general adequate.

Dates of visits: April, 1909 ; December, 1909.

(4) CHICAGO COLLEGE OF MEDICINE AND SURGERY. Organized 1901, and since 1902 the medical department of Valparaiso (Indiana) University ; up to 1905 an eclectic institution.

Entrance requirement: A high school education or its equivalent, interpreted to include anything that the state board will accept.

Attendance: The school had an enrolment of 315 in 1907–8, and of 366 in 1908–9, the senior class of the former year numbering 95, the freshman 69. This disproportion is largely due to the fact that advanced standing has been indiscriminately granted to students who had previously attended low-grade institutions, some of them now defunct. Credit has been allowed to former students of even the worst of the Chicago night schools.

Teaching staff: The school has a faculty of 71, of whom 37 are professors. There are no full-time teachers, though some of the scientific branches are taught by full-time teachers of Valparaiso University, who come to the Chicago department on certain days weekly.

Resources available for maintenance: Fees, amounting to $43,430 (estimated).

Laboratory facilities: The equipment throughout is ordinary, the usual laboratories being provided. There are few teaching accessories.

Clinical facilities: Clinical facilities are inadequate, being limited in the main to an adjoining hospital of 75 beds, of which one-fourth can be used for teaching, and to the Cook County Hospital, on the staff of which the school has two representatives.

The dispensary has a fair attendance and is in some respects well organized.

Date of visit: April, 1909.

(5) BENNETT MEDICAL COLLEGE. Organized 1868, and up to 1909 an eclectic school. A stock company, practically owned by the dean of the school: "there are enough others to legalize the thing."

Entrance requirement: Nominal compliance with the Illinois law on the subject. A pre-medical department,— Jefferson Park Academy,— recruited by solicitors, has been organized by way of feeding the medical school. A vigorous advertising and soliciting system is operated.

Attendance: 181 ; about one-half from Illinois.

Teaching staff: 42, of whom 21 are professors.

Resources available for maintenance: Fees, amounting to $19,380 (estimated).

Laboratory facilities: The school building is in wretched condition. One badly kept room is devoted to anatomy ; it contained a few cadavers as dry as leather; another, in similar condition, is given to chemistry. There is slight provision for pathology and bacteriology; equipment for physiology is sufficient only for simple demonstrations. There are no teaching accessories worthy of mention.

Clinical facilities: These comprise a pay hospital of 45 beds, in which it is claimed that 20 are made available for teaching use by means of free medical (not hospital) services ; and two places on the Cook County Hospital staff. The clinical facilities are utterly inadequate.

There is a small dispensary.

The institution is frankly commercial. Its change of name (dropping "eclectic") is a business move.

Date of visit: April, 1909.

(6) AMERICAN MEDICAL MISSIONARY COLLEGE. Organized 1895. This school gives the bulk of its instruction at Battle Creek, Michigan, which see for complete account.

(7) JENNER MEDICAL COLLEGE. Organized 1892. A night school, occupying three upper floors of a business house. An independent institution.

Entrance requirement: Nominal compliance with state law. A one-year pre-medical class is operated by way of satisfying the law.

Attendance: 112.

Teaching staff: 37, of whom 28 are professors.

Resources available for maintenance: Fees, amounting to $12,880 (estimated).

Laboratory facilities: The equipment consists of a meager outfit for chemistry, a somewhat better equipment for physiology, though no animals were to be seen, and a slight outfit for pathology and bacteriology. Anatomy is taught by lectures "with the cadaver" from the beginning of the year until May 15, after which there is "dissecting until the close of the year."

Clinical facilities: Clinical facilities are practically nil,— one or two night clinics being all that the school claims to offer. The school once had access to Grace Hospital, a private institution of 30 beds; but it has recently been turned out for failure to pay for the privilege.

The dispensary attendance varies from two to ten, four nights weekly. No particular rooms for dispensary purposes are provided: "patients are taken right into the rooms where the classes are."

An out-and-out commercial enterprise. The instruction is plainly a quiz-compend drill aimed at the written examinations set by the state board of Illinois and of other states. The possibility of teaching medicine acceptably in a night school is discussed below (p. 216, note).

Date of visit: April, 1909.

(8) ILLINOIS MEDICAL COLLEGE. Organized 1894. ⎫
(9) RELIANCE MEDICAL COLLEGE. Organized 1907. ⎭

These two schools are bracketed because they are only different aspects of one enterprise worked in two shifts, one body of students attending by day, the other by night. The plant is thus in "continuous performance." It is owned by its president, who is in the main assisted in the scientific branches by recent college graduates, to whom small sums are paid; in the clinical branches by young physicians who tender their services gratis in order to "work up their business." The day school is affiliated with Loyola University.

Entrance requirement: Of the kind usual in Illinois commercial medical schools. A pre-medical class, running three hours each night, covers in one year the work of two high school years. A boy who is engaged all day in trade can thus "finish" two years' English, Latin, and mathematics at night in a single session. It is probable that the pre-medical course will be lengthened to two such years, "equivalent" to an entire high school course according to the "Illinois idea."

Attendance: Reliance Medical College, 83; Illinois Medical College, 69.

Teaching staff: The night medical school (Reliance) has a faculty of 44, 23 being professors; the day branch (Illinois Medical) has a faculty of 73, 38 being professors.

Resources available for maintenance: Fees, amounting to $9945 (Reliance, estimated); $9175 (Illinois, estimated).

Laboratory facilities: The equipment conforms to legal stipulations: there is a library, the beginnings of a museum, an ordinary dissecting-room, a small amount of apparatus for physiology, and fair laboratories, as things go, for chemistry, histology, pathology, and bacteriology. The laboratories are in good condition and are really used.

Clinical facilities. Day students: Some eight or ten hours weekly for junior and senior classes in scattered hospitals; work almost wholly surgical; one to two hours daily in the dispensary in the college building. Students see no contagious diseases; obstetrical work is all out-patient. *Night students:* About six hours weekly at the Cook County Hospital between 6.30 and 9.30 p.m., opportunities being limited to looking on at surgical work; dispensary, nightly. The night students see no children's diseases, no acute medical diseases at the bedside, no contagious diseases.

Dates of visits: April, 1909; December, 1909.

(10) NATIONAL MEDICAL UNIVERSITY. A night school, organized in 1891 as "homeopathic," which word was subsequently dropped. Ostensibly the medical department of the "Chicago Night University," which claims departments of arts, law, dentistry, pharmacy, etc. The school appears to be owned by the "dean."

Entrance requirement: Entrance is on the same basis as in other night schools; a "preparatory department" is also in operation.

Attendance: 150. "Free transportation from Chicago to Vienna by way of New York, London, Paris," etc., is offered to any graduate who has for "three years or more paid regular fees in cash."

Teaching staff: 36.

Resources available for maintenance: Fees, amounting to $22,500 (estimated).

Laboratory facilities: The school occupies a badly lighted building, containing nothing that can be dignified by the name of equipment. There had been no dissecting thus far (October to the middle of April), anatomy being didactically taught. Persistent inquiry for the "dissecting-room" was, however, finally rewarded by the sight of a dirty, unused, and almost inaccessible room containing a putrid corpse, several of the members of which had been hacked off. There is a large room called the chemical laboratory, its equipment "locked up," the tables spotless. "About ten" oil-immersion microscopes are claimed—also "locked up in the storeroom." There is not even a pretense of anything else. Classes in session were all taking dictation.

Clinical facilities: The top floor is the "hospital:" it contained two lonely patients. Access to a private hospital two miles distant is also claimed.

Recently this school has been declared by the Illinois State Board of Health as "not in good standing." The same action was taken once before, but was afterwards revoked; just why, it is impossible to find out; for the school was after the revocation just exactly what it was at the time of its suspension; and it is the same to-day.

Date of visit: April, 1909.

(11) COLLEGE OF MEDICINE AND SURGERY: PHYSIO-MEDICAL. Organized 1885. An independent school.

Entrance requirement: Such as satisfies the present interpretation of the law. A diligent search in the office desk and safe failed to discover any credentials of students now in the school.

Attendance: 33.

Teaching staff: 42, of whom 33 are professors.

Resources available for maintenance: The school has no resources but fees, amounting to $2935 (estimated).

Laboratory facilities: The equipment is very meager.

Clinical facilities: Clinical facilities amount to little: there were in the hospital last year 167 patients, over one-half surgical; there is an annual attendance of 250 in the dispensary.

Date of visit: April, 1909.

(12) HERING MEDICAL COLLEGE. Homeopathic. Organized 1892. This school teaches homeopathic doctrine in its original purity.

Entrance requirement: "High school or equivalent."

Attendance: 32.

Teaching staff: 44, of whom 30 are professors.

Resources available for maintenance: Fees, amounting to $3360 (estimated).

Laboratory facilities: The equipment is very meager.

Clinical facilities: These are very limited. Students are not admitted to the adjoining hospital. There is a small dispensary.

Date of visit: April, 1909.

(13) HAHNEMANN MEDICAL COLLEGE. Homeopathic. Organized 1859. An independent institution.

Entrance requirement: "High school or equivalent."

Attendance: 130.

Teaching staff: 84, of whom 38 are professors.

Resources available for maintenance: Fees, amounting to $14,300 (estimated).

Laboratory facilities: The school occupies a building wretchedly dirty, excepting only the single laboratory, fairly equipped, devoted to pathology and bacteriology. The equipment covers in a meager way also anatomy, physiology, histology, chemistry.

Clinical facilities: In the adjoining hospital there are accommodations in the wards for 60 beds, but there are no ward clinics. The superintendent is a layman who "does not believe in admitting students to the wards. There is no regular way for them to see common acute diseases," as only amphitheater clinics are held. Hospital internes do all the obstetrical work; students "look on." The school also holds two appointments on the surgical side in the Cook County Hospital.

There is a fair dispensary.

Date of visit: April, 1909.

(14) LITTLEJOHN COLLEGE OF OSTEOPATHY. An undisguised commercial enterprise.

Entrance requirement: Nominal.

Attendance: 75.

Teaching staff: 43.

Resources available for maintenance: Fees, and income from patients.

Laboratory facilities: Practically none. At the time of the visit, some rebuilding was in progress, in consequence of which even such laboratories as are claimed were, except that of elementary chemistry, entirely out of commission and likely to remain so for months: but "teaching goes on all the same." Class-rooms were practically bare, except for chairs and a table.

Clinical facilities: The Littlejohn Hospital,—a pay institution of 20 beds, mostly surgical,—which can be of little use. It was claimed, too, that "medicine and surgery are taught in the school," and color is lent to the statement by the presence on the faculty of physicians teaching materia medica, etc.

Date of visit: December, 1909.

(15) THE POSTGRADUATE MEDICAL SCHOOL AND HOSPITAL. A stock company.

Teaching staff: 98.

Resources available for maintenance: Fees.

Laboratory facilities: A good working clinical laboratory.

Clinical facilities: The school offers clinical instruction in its own hospital, containing a small number of beds, and in other Chicago institutions. The instruction is attended by physicians for periods varying from a few weeks to a year.

Date of visit: April, 1909.

(16) CHICAGO POLYCLINIC. A postgraduate institution organized as a stock company. Offers special courses to graduated physicians.

Attendance: Perhaps 30 at any given time; a total of 350 in the course of a year.

Teaching staff: 92, 30 being professors, 62 of other grade.

Resources available for maintenance: Fees.

Laboratory facilities: A small clinical laboratory, the instruction in technique being given by a first-year student in one of the night schools; in the absence of the instructor, he also conducts classes.

Clinical facilities: The main reliance is the Polyclinic Hospital of 80 beds, two-thirds of them surgical.

Date of visit: December, 1909.

(17) CHICAGO EAR, EYE, NOSE, AND THROAT COLLEGE. A stock company offering courses in certain specialties.

Attendance: 20 on average; average period of residence, two months; a few remain six to twelve months.

Teaching staff: 22.

Resources available for maintenance: Fees.

Facilities: A fairly equipped dispensary with a daily attendance of 15 to 20 new patients; a hospital with 10 ward beds, empty at time of visit, "but full a week ago." The work is all immediately practical; there are no facilities for fundamental or intensive instruction or effort.

Date of visit: December, 1909.

(18) ILLINOIS POSTGRADUATE SCHOOL. A stock company.

Entrance requirement: The M.D. degree.

Attendance: 6 to 8 at any given time.

Teaching staff: 36, of whom 26 are professors, 10 of other grade.

Resources available for maintenance: Fees.

Laboratory facilities: Practically none.

Clinical facilities: The school offers courses at the West Side Hospital, a private institution of 86 beds occupied mostly by surgical cases. There is a large dispensary.

Date of visit: December, 1909.

General Considerations

THE city of Chicago is in respect to medical education the plague spot of the country. The state law is fairly adequate, for it empowers the board of health to establish a standard of preliminary education, laboratory equipment, and clinical facilities, thus fixing the conditions which shall entitle a school to be considered reputable. In pursuance of these powers, the board has made the four-year high school or its equivalent the basis, and has enumerated the essentials of the medical course, including, among other things, clinical instruction through two annual terms.

With the indubitable connivance of the state board, these provisions are, and have long been, flagrantly violated. Of the fourteen undergraduate medical schools above described, the majority exist and prepare candidates for the Illinois state board examinations in unmistakable contravention of the law and the state board rules. These schools are as follows: (1) Chicago College of Medicine and Surgery (Valparaiso University), (2) Hahnemann Medical College, (3) Hering Medical College, (4) Illinois Medical College, (5) Bennett Medical College, (6) Physio-Medical College of Medicine and Surgery, (7) Jenner Medical College, (8) National Medical University, (9) Reliance Medical College, (10) Littlejohn College of Osteopathy. Of these, only one, the National Medical University, has been deprived of "good standing" by the state board. Without exception, a large proportion of their attendance offers for admission an "equivalent," which is not an equivalent in any sense whatsoever; it is nevertheless accepted without question by the state board, though the statute explicitly states that it can exact an equivalent by "satisfactory" examination. In the case of the night schools,[1] for instance, one or two years' requirements are satisfied

---

[1] Even supposing the night schools enforced an entrance standard and actually provided laboratories and hospitals of the right kind, the teaching of anything but didactic medicine at night is practically impossible, because : (1) The time is too limited. The day school is in operation all day long and the student has his evenings for study ; the night school can at most secure three or four hours when the student is already physically fatigued. (2) Laboratory work by artificial light is bound to be unsatisfactory, even if the lighting is good, which is not usually the case. (3) Hospital clinics, operations, etc.. must be very limited at night, when the interest of the patient requires that he be allowed to rest. Children's diseases cannot be studied at night at all. (4) The situation is rendered even more absurd by the fact that, in addition to all these handicaps, the night school student frequently has to make up some conditions in preliminary studies.

by "coaching" one night a week in each of the several subjects : one evening is devoted to Latin, the next to English, the next to mathematics. There is absolutely no guarantee that the candidate accepted on the equivalent basis has had an education even remotely resembling the high school training which the Illinois law intends as the minimum upon which it will recognize a candidate for the physician's license. If the state board should—as in duty bound—publicly brand these schools as "not in good standing" by reason of their failure to require a suitable preliminary education of their students, their graduates would be immediately excluded from practice in Illinois ; adjoining states would rapidly follow suit, with the result that the schools would shortly be exterminated. Fortunately, the case against them does not rest alone on the question of entrance requirements : for not a single one of the schools mentioned furnishes clinical opportunities in proper abundance, and some of them even fail to provide the stipulated training in other branches, e. g., anatomy. An efficient and intelligent administration of the law would thus reduce in short order the medical schools of Chicago to three, Rush, Northwestern, and the College of Physicians and Surgeons.[1] In the matter of entrance requirements, Rush alone is secure. The College of Physicians and Surgeons rests on the high school or equivalent basis; if a scholastic equivalent, such as would be acceptable to the academic department of the state university, is insisted on, the registration will be seriously diminished. Northwestern is in a similar plight: it requires now a high school education or equivalent, followed by a year of college which it does not get. If its standard were enforced, its present attendance would be considerably reduced. At both Northwestern and the College of Physicians and Surgeons the inequality and incapacity of the present student body are frankly conceded. "The facilities are better than the students," said a professor at the former; "the admission machinery does n't stop the unfit," said a professor at the latter. That both these schools will be driven by internal and external forces to a higher level, actually enforced, is inevitable. When that happens, their attendance will materially shrink; and as higher standards will check the invasion of medical schools by drifting waverers, and will tend to keep the number of doctors in more nearly normal relation to the needs of the population, it is not likely that either school will again attain its former size. This consideration is rendered additionally important because it portends a marked reduction in income through fees, upon which both schools still depend.

In the matter of teaching facilities, the three schools under discussion satisfy the law; but they satisfy the aspirations of their faculties only in varying degrees. The scientific work of the University of Chicago, relied on by Rush, is excellent; the provision made by Northwestern and the College of Physicians and Surgeons is distinctly inferior to it. Assuming that Northwestern will rise to an actual one or two year college basis, it must provide correspondingly increased facilities both for the higher grade students and for the more productive teaching body which these students will

[1] For the American Medical Missionary College, see "Michigan."

demand. There are, for instance, several full-time instructors, but they are without an adequate force of assistants. The needs of the College of Physicians and Surgeons are much greater. Its laboratory facilities and equipment are inadequate even for the present student body; and it has barely begun the development of a full-time teaching staff in the scientific branches. Both these schools face an era of increased investment in plant and of considerably augmented running expenses, coinciding with a period of reduced income from tuition fees.

On the clinical side, Rush and Northwestern do not differ substantially; the College of Physicians and Surgeons is somewhat inferior. Both Rush and Northwestern have an exclusive staff connection with certain hospitals. Their hospital situation is therefore, as things go in this country, tolerable. They command a sufficient number of cases, subject, however, to two defects that will be more acutely felt as clearer ideals become dominant in medical education: (1) they are not in position freely to import clinical teachers, nor (2) can they in general discontinue a professorial appointment without to the same extent abridging their clinical resources; none of them completely controls, even in a single hospital, the conditions under which clinical instruction is given.[1]

The Cook County Hospital is common to all three. Its relations to the medical schools have been subject to variation and disturbance. The institution is conducted by a lay warden, who, though a politician, is now friendly to the schools. At present, the staff is selected by civil service examination every six years. Rush now holds twice as many appointments as either of the other two schools, a discrepancy that may be either emphasized, obliterated, or reversed at the next examination. The main clinical facilities of the several schools are thus precarious. They are also limited: a recent unpleasantness—due, according to one version, to a quarrel between certain doctors and some nurses who objected to the careless way in which the doctors replaced the bed sheets—has resulted in the exclusion of students from the wards. Patients are exhibited in rooms. The incident involves serious limitations upon teaching methods, and illustrates the uncertainty which attaches to mere privileges and courtesies. Cases cannot be assigned for intensive study to particular students; hospital residents make the records and do the clinical laboratory work. The undergraduate student can see conditions in abundance; he cannot at close range observe processes in development. The Cook County Hospital is therefore, from a strictly educational point of view, not a laboratory in which beginners can be trained in a thorough technique. It is, however, immensely valuable as a storehouse of illustrative material for students who have elsewhere received a satisfactory preliminary discipline.

None of the supplementary hospitals used by the schools cures these defects. They

---

[1] Rush comes nearest to desirable conditions at Presbyterian Hospital, for staff appointments there are by contract completely controlled by its faculty. But it is provided that "no patient shall be made the subject of clinical instruction without his or her consent."

are too small; their purpose is only secondarily educational; friction is liable to arise over efforts to retain patients for teaching purposes; the students remain more or less outsiders.

The modernization of medical education in Chicago requires, then, that two of the three schools in question should greatly strengthen their laboratory instruction, and that all three should strengthen their clinical instruction. The number of students to be provided for is a factor in determining a definite line of procedure. Rush has on its two-year college basis 488 students; Northwestern had in its first-year class, on a very loosely enforced one-year college basis, 66; the inevitable two-year standard will greatly reduce this number. Should the College of Physicians and Surgeons go to the two-year college standard,—an inevitable development if it lives,— it would suffer similarly. It seems fair to estimate, then, that the actual number of medical students in Chicago on a two-year college basis will not be too large to be cared for in a single school adequately equipped with laboratories and hospital. As medical education on the proper basis cannot be attempted outside a university, and as none of the three universities now teaching medicine in Chicago is likely to abandon the field to the others, it is suggested in the interest of efficiency and economy that (1) each of the three universities continue to provide—like the University of Chicago—the instruction of the first two years; (2) all three universities combine to form a clinical department under joint management, the first step towards which would be a concerted effort to procure a proper hospital for the use of third and fourth year men. The sum necessary to procure three such hospitals is so large that it is highly improbable that as separate institutions the schools can acquire separate and adequate clinical departments. Inasmuch as there is no demand for graduates exceeding the capacity of one clinical school, it would be sheer extravagance to equip three on the basis proposed. The Cook County and other hospitals would, on the suggested arrangement, play the part for which they are exactly suited in furnishing illustrative material for advanced students whose discipline had been elsewhere looked to, and in making possible the development of instruction for graduates in all the specialties,—a form of opportunity for which, just for lack of differentiation and organization, our physicians are still forced to go abroad. A great opportunity is thus fairly within the grasp of Chicago: the conditions to its realization are honesty and intelligence on the part of the state authorities, and coöperation between the three great universities of the state. The execution of this plan might set the country at large to thinking on the wisdom and necessity of coördinating our educational enterprises. Everywhere, thus far, our higher education has worn a competitive aspect. Some good has been thus accomplished; but now that local or numerical competition can be replaced by scientific and scholarly competition, to which the entire country and indeed the civilized world are parties, we begin to realize the waste and demoralization due to institutional competition. It is difficult to see how the state of Illinois, which in the interest of public health ought to be a factor in medical education, can make an effective contribution thereto except by coöperation with the Chicago schools. Should the state seek to develop its own school in Chicago with the inevitable low tuition fees, great friction must result. Much preferable to conflict would be the withdrawal of the state from participation in clinical instruction altogether, content in that event with a half-school at Urbana, strengthened, be it hoped, by state laboratories of public health. The entire situation presents a rare opportunity for educational statesmanship.

INDIANA

Population, 2,808,115. Number of physicians, 5,036. Ratio, 1 : 558.

Number of medical schools, 2.

BLOOMINGTON-INDIANAPOLIS: (*Population:* Bloomington, 8,902; Indianapolis, 249,426).

(1) INDIANA UNIVERSITY SCHOOL OF MEDICINE. Started at Bloomington, 1903, it first gave two years' work at Bloomington, 1905, and the entire course at Indianapolis, 1909, through absorption of the local school. The double department is an organic part of the state university.

Entrance requirement: One year of college work.

Attendance: 266, 94 per cent from Indiana.

Teaching staff: 175, of whom 99 are professors. The laboratory branches at Bloomington are taught by full-time teachers, some of whom will for a while divide their time between Indianapolis and Bloomington. The Indianapolis teachers are otherwise all practitioners.

Resources available for maintenance: Both departments will be hereafter supported out of the general funds of the university, as the Bloomington department has hitherto been,—at a heavy loss, of course. Fees (amounting at Indianapolis and Bloomington together to $31,240) are paid into the university treasury.

Laboratory facilities: At Bloomington separate laboratories with good equipment are provided for pathology and bacteriology, physiology and pharmacology, and anatomy,—the last-named strong in histology and neurology. Embryology is taught in the department of biology, physiological chemistry in the department of chemistry. Books and periodicals are accessible.

At Indianapolis the laboratories of the absorbed school were limited, but the university has already taken some steps to bring them up to the level of the Bloomington department.

Clinical facilities: Clinical instruction will be given at Indianapolis alone. The city dispensary is under control of the school faculty and has just been placed in charge of a man of modern training. The attendance has been good. The City Hospital staff is appointed by the board of health on nomination of the university. The facilities are fair, but they have been used to little advantage in the past. There is no pavilion for contagious diseases.

Date of visit: December, 1909.

VALPARAISO: *Population,* 6280.

(2) VALPARAISO UNIVERSITY. This institution offers first two years at Valparaiso and all four in Chicago. (*See Chicago College of Medicine and Surgery.*) The two-year department was organized in 1901.

Entrance requirement: A high school course or its equivalent.

Attendance: 25.

Teaching staff: Two instructors conduct the classes in physiology, pathology, bacteriology, and anatomy, in the medical building. Chemistry, materia medica, and pharmacy are taught by men who give courses in these same branches to other students. The pathologist spends one-third of his time in the Chicago department.

Resources available for maintenance: Fees only.

Laboratory facilities: There is a simple but good equipment for teaching the necessary branches in an elementary form, pathology being perhaps the weakest by reason of the small amount of gross material available. The time of the teachers is consumed in routine work.

Date of visit: December, 1909.

General Considerations

THE situation in the state is, thanks to the intelligent attitude of the university, distinctly hopeful, though it will take time to work it out fully. The university has just secured complete control of the Indianapolis school. The state board has already come to its help by making the two-year college standard, in force at the university in 1910, the legal minimum for practice within the state. This places medical education in Indiana, as it already is in Minnesota, in the hands of the state university. The Bloomington department has been of such a character that it was easily possible to make it worthy of college-bred students, but the detachment of its teachers for regular service at Indianapolis should not long continue. While it is highly important that close relations be encouraged, it is necessary to accomplish this by progressively strengthening the Indianapolis end.

The Indianapolis school has been of the ordinary local type of the better sort. In order to make the school attractive to highly qualified students, it will be necessary (1) to employ full-time men in the work of the first two years, (2) to strengthen the laboratory equipment, (3) greatly to improve the organization and conduct of the clinical courses. The trustees have formally committed themselves to this policy. It would appear necessary for some years to regard the needs of the Indianapolis department as a first lien on the increasing income of the university, if the university is to make good the ideals indicated by its entrance requirement. It can do Indiana no greater service in any direction. That done, Indiana will be one of the few states that have successfully solved the problem of medical education.

IOWA

Population, 2,192,608. Number of physicians, 3,624. Ratio, 1 : 605.
Number of medical schools, 4.

DES MOINES: *Population*, 89,113.

(1) DRAKE UNIVERSITY COLLEGE OF MEDICINE. Organized in 1882 as an independent school, it became a university department in 1900.[1]

Entrance requirement: A four-year high school education.

Attendance: 106.

Teaching staff: 16 professors and 29 of other grade; total, 45. There are no whole-time teachers. Student assistants are employed in the laboratories.

Resources available for maintenance: The school is practically dependent on its fees, the volume of which is not large,—for the funds of the university are too slender to permit any considerable allotment to the medical department. The total budget of the department was $12,417, of which $9505 came from student fees, $1239 from interest.

Laboratory facilities: Modest laboratories, whose condition speaks well for the conscientiousness of those in charge, are provided for chemistry, anatomy, pathology, and bacteriology. The provision for physiology is somewhat more slender.

Clinical facilities: The school conducts clinics by courtesy at two hospitals, where instruction is given in a demonstrative way for some twelve to fifteen hours weekly. The opportunities are in every respect inadequate: the time is too short, the amount of material available too little, and the opportunities open to students too limited. A fair amount of obstetrical work is obtained.

The school owns and controls a small dispensary, fairly well equipped and painstakingly conducted.

Date of visit: April, 1909.

---

[1] As this report goes to press, it is announced that a fund of $100,000 has been subscribed with which to improve this school.

(2) STILL COLLEGE OF OSTEOPATHY. Organized 1898. An independent school.

Entrance requirement: Less than a common school education.

Attendance: 115.

Teaching staff: 15, of whom 13 are professors.

Resources available for maintenance: Fees, amounting to $17,250 (estimated).

Laboratory facilities: These are mainly limited to signs. "Anatomy" is painted prominently on a door which, on being opened, reveals an amphitheater; "Physiology" on a door which, on being opened, reveals a class-room with an almost empty bookcase, but no laboratory equipment; the key to "Histology" could not be found; "Chemistry" proved to be a disorderly elementary laboratory with some slight outfit for bacteriology besides. The dissecting-room was inadequate and disorderly.

Clinical facilities: The school makes no pretense of having hospital facilities. The catalogue states: "Cases"—pay cases of course—"needing hospital service are placed in the hospitals of the city,"—where the students cannot see them. The catalogue says of the infirmary: "The patient in no way comes in contact with the college clinic."

Everything about the school indicates that it is a business. One is therefore not surprised to find the following advertisement in the local newspaper: "Have your case diagnosed at Still College of Osteopathy, 1442 Locust Street." (Des Moines *Register and Leader,* Nov. 3, 1909.)

Date of visit: April, 1909.

IOWA CITY: *Population, 9007.*

(3) STATE UNIVERSITY OF IOWA COLLEGE OF MEDICINE. Organized 1869. An organic department of the state university.

Entrance requirement: One year of college work.

Attendance: 267, 87 per cent from Iowa.

Teaching staff: 32, of whom 12 are professors. The laboratory instructors devote full time to their work; the clinical teachers are practitioners, some of them non-resident: the professor of surgery resides at Sioux City, the professor of gynecology, who is likewise dean of the department, at Dubuque.

Resources available for maintenance: The department is supported by state appropriations. Its income from fees is $13,707; its budget, $35,216; the university hospital budget is $33,745. Chemistry, general expense (light, heat, etc.), and a share of expense of general administration are not included in these figures.

Laboratory facilities: The equipment and instruction in the scientific branches are, in general, good. This is particularly true of anatomy, which is admirably cared for. The departments of pathology and physiology lack a sufficient number of skilled assistants. An excellent museum and books are at hand.

Clinical facilities: The university hospital is, as it now stands, too small; the amount of material available in medicine, obstetrics, and contagious diseases has been very limited. An appropriation of $75,000 has, however, been made for the purpose of increasing the hospital capacity. The methods of clinical teaching hitherto pursued have not been entirely modern, mainly for lack of proper organization and material. Supplementary clinical material is obtainable at the Sisters' Hospital and the Tuberculosis Sanitarium.

The dispensary is just in process of development. The dispensary clinic is so far largely limited to the eye, ear, nose, and throat.

Date of visit: November, 1909.

(4) STATE UNIVERSITY OF IOWA COLLEGE OF HOMEOPATHIC MEDICINE. Organized 1877. An organic department of the state university.

Entrance requirement: A four-year high school education.

Attendance: 42, 83 per cent from Iowa.

Teaching staff: 10 professors and 15 of other grade. The professor of materia medica and therapeutics, who is likewise dean of the department, resides at Des Moines, the professor of theory and practice at Davenport.

Resources available for maintenance: The department is supported by state appropriations. Its income from fees is $1864, its budget is $5453, its hospital budget is $7847. The school budget does not include expense incurred for laboratory instruction for a reason that the next paragraph will explain.

Laboratory facilities: Homeopathic students receive their laboratory instruction together with regular students of medicine, though there is now a difference of one year of college work and there will be next year a difference of two such years in their preparation, unless a resolution adopted by the board of education establishing the same basis of admission in the two departments becomes effective before that time.

Clinical facilities: The department possesses a hospital of 35 beds, quite inadequate to its purpose. The dispensary is correspondingly slender. Operating during part of last year, it received only 134 cases, of which 101 were diseases of the eye, ear, nose, and throat.

Date of visit: April, 1909.

General Considerations

IOWA is a state in which there are now between two and three times as many doctors as are really needed. The population of the state is increasing slowly, if at all. There is, then, from the standpoint of the public interest no reason why a great number of physicians should be produced; there is no reason why any physician should be graduated unless his entrance into the profession will actually improve it. Further dilution would be unpardonable.

Of the four medical schools in the state none is at this time satisfactory. The osteopathic school at Des Moines is a disgrace to the state and should be summarily suppressed. In the absence of police power to terminate its career in this way, its graduates, undertaking as they do to treat all sorts of diseases, should be compelled to meet whatever standards are applied to other practitioners. The medical department of Drake University and the homeopathic department of the state university are well intentioned but feeble institutions that only a large outlay could convert into acceptable and efficient schools. Elevation of standards will probably embarrass rather than aid; for the urgent necessity of additional outlay will coincide with a decrease in the revenues on which Drake, at least, wholly depends. It would be the part of wisdom to retire from a contest to which the institution is clearly unequal; at any rate, it ought to be content to limit its endeavor to the work of the first two years.

The homeopathic department of the state university has now a small attendance on a relatively low entrance basis. As its students receive their scientific instruction with the classes now on a one-year, and hereafter to be on a two-year, college basis, it is clear that the entrance standard of the homeopathic department must be correspondingly elevated. The already slender enrolment is therefore destined still further to shrink. For so small a body of students the state is not likely to provide increased clinical facilities and a resident faculty of its own. Wisdom would therefore counsel the adoption in Iowa of the Minnesota plan: the two medical departments of the state university should be consolidated, with a provision for special teaching in materia medica and therapeutics for students who desire the homeopathic diploma.

The two university hospitals could thus be added together; the smaller would perhaps be devoted to obstetrics; the larger, with the additional wing now to be added, would provide comfortably for general medical and surgical clinics. The creation of a strong resident faculty, and the adoption of a liberal and enlightened policy in dealing with the sick poor of the state, would place Iowa City in position to duplicate the honorable record which the University of Michigan has, under similar circumstances, made at Ann Arbor.

KANSAS

Population, 1,663,438. Number of physicians, 2650. Ratio, 1: 628.
Number of medical schools, 3.

LAWRENCE–ROSEDALE: (*Population:* Lawrence, 13,678; Rosedale, 3270— suburb of the two Kansas Cities, population, 286,074).

(1) UNIVERSITY OF KANSAS SCHOOL OF MEDICINE. The Scientific Department, at Lawrence, was organized in 1899; the Clinical Department, at Rosedale, was organized by merger with a local school in 1905.

Entrance requirement: Two years of college work.

Attendance: 89, 79 from Kansas, 8 from Missouri.

Teaching staff: At Lawrence, anatomy, physiology, and bacteriology are taught by teachers whose instruction is confined to medical students; but the professor of anatomy is also professor of gynecology at Rosedale and practises his specialty. The pathologist is expected to eke out his income by outside work. Physiology, chemistry, and pharmacy are taught in general laboratories devoted to those subjects. The medical classes are not always separate.

At Rosedale there is a teaching staff of 63, of whom 24 are professors. Two of them devote their whole time to teaching pathology, bacteriology, and clinical pathology. A third, the dean of this end, likewise gives his entire time to the school and hospital.

Resources available for maintenance: The medical school shares in the general funds of the university. The budget for the current year is about $17,000 for the Scientific Department, and $23,000 for the Clinical Department. Income in fees, $5030.

Laboratory facilities: The laboratories for anatomy, chemistry, and physiology are good and in active operation. Pathology and bacteriology are, so far, less highly developed. Books and current scientific periodicals are accessible.

Clinical facilities: The Clinical Department has a small hospital of 35 beds, not used, however, to the best advantage, partly because the faculty is not composed of men whose training has been modern, partly because, being practitioners, they cannot devote time enough to teaching. The school enjoys additional privileges of the usual kind at a Catholic hospital in Kansas City, Kansas, and at the City Hospital in Kansas City, Missouri. The obstetrical work is mainly out-patient; contagious diseases are rarely seen. On the whole, far too little clinical material under proper control is offered. An excellent building, well equipped, devoted to pathology, clinical pathology, and bacteriology, adjoins the university hospital. It contains a few books and some current periodicals.

Two dispensaries are available, one at the Rosedale building, not used for teaching until this year; the other, the so-called North End Dispensary, where a fair amount of material has hitherto been handled in an incredibly slipshod manner.

Each of the two parts of the university school of medicine has its own dean; for all practical purposes, the university conducts two half-schools.

Date of visit: November, 1909.

(2) WESTERN ECLECTIC COLLEGE OF MEDICINE AND SURGERY. Organized 1898. A stock company.

Entrance requirement: Nominal.

Attendance: 21.

Teaching staff: 32, of whom 30 are professors, 2 of other grade.

Resources available for maintenance: Fees, amounting to perhaps $1600 this year.

Laboratory facilities: These comprise a few small, indescribably dirty and disorderly rooms, containing three microscopes, a small amount of physiological apparatus, some bacteriological stains, a few filthy specimens, and meager equipment for elementary chemistry, but no running water. All laboratory work is conducted by one teacher, who serves in the same capacity in the local osteopathic and homeopathic schools and does commercial work besides. No anatomy was going on at the time of the visit, as dissection runs only from January 3 to March 12.

Clinical facilities: Practically none. A wretched room is called the "Dispensary," and an attendance of "about three a day" is claimed; it is hoped that this "can be worked up to six a day." The catalogue states that "clinics are held weekly at the Kansas City, Missouri, General Hospital," but the statement is denied by the superintendent of the hospital.

Date of visit: November, 1909.

TOPEKA: *Population,* 45,143.

(3) KANSAS MEDICAL COLLEGE. Established 1890. Since 1902 the medical department of Washburn College, which teaches chemistry to the medical students, but is without control of appointments in the medical faculty.

Entrance requirement: A four-year high school course or its equivalent.

Attendance: 65, 92 per cent from Kansas.

Teaching staff: 47, 31 being professors. There are no instructors giving their whole time to the school, except in so far as chemistry, above mentioned, is concerned.

Resources available for maintenance: Practically only fees, amounting to $4876 a year.

Laboratory facilities: The school occupies a three-story building, on the upper floors of which there have been improvised laboratories for pathology and bacteriology. They contain the necessary equipment for routine teaching, but are poorly kept. There is a small amount of apparatus for physiological demonstrations. The dissecting-room is indescribably filthy; it contained, in addition to necessary tables, a single, badly hacked cadaver, and was simultaneously used as a chicken yard.[1] There is no museum, only a few old books, some charts, a few models, etc.

[1] This is explained as follows : " It had not been in use for eight months or so and would not be in use

Clinical facilities: A total of eleven hours a week of clinical instruction, only nine of which can be attended by any one student, is offered at four different hospitals. The opportunities, limited as they are, are largely surgical. The feeling towards the school is unusually cordial, but the hospitals lack the necessary equipment and organization for effective teaching.

At the time the school was visited a small room was used for a dispensary; the attendance was slight; there was no equipment at all. Recently larger quarters have been provided.

Date of visit: November, 1909.

General Considerations

RECENT action making a year of college work the minimum preliminary to practise in Kansas will wipe out the eclectic school at Kansas City and the Topeka school, both of which would, however, die out even on the present standard. The future of medical education in the state, therefore, very properly lies with the state university. This institution has shown the desire to provide instruction of high grade by raising its entrance requirements until they now call for two years of college work; but it did not realize that it was incumbent upon it to improve facilities and instruction at the same time. Great efforts must therefore be made to hasten their development, for the higher entrance requirement is already in force. The school is now a divided school. It would be a simple matter to develop the laboratory end at Lawrence; it will be difficult and expensive to develop the clinical end at Rosedale correspondingly; and still more difficult, to establish effective coöperation between the severed halves of the department. The needs of a university medical department are so great that the university will find it necessary to refrain from many other projects, pending the upbuilding of a creditable school of medicine. It is therefore unfortunate that the educational funds of the state have been already to some extent needlessly consumed in the duplication of engineering and normal departments within the several state institutions. No comprehensive and well coördinated scheme of state educational development has been worked out. It would seem essential in the first place to demarcate the respective provinces of the several state institutions, so that each would care for certain interests without trespassing on the ground reserved to the others. That done, medicine would fall to the state university and would include a public health laboratory. Certain fundamental questions respecting the location, organization, and general scope of the entire department would next require to be settled. Thereafter, the plan adopted could be realized unit by unit, year by year.

until cold weather. [It was then the middle of November.] The cadaver happened to be there because of the private studies of one of the professors, who put it there for his own convenience. In the same way, because the room was not in public use and would not be for some time, another member of the faculty stored there, for use in embryology, the coop of live chickens."

KENTUCKY

Population, 2,406,859. Number of physicians, 3708. Ratio, 1 : 649.
Number of medical schools, 3.

LOUISVILLE: *Population, 240,160.*

(1) UNIVERSITY OF LOUISVILLE MEDICAL DEPARTMENT. Organized 1837, it has recently
absorbed four other schools. Until lately the university was limited to loosely
aggregated schools of law and medicine; latterly an academic department without
endowment has been started.

Entrance requirement : Less than a high school education. Examples were found of
students admitted from two-year high schools or less.

Attendance : 600.

Teaching staff : 90, of whom 40 are professors. The distribution of the chairs is significant : the major medical staff contains twelve names, six of them professors ; surgery, twelve names, all professors. The laboratory branches are in marked contrast:
two names make the major staff in physiology, one in chemistry, one in pathology
and bacteriology. There are four whole-time professors of modern training in the
scientific departments. Assistants, some of them also giving entire time to the
school, are provided.

Resources available for maintenance : Fees, amounting to $75,125.

Laboratory facilities : Teaching laboratories are provided for chemistry, pathology,
bacteriology, physiology, and pharmacy. They are inadequate in appointments and
teaching force for the thorough teaching of the fundamental sciences to so large
a student body. A separate building has just been set apart for anatomy, operative surgery, and the city morgue.

Clinical facilities : The school has a hospital of 50 beds, with an average of 30 patients, two-thirds of the cases being surgical, and not all available for teaching.
Obstetrical cases are rare, but there is an out-patient obstetrical service. At the
City Hospital eight amphitheater clinics are held weekly for classes containing
from 100 to 300 students. There are no regular ward classes. The obstetrical ward
is not open to students ; there is no pavilion for contagious diseases. The hospital
facilities are therefore poor in respect to both quality and extent : unequal to the
fair teaching of an even smaller body of students, they are made to suffice for the
largest school in the country.

The school dispensary has an average daily attendance of over one hundred.
It is regularly used for teaching on the section method.

Date of visit : December, 1909.

(2) SOUTHWESTERN HOMEOPATHIC MEDICAL COLLEGE. Organized 1892. An independent school.

Entrance requirement: The same as that of the University of Louisville Medical Department.

Attendance: 13.

Teaching staff: 27, 12 being professors.

Resources available for maintenance: Fees, amounting to $1100.

Laboratory facilities: There is no outfit worth speaking of in any department; the building is wretchedly dirty, especially the room said to be used for anatomy. There is nothing to indicate recent dissecting.

Clinical facilities: The school gets one-fifth of the patients admitted to the City Hospital and can use them for demonstrative purposes.
There is no organized dispensary.

Date of visit: January, 1909.

(3) LOUISVILLE NATIONAL MEDICAL COLLEGE (Colored). An independent school, organized 1888, now affiliated with the colored State University.

Entrance requirement: Less than high school education.

Attendance: 40.

Teaching staff: 23, of whom 17 are professors.

Resources available for maintenance: Fees, amounting to $2560.

Laboratory facilities: Nominal.

Clinical facilities: A small and scrupulously clean hospital of 8 beds is connected with the school.

Date of visit: January, 1909.

General Considerations

THE situation in Kentucky is a simple one. The homeopathic school is without merit. Its graduates deserve no recognition whatsoever, for it lacks the most elementary teaching facilities. The University of Louisville has a large, scattered plant, unequal to the strain which numbers put upon it. In the old days, Louisville, with a half-dozen "regular" schools, was a popular medical center, to which crude boys thronged from the plantations. The schools offered little beyond didactic teaching. Now, they have been arithmetically added together; the resulting school is indeed superior on the laboratory side to any of its component parts; but there are radical defects for which there is no cure in sight. The classes are unmanageably huge; the laboratories overcrowded and undermanned; clinical facilities, meager at best, broken into bits in order to be distributed among the aggregated faculty. To carry the school at all, a large attendance is necessary; but a large attendance implies a low standard. The situation is thus practically deadlocked.

The outlook is not promising; for there is no indication of such support, financial or academic, as would be required in order to reconstruct the institution on acceptable lines. Elsewhere a strong college or university has been in reach: as, for example, across the Ohio, Indiana University has just now put its hand to the plow and will not turn back. But in Kentucky the state university is totally unequal to the task. It labors under the initial disadvantage of being situated in another town,— not the less a disadvantage because capable of being overcome; more serious, however, is its educational ineptitude. It has never been an active educational factor, and having now chosen a politician, without educational qualification or experience, as its president, its immediate future promises little. From the existing so-called academic department of the University of Louisville neither aid nor ideals can come. It is quite without resources. We have indeed progressed too far in our social and educational development to use the word "university" for an enterprise of this kind. Classes in literature, languages, and elementary science may indeed be organized by volunteer teachers, in hours left open by their regular engagements, or by instructors supported from year to year by subscription; they may discharge a highly useful office in any community, but they ought to be called by their right name. An academic department of a university they are not: why should they not be described as a people's institute, or by some other designation calculated to indicate their actual character?[1] The loose use of the words "college" and "university" prolongs educational chaos; it hinders the apprehension of genuine and fundamental educational distinctions. Assuredly, an institute of the type described cannot dominate or transform a hitherto independent group of medical schools.

LOUISIANA

Population, 1,618,358. Number of physicians, 1798. Ratio, 1 : 900.
Number of medical schools, 2.

NEW ORLEANS: *Population, 332,169.*

(1) MEDICAL DEPARTMENT OF THE TULANE UNIVERSITY OF LOUISIANA. Organized in 1834, the school affiliated with the University of Louisiana in 1845, and with Tulane in 1884, at which date the University of Louisiana became Tulane University. In 1902 it assumed its present status as an organic part of the university.

Entrance requirement: A four-year high school education or its equivalent, administered by the academic authorities. The actual standard is somewhat below the nominal standard, though gradually rising towards it.

[1] These comments apply with equal force to Toledo.

Attendance: 489.

Teaching staff: 75, of whom 17 are professors. The laboratory branches are in charge of five men, who give their entire time to teaching and investigation.

Resources available for maintenance: Endowment funds, aggregating about $900,000, yield an income of $26,000 annually; fees amount to $67,500. The budget of the department amounts to $101,781.

Laboratory facilities: New and excellent laboratories are provided for the work of the first and second years. The professors in charge represent modern ideals, and are enthusiastically engaged in reconstructing the entire school on progressive lines. The anatomical museum is one of the best in the country. The library is small.

Clinical facilities: The school enjoys unusual privileges and opportunities in the Charity Hospital, an institution of 1050 beds. Recently an additional ward for surgery and gynecology has been added, full control of the services being vested in the Tulane faculty by the terms of the gift. The abundant material is freely used by the medical faculty, though certain defects of organization, equipment, and relationship must be corrected in order to render the situation ideal. The main point, however, is secure, for the position of the medical school in the hospital is ensured through legislative enactment. The professorship in medicine has recently been filled by importation without any friction whatsoever.

The dispensary service is adequate.

Postgraduate instruction in specialties is offered by the New Orleans Polyclinic, affiliated with the Tulane University.

(2) FLINT MEDICAL COLLEGE (Colored). Organized in 1889, it is a department of New Orleans University, which is managed by the Freedman's Aid Society of the Methodist Episcopal Church, North.

Attendance: 24.

Teaching staff: 15, of whom 6 are professors. All are practitioners.

Resources available for maintenance: Tuition fees, $1300 (estimated), and small appropriations voted by the Freedman's Aid Society constitute the income. The entire budget, including that of the hospital adjoining, is less than $10,000 annually.

Laboratory facilities: There is scant equipment in anatomy, chemistry, pathology, and bacteriology. The rooms are in poor condition.

Clinical facilities: The school controls a hospital of 20 beds, with an average of 17 patients monthly, and a dispensary with an average daily attendance of one or two.

Date of visit: January, 1909.

General Considerations

THE medical department of Tulane University is one of a very few existing southern schools that deserve development. The south is in general overcrowded with schools with which nothing can be done; for they are conducted by old-time practitioners, who could not use improved teaching facilities if they were provided. The case is different at Tulane. Its recent reorganization has put imported men of modern training and ideals in charge of the most important departments, laboratory and clinical. There is no question that if properly supported, they will quickly bring the institution to a position of commanding influence. To achieve this result, the school must be freed of the necessity of so largely relying upon fees for its support. For once rendered by endowment comparatively independent, it can use its superior opportunities as a lever to brace up the general educational situation of the southern states. It could compel those seeking these opportunities to improve their preparation at least to the full limit of local possibilities. The urgent need of the south is an object lesson in medical education, such as will prominently embody what is sound and desirable; and such an object lesson the medical department of Tulane could readily be made: it possesses already the laboratories and the hospital; it requires only the means that will enable it to utilize them fully.

Flint Medical College is a hopeless affair, on which money and energy alike are wasted. The urgent need in respect to the medical education of the negro is concentration of resources slender at best on a single southern institution. Much the most favorably situated for this purpose is Meharry Medical College at Nashville.

MAINE

Population, 724,508. Number of physicians, 1198. Ratio, 1: 600.
Number of medical schools, 1.

BRUNSWICK–PORTLAND: (*Population:*[1] Brunswick, 2321; Portland, 58,512).

MEDICAL SCHOOL OF MAINE. Organized 1820. A divided school, being the medical department of Bowdoin College.

Entrance requirement: Four-year high school diploma or equivalent, ascertained by examination, conducted, however, under the auspices of the medical school, not by Bowdoin College, and below the college standard. Certificates are accepted far below standard in value.

Attendance: 81, 86 per cent from Maine.

Teaching staff: 35, 14 being professors, 21 of other grade.

[1] Census Bureau without data.

Resources available for maintenance: From endowment, $7600; from fees, $8100; total, $15,700.

Laboratory facilities: The laboratory branches are taught in the medical school building at Brunswick with the exception of chemistry, which is well provided for in the college laboratories; the equipment covering physiology, bacteriology, and pathology is slender. There is nothing in pharmacology at all. There are no whole-time teachers in the scientific branches. The professor of anatomy is non-resident; his main duty is lecturing, the dissecting-room being supervised by recent graduates, engaged in practice. "The professor looks in occasionally." The professor of pathology is physical director of Bowdoin College. The professor of physiology is non-resident.

Clinical facilities: Clinical instruction is given at Portland by teachers who have little commerce with the laboratories at Brunswick. The chief clinical reliance of the school is the Maine General Hospital, where instruction is given principally in the amphitheater, as a majority of the cases are surgical. Obstetrical work is not to be counted on. Internes do the clinical laboratory work and make up case histories. The records are indexed only by name of the patient. Additional clinical material is obtained at the Eye and Ear Infirmary, Children's Hospital, etc.

Students spend also a small amount of time at a thoroughly wretched city dispensary, where the cases are few, where no records are kept, and where not even copies of prescriptions are filed. The dispensary does not own a microscope.

A course in clinical microscopy is given at the college building in Portland. "Urine and sputum are gathered, and students are told about the cases from which they come." Neither end of this school meets the requirements for the teaching of modern medicine. *

Date of visit: October, 1909.

[*For general discussion see* "*New England,*" p. 261.]

MARYLAND

Population, 1,319,132. Number of physicians, 2012. Ratio, 1: 658.
Number of medical schools, 7.

BALTIMORE: *Population, 588,475.*

(1) MEDICAL DEPARTMENT OF THE JOHNS HOPKINS UNIVERSITY. Established 1893. An organic university department.

Entrance requirement: The bachelor's degree, representing specific attainments in chemistry, physics, biology, German, and French.

Attendance: 297.

Teaching staff: 112, of whom 23 are professors. All the laboratory teaching is conducted by instructors who give their entire time to teaching and research; the heads of the clinical departments are salaried teachers attached to the Johns Hopkins Hospital.

Resources available for maintenance: The income from tuition fees is $60,542, that from endowments $19,687, making a total of $80,229. The budget calls for $102,429, not including salaries of the clinical faculty and other items carried by the Johns Hopkins Hospital, which is thus actually an integral part of the medical school. The productive hospital endowments now aggregate $3,632,289, not including the bequests for the Phipps Psychiatric Clinic and the Harriet Lane Johnson Home for Children.

Laboratory facilities: These facilities are in every respect unexcelled. As the institution has been from the beginning on a graduate basis, teaching and research have been always equally prominent in its activities.

Clinical facilities: The Johns Hopkins Hospital and Dispensary provide practically ideal opportunities. The medical staff of the hospital and the clinical faculty of the medical school are identical; the scientific laboratories ranged around the hospital are in close touch with clinical problems, immediate and investigative. The medical school plant is thus an organic whole, in which laboratories and clinics are inextricably interwoven. Recent foundations have greatly augmented the original hospital plant in the direction of psychiatry, pediatrics, and tuberculosis. Three hundred and eighty-five beds under complete control are now available.

The dispensary is largely attended, and is admirably conducted from the standpoint of both public service and pedagogic efficiency.

Date of visit: December, 1909.

(2) COLLEGE OF PHYSICIANS AND SURGEONS. Established 1872. An independent institution.

Entrance requirement: Less than a high school education.

Attendance: 252.

Teaching staff: 59, of whom 21 are professors, 38 of other grade. One teacher devotes his entire time to medical instruction.

Resources available for maintenance: Fees, amounting to $39,000.

Laboratory facilities: Ordinary working laboratories are provided for bacteriology, histology, and pathology, including surgical pathology; the chemical laboratory provides satisfactorily for general chemistry. The dissecting-room is fair, as far as it goes. There is no experimental pharmacology and no student work in experimental physiology. The museum consists of several hundred specimens; the library, of which there is a librarian in charge, of perhaps 1500 volumes and a few current periodicals. The undeveloped character of the laboratories is due, (1) to the payment of faculty dividends; (2) to the application of current fee income to the discharge of building debts.

Clinical facilities: The school completely controls the adjoining hospital, of which some 210 beds, including a maternity ward, are available for teaching. Wardteaching on the section plan is in use. The clinical laboratory is open to the students.

The dispensary occupies an excellent suite of rooms; the attendance is ample.

Date of visit: March, 1909.

(3) UNIVERSITY OF MARYLAND SCHOOL OF MEDICINE. Organized 1807. Essentially an independent institution with a university charter, though nominally the medical department of St. John's College (Annapolis).

Entrance requirement: Less than a high school education.

Attendance: 316.

Teaching staff: 61, of whom 24 are professors, 37 of other grade.

Resources available for maintenance: Fees, amounting to $44,530 (estimated), out of which dividends are paid to the faculty and a large mortgage debt carried.

Laboratory facilities: Good undergraduate laboratories adequate to routine teaching are provided in two poorly kept buildings for the following subjects: chemistry, physiology, including physiological chemistry and histology, pathology and bacteriology. Anatomy is poor. There is a small museum. In a separate building is a large and interesting library, but it is open only two hours each day.

Clinical facilities: The school controls its own hospital, opposite the laboratory buildings, about 140 beds being available for teaching. The hospital records are well kept, senior students who pay for the privilege serving as clinical assistants. A separate maternity ward furnishes obstetrical work in abundance.

The dispensary is large, properly equipped, and well kept.

Date of visit: March, 1909.

(4) BALTIMORE MEDICAL COLLEGE. Organized 1881. An independent institution.

Entrance requirement: Much less than a four-year high school education. Advanced standing is freely granted to failed students dropped from other schools.

Attendance: 392.

Teaching staff: 63, of whom 20 are professors, 43 of other grade. There are no teachers giving entire time to medical instruction.

Resources available for maintenance: Fees, amounting to $33,424.

Laboratory facilities: The school possesses a new and very attractive laboratory building. It is well equipped for undergraduate instruction in chemistry and pathology; inadequately for physiology and bacteriology. A large room with ample material provides for dissecting.

Clinical facilities: The school has the use of about 122 beds in a hospital which it built and has leased to the Sisters of Charity; it has access to several other institutions besides.

A suite of poorly kept rooms is set aside for a dispensary. The attendance is ample.

Date of visit: March, 1909.

(5) WOMAN'S MEDICAL COLLEGE OF BALTIMORE. Organized 1882. An independent institution.

Entrance requirement: Less than a high school education.

Attendance: 22.

Teaching staff: 31, of whom 18 are professors, 13 of other grade.

Resources available for maintenance: Fees, amounting to $2000.

Laboratory facilities: Small laboratories, scrupulously well kept, show a desire to do the best possible with meager resources: pathology, bacteriology, embryology, chemistry, and anatomy are thus taught.

Clinical facilities: These are quite insufficient: across the street from the school is a hospital with 17 beds; supplementary material is obtained at several institutions through staff connections.

A suite of rooms in the college building is devoted to dispensary purposes. There is a fair attendance.

Date of visit: March, 1909.

(6) MARYLAND MEDICAL COLLEGE. Organized 1898. An independent institution.

Entrance requirement: Nominal.

Attendance: 95. Almost one-half the school is in the senior class.

Teaching staff: 39, of whom 21 are professors, 18 of other grade.

Resources available for maintenance: Fees, amounting to $7460 (estimated).

Laboratory facilities: The school building is wretchedly dirty. Its so-called laboratories are of the worst existing type: one neglected and filthy room is set aside for bacteriology, pathology, and histology: a few dirty test-tubes stand around in pans and old cigar-boxes. The chemical laboratory is perhaps equal to the teaching of elementary chemistry. The dissecting-room is foul. This description completely exhausts its teaching facilities. There is no museum or library and no teaching accessories of any sort whatsoever.

Clinical facilities: The college faculty own and conduct a hospital within a few blocks. It is essentially a private institution, of no great value to students. Less than 50 beds are free.

The dispensary claims a fair attendance.

Date of visit: March, 1909.

(7) ATLANTIC MEDICAL COLLEGE. Organized 1891 as an independent homeopathic institution. Having "passed through many vicissitudes," it is now non-sectarian.

Entrance requirement: Nominal.

Attendance: 43, of whom 31 are in the senior class, 1 in the freshman class. Of 21 graduates, class of 1908, almost all had failed at other schools or before the regular state board before entering the Atlantic Medical College, on graduation from which they could appear before the Homeopathic State Board of Maryland, "reputed to be a much easier board to pass."

Teaching staff: 47, of whom 12 are professors, 35 of other grade. Two members of the teaching staff were graduated in the class of 1908, above mentioned, after having failed before the regular state board; a third instructor, also a graduate of 1908, entered this school after failure at the local College of Physicians and Surgeons.

Resources available for maintenance: Fees, amounting to $3905 (estimated).

Laboratory facilities: The school occupies a filthy building, in which are to be found an elementary chemical laboratory, a small room assigned to pathology, bacteriology, and histology, equipment being scant and dirty, an ordinary dissecting-room, a lecture-room with half a skeleton, a small amount of imperfect physiological apparatus with a few frogs, and a few cases of books, mostly old and useless.

Clinical facilities: These are claimed at a small private hospital several miles off. They can at best be hardly more than nominal.

The basement of the college building is used for a dispensary.

Date of visit: March, 1909.

General Considerations

THERE are seven medical schools in Maryland, a state whose population increases slowly and in which there are between two and three times as many physicians as it now requires. Of these seven schools, two belong to the worst type of American medical school, viz., the Atlantic Medical College and the Maryland Medical College. That such unconscionable concerns should at this day continue to flourish is a blot upon the state of Maryland and the city of Baltimore.

Two more of the seven schools, the Baltimore Medical College and the Woman's

Medical College, are weak; two others, the College of Physicians and Surgeons and the University of Maryland, are large commercial enterprises, whose financial responsibilities are far too extensive for their capital or fee income; the sums annually applicable to debts in order to simplify their position, or to maintenance in order to improve their teaching, are reduced by the payment of substantial dividends to practitioner teachers. Education is thus overshadowed by business. Entrance standards are low, the full-time teacher is practically unknown, the laboratories are slovenly, the atmosphere depressing.

Like Pennsylvania, Maryland has granted lump sums to private corporations engaged in charitable work. The larger ones of the six medical schools mentioned have thus combined to obtain from the state money enough to build and partly to support their hospitals. Should the state ever conduct its philanthropic business intelligently, these irresponsible methods would stop; and with them, the medical schools which they have helped to float. The Johns Hopkins Medical School, for which neither the state of Maryland nor the city of Baltimore has ever done anything, is thus the only medical school in Maryland that either ought to or can live, and to its development greatly increased means should be freely devoted.

If, meanwhile, a combination of the better independent schools of Baltimore were effected, much of their property could be disposed of, the equity being used to equip the resulting institution. A single independent school might thus have a brief and not discreditable career. In the end, however, the independent schools will pass away, in Maryland as elsewhere. To their present hospitals the Johns Hopkins would become the heir, thus greatly strengthening its clinical resources. At this date the Johns Hopkins University is the only academic institution in the state capable of conducting a modern medical school. It would be safe, interesting, and instructive to leave medical education in Maryland for a decade or two wholly in its hands. The state will not meanwhile lack for doctors; it is already overcrowded.

The prerequisite to any reconstruction of the Baltimore situation is the revision of the state law. The country affords no more conclusive proof of the viciousness of the two-board system. Not only is neither state board empowered to enforce a preliminary educational requirement, but candidates refused by the "regular" board subsequently succeed before the homeopathic board. This underground traffic is responsible for the existence of the Atlantic Medical College, a homeopathic school that has rendered itself an attractive haven of refuge to rejected "regular" students by dropping the significant word from its title.

MASSACHUSETTS

Population, 3,162,347. Number of physicians, 5,577. Ratio, 1 : 567.
Number of medical schools, 5.

BOSTON: *Population, 629,868.*

(1) MEDICAL SCHOOL OF HARVARD UNIVERSITY. Organized 1782. An integral department of Harvard University.

Entrance requirement: The student has a choice between the bachelor's degree or certain definite requirements in science and modern languages representing two years of undergraduate work, provided that in the latter case a higher passing mark is required for graduation. In the present year, out of a first-year class of 62, 60 entered with the bachelor's degree.

Attendance: The total enrolment is 285; about 69 per cent from New England, 53 per cent from Massachusetts.

Teaching staff: 173, of whom 23 are professors; laboratory instructors as a rule devote their entire time to the department.

Resources available for maintenance: The department has an endowment of $3,326,-961; the fees are merged in the general income of the school. The annual budget is $251,389, of which $72,037 are derived from tuition fees.

Laboratory facilities: The laboratories are unexcelled in equipment and organization, in respect to both teaching and research.

Clinical facilities: Abundant clinical material is available at the Massachusetts General Hospital, the City Hospital, and elsewhere. But serious restrictions are felt in two directions: (1) While the university is free to secure laboratory men wherever it chooses, it is practically bound to make clinical appointments by seniority, in accordance with the custom prevailing in the hospital which it uses, or to leave its professor without a hospital clinic. In general it follows that the heir to the hospital service is heir to the university chair. In consequence there is a noticeable lack of sympathy between the laboratory and the clinical men. They do not represent the same ideals. There is no question but that an institution of this rank ought to work in the most intimate coöperation with a hospital; and that, if such were the case, the same principles would obtain in selecting clinical teachers as prevail elsewhere in the university. (2) The extent to which hospital material can be utilized is also limited, though less in surgery than in medicine. The teaching is in the main of the demonstrative character. Something more intimate is possible in a limited way with fourth-year students. The hospital services with one exception rotate at the end of periods of four months.

The school is now installing its own dispensary, likely to be of great value in its clinical instruction.

Date of visit: October, 1909.

(2) TUFTS COLLEGE MEDICAL SCHOOL. Organized 1893. Administratively an integral department of Tufts College, though actual scientific intercourse is not intimate.

Entrance requirement: Below an actual four-year high school course, since certificates of uncertain value have been accepted and examinations used cover less than half a high school course. This is the less defensible as 97 percent of the total enrolment come from New England.

Attendance: The attendance is 884; 97 per cent from New England, 80 per cent from Massachusetts.

Teaching staff: 108, of whom 88 are professors. There are five full-time professors and five full-time assistants in pathology, histology, physiology, and chemistry.

Resources available for maintenance: The school relies on its fees, amounting to $59,098, repaying out of them large advances for buildings made out of the general income of the college.

Laboratory facilities: The laboratories are entirely adequate to the teaching work of the school.

Clinical facilities: For medical clinics the school is confined to the Boston City Hospital and the Boston Dispensary, which furnish abundant material under the usual more or less imperfect control. The Carney Hospital provides considerable additional work in surgery; the specialties are cared for in other institutions. The school is thus clinically handicapped in exactly the same way as Harvard, but to a greater degree by reason of its being restricted in its medical clinics to a single municipal hospital and dispensary. Its range of choice in the matter of clinical professors is limited by the same considerations.

Date of visit: October, 1909.

(8) BOSTON UNIVERSITY SCHOOL OF MEDICINE. Homeopathic. Organized 1878. The University connection is nominal.

Entrance requirement: A certificate of graduation from an approved four-year high school, or examination; the examination is not set by the university, but by the medical school, and is markedly below the four-year high school standard.

Attendance: Total enrolment, 90; 88 per cent from New England, about 60 per cent from Massachusetts.

Teaching staff: 64, 29 being professors.

Resources available for maintenance: The institution is mainly dependent on fees ($12,762, estimated), but these have been consistently used to develop its facilities.

Laboratory facilities: In striking contrast with schools in which, whatever the claim, fees have not been so used, this school has an excellent building, admirably kept and well equipped, and attractive laboratories for pathology, bacteriology, physiology, chemistry, and anatomy. There is no experimental pharmacology. It possesses a library in charge of a permanent librarian, a beautifully mounted collection of pathological material, an excellent refrigerator plant, and other features indicative of intelligent and conscientious effort.

Clinical facilities: The school adjoins a hospital of some 230 beds, of which 125 are available for amphitheater and ward clinics. The material is fairly abundant and varied; but students do not make laboratory examinations for the patients whom they see in the wards. A pavilion for contagious diseases is also accessible. Connected with the hospital is a large, thoroughly modern, and systematically conducted dispensary, in which laboratory work and physical examination are more closely connected.

Date of visit: October, 1909.

(4) COLLEGE OF PHYSICIANS AND SURGEONS. Organized 1882. An independent institution.

Entrance requirement : Vague.

Attendance : 172, called in the catalogue " matriculates and applicants."

Teaching staff: 30 professors and 15 lecturers.

Resources available for maintenance : Fees, amounting to $10,000 (estimated). A reduction of 20 per cent is made to students who pay in advance for the entire four years.

Laboratory facilities : These facilities are wretched : ill-lighted, dirty, and poorly equipped so-called laboratories are provided for anatomy, pathology, etc.

Clinical facilities : The clinical resources are dubious. The catalogue attempts to convey the idea (p. 21) that the school has the same opportunities as Harvard and Tufts ; as a matter of fact, no member of the faculty of the College of Physicians and Surgeons has a staff appointment in the City Hospital, and teaching there is utterly impossible otherwise. The same is true of the wards of the Massachusetts General Hospital. At both institutions anyone, whether a student or not, may attend the public amphitheater clinics once weekly. But as these are freely open to the public and are of little or no value, they are hardly to be counted as teaching facilities. A limited attendance is required at a miserable dispensary, more than an hour's journey from the college building.

Date of visit : October, 1909.

CAMBRIDGE : *Population,* 102,982.

(5) MASSACHUSETTS COLLEGE OF OSTEOPATHY. Established 1897. An independent institution.

Entrance requirement : Vague.

Attendance : 90.

Teaching staff: 34, of whom 19 are professors.

Resources available for maintenance: Fees, amounting to $11,400 (estimated).

Laboratory facilities: The school occupies a neatly kept building, in which are provided one poorly equipped laboratory in common for pathology and bacteriology, and another, similar in character, for chemistry and urinalysis, and an anatomical room. It possesses neither museum nor library. Instruction at the school building is limited to lectures, recitations, and "laboratory" work.

Clinical facilities: No "treatment" is administered in the school building. For that the students resort in their last year to the Chelsea Hospital, a pay institution of 10 to 15 beds, more than one hour's journey from the college building. Pathology is taught in the same year.

Date of visit: October, 1909.

[*For general discussion see "New England," p. 261.*]

MICHIGAN

Population, 2,666,308. Number of physicians, 4109. Ratio, 1: 649.
Number of medical colleges, 5.

ANN ARBOR: *Population, 14,734.*

(1) UNIVERSITY OF MICHIGAN DEPARTMENT OF MEDICINE AND SURGERY. Organized in 1850. An integral part of the university.

Entrance requirement: Two years of college work, including sciences strictly enforced.

Attendance: 389, 45 per cent from Michigan.

Teaching staff: 63, of whom 22 are professors. The laboratory work is wholly in charge of full-time instructors; but assistants in adequate number are lacking. The clinical teachers are salaried and owe their first duty to the school.

Resources available for maintenance: The school and the university hospital are supported mainly by state appropriation. The budget of the school is $83,000, that of the hospital, $70,000. Endowments to the extent of $175,000 carry a part of this charge. The income in fees is $34,093.[1]

Laboratory facilities: Excellently equipped laboratories are provided for all the fundamental branches; the men in charge are productive scientists as well as competent teachers. There is a large library, a good museum, and other necessary teaching aids.

Clinical facilities: The school is fortunate in the possession of its own hospital, every

[1] Including laboratory fees paid by students registered in the homeopathic department; see (2).

case in which can be used for purposes of instruction. A liberal policy has largely overcome the disadvantages of location in a small town; for the clinical material is in the departments of surgery, psychiatry, and various specialties, of sufficient amount; it is fair in medicine, increasing in obstetrics. The thoroughness and continuity with which the cases can be used to train the student in the technique of modern methods go far to offset defects due to limitations in their number and variety.

Date of visit: March, 1909.

(2) UNIVERSITY OF MICHIGAN HOMEOPATHIC COLLEGE. Organized 1875. An organic department of the university.

Entrance requirement: A four-year high school education.

Attendance: 80, 88 per cent from Michigan.

Teaching staff: 26, of whom 15 are professors.

Resources available for maintenance: The school and its hospital are supported by state appropriations. Its budget is $16,400; that of its hospital, $31,000. The income in fees is $4515.

Laboratory facilities: The students receive their laboratory instruction in common with the students of the Department of Medicine and Surgery, despite the fact that there is a difference of two years of college work in their preparation.

Clinical facilities: The college has its own hospital of about 100 beds, where clinical instruction is given according to homeopathic principles.

Date of visit: March, 1909.

BATTLE CREEK: *Population, 25,862.*

(3) AMERICAN MEDICAL MISSIONARY COLLEGE. Organized 1895. An independent institution. A divided school, part of the work being given in Chicago, part at Battle Creek. No year is given entire at either place.

Entrance requirement: A four-year high school course or its equivalent. Christians only are admitted. The Chicago teachers are all practitioners; the Battle Creek teachers are connected with the Battle Creek Sanitarium as laboratory workers or physicians.

Attendance: 75.

Teaching staff: 81, of whom 22 are professors, 9 of other grade.

Resources available for maintenance: Income from endowment of $200,000 and fees.

Laboratory facilities: Anatomy is given in Chicago, where the student spends six weeks during each of the first three years and 30 weeks of the fourth year. The other laboratory courses are given at Battle Creek by the laboratory men and physicians connected with the Battle Creek Sanitarium. Indeed, the school and the sanitarium are inextricably interwoven. Students assist in the laboratories and treatment-rooms. Their laboratory training thus takes on a decidedly practical character. But this has its disadvantages; for the sanitarium is devoted to the application of certain ideas rather than to untrammeled scientific investigation. Disciples rather than scientists are thus trained. The outfit is adequate for routine work, with abundant practical illustration in chemistry, pathology, bacteriology, and histology. In physiology and pharmacology the provision is slighter.

Clinical facilities: Of the last year, 30 weeks are spent in Chicago, where the students attend St. Luke's Hospital, one or two other institutions, and a dispensary in the school building. For additional clinical teaching they depend on Battle Creek: in the sanitarium they see an abundance of chronic and surgical cases; acute cases are rare, and are accessible chiefly when physicians can ask students to accompany them on their rounds. The clinical laboratory is closely correlated with bedside work. By assisting in the sanitarium and out, the student gets an unusually close experience as far as it goes, but, once more, under the limitations of the therapeutic theories approved by the sanitarium authorities; a critical and investigative spirit is not cultivated.

The instructors of the divided parts of the school form practically separate faculties.

Date of visit: February, 1910.

DETROIT: *Population, 393,536.*

(4) DETROIT COLLEGE OF MEDICINE. Organized by merger 1885. An independent institution.

Entrance requirement: A four-year high school diploma or its equivalent, actually enforced.

Attendance: 161, 70 per cent from Michigan (16 per cent from Canada).

Teaching staff: 104, of whom 25 are professors and 79 of other grade. There are no full-time teachers.

Resources available for maintenance: Fees only, amounting to $22,000 (estimated).

Laboratory facilities: The school is provided with separate laboratories, each with ordinary routine equipment, for the following subjects: chemistry, anatomy, physiology, pathology, clinical microscopy, histology, and bacteriology. There is a slight additional equipment in the way of museum, charts, books, and other teaching adjuncts.

Clinical facilities: The school has access on the usual terms to several hospitals, staff members of which hold positions on the school faculty. The hospital service rotates every three months. At one hospital 100 available beds are perhaps equally divided between medicine and surgery; elsewhere surgery greatly predominates. Obstetrical work is mainly furnished by the Woman's Hospital and by an out-patient department just started. Post-mortems are hard to get. The dispensary service is fair.

Date of visit: December, 1909.

(5) DETROIT HOMEOPATHIC COLLEGE. Organized 1899. An independent school.

Entrance requirement: A four-year high school course or its equivalent.

Attendance: 34.

Teaching staff: 35, of whom 17 are professors, 18 of other grade.

Resources available for maintenance: Fees, amounting to $3010 (estimated).

Laboratory facilities: These are wretched. There is an ordinary laboratory for chemistry; another, much less than ordinary, for bacteriology. The pathological room contained a few dozen specimens in utter disorder; the anatomical room contained a single cadaver. The teaching-rooms are bare, except for chairs and tables; the building is poorly kept. The dean and the secretary have their offices "downtown."

Clinical facilities: The school has access to Grace Hospital, the wards of which contain 56 beds, mostly surgical. Clinics are held two days weekly. The hospital authorities are well disposed towards the school, but the "boys don't take advantage of their opportunities."

There is a dispensary at the school building. It is incredibly bad. Prescriptions are found written on scraps of paper, unnumbered. There are no systematic records.

Date of visit: December, 1909.

General Considerations

MICHIGAN is fortunate in the possession of an alert state board, which enforces with vigor the high school requirement, and may perhaps be counted on to advocate an advance of the state practice standard to meet the educational standard of the state university. As the state furnishes a thoroughly admirable education at relatively slight expense, there is no reason why it should keep the practice of medicine open to low-grade physicians, whether trained within or without its borders. Sound policy would quickly close the two homeopathic schools and, in all probability, the Detroit College of Medicine. To the credit of the latter institution, however, be it said that its officers have heartily coöperated with the state board in the enforcement of a genuine high school standard.

The real problem now agitating the state concerns the medical department of the state university at Ann Arbor. The defects of Ann Arbor as the seat of a medical school have been touched on in these pages. There is no question that, if the entire state university were at Detroit, the medical department would be better off. But this is by no means equivalent to urging that it be detached or split. The entire detached school is now on trial at Galveston, Indianapolis, New York. It would be well to watch the outcome of those experiments before trying any others. It is already clear that if a university department of medicine is to be genuinely productive, the remote department requires most generous support; for much that is provided at the seat of the university for other departments will have to be duplicated. To create the university spirit in a distant institution is almost like developing a second — though much less expensive—university.

An alternative suggestion looks to the removal to Detroit of part or all of the clinical instruction. If part is removed, clinical teachers must oscillate backward and forward between Detroit and Ann Arbor. Where would the productive clinical teacher have his workshop? Nowhere, in all likelihood. If the entire clinical department is removed, the split school faces the conditions we encounter in Nebraska, California, and Kansas. Once more, let us wait for the successful operation of one of these divided schools before multiplying unpromising experiments. Meanwhile, the state can by increased liberality almost at will develop the medical clinic of the university hospital. Agitation in favor of splitting or removing it may proceed from several considerations,—it is not inspired by sound scientific or educational ideas.

For, Ann Arbor has itself proved what the experience of Germany had previously demonstrated,—that a school of medicine can be developed in a small university town. The ideals are there; the contiguous departments are there; there is an absence of the distractions which have thus far proved so damaging to city clinicians. A faculty of distinction, with a hospital well equipped for the care of the sick, and for teaching and research, can successfully overcome the most serious difficulties of the situation. The problem can be solved by intelligent organization and liberal support. Gaps may indeed remain in the student's experience. But if he has been well drilled in technique and method, his defects will be readily cured by a hospital year. The solution for Michigan may therefore come, as has been proposed, through an effective affiliation of the hospitals of the state with the school of medicine of the state university. The hospitals would profit by a connection of this kind, and they would assist by becoming factors in the education of the future physicians of the state.

MINNESOTA

Population, 2,162,726. Number of physicians, 2204. Ratio, 1 : 981.
Number of medical schools, 1.

MINNEAPOLIS–ST. PAUL: *Population*, 552,211.

(1) UNIVERSITY OF MINNESOTA COLLEGE OF MEDICINE AND SURGERY. Organized in 1883, it has step by step absorbed all other medical schools in the state, including (1909) the homeopathic department of the university. Elective courses in homeopathic

materia medica and therapeutics are offered on condition that students following them shall receive the degree of Doctor of Medicine in Homeopathy.

Entrance requirement: Two years of college work, specifically including the fundamental sciences and a modern language.

Attendance: 174 , 83 per cent from Minnesota.

Teaching staff: 49 professors and 71 of other grade,—total, 120.

Resources available for maintenance: State appropriations. The budget calls for $71,336. The income from fees is $16,546.

Laboratory facilities: Excellent, exceedingly attractive, and well organized laboratories are provided for all the scientific branches. The State Laboratory of Public Health is practically part of the school plant. The instruction is in charge of full-time teachers, generously supplied with books, apparatus, and material.

Clinical facilities: The school has hitherto relied on the municipal hospitals and unpaid clinical teachers, with the usual results. Teaching opportunities were both limited in extent and precarious in character. These institutions are in fact not organized, equipped, or conducted with educational requirements in mind. An appropriation has now been made to build a teaching hospital; and a small temporary hospital has been started. Simultaneously, the clinical teaching has been reorganized by placing the chiefs in medicine and surgery respectively on salaries that command the interest and effort of active teachers. The same policy must be applied generally throughout the clinical department.

The dispensary, well attended and long loosely conducted, has recently been reconstructed along the same lines.

Date of visit : May, 1909.

General Considerations

MINNESOTA is perhaps the first state in the Union that may fairly be considered to have solved the most perplexing problems connected with medical education and practice except as to osteopathy. It has indeed still to realize its plans for an adequate clinical establishment of modern character; but there is little doubt that this is only a question of time,—and of a short time, at that. Meanwhile medical education has, with the active coöperation of the state board, been concentrated in the hands of the university, fortunately situated in the heart of the largest community of the state; the state has got rid of rival schools, regular and sectarian, the latter by a perfectly fair provision for separate instruction in sectarian dogmas for any student who is willing to accept a diploma qualified so as to mark that fact. Since all else—anatomy, physiology, surgery—are common to and the same for all " schools " of medicine, there is one standard of admission to the department, one quality of instruction, one examination for the degree for all alike. Finally, the educational preliminary qualification of the state medical school has become the practice preliminary of the state. In future, any person desiring to practise medicine in Minnesota must get as good an education — preliminary and professional — as the state furnishes and requires of its own sons : a regulation both fair and wise, whether viewed from the standpoint of the student or from the broader standpoint of public interest, to which all else is properly subordinate. Henceforth, the success of the school will depend largely on the generosity of the state in developing the clinical teaching, and on the character of the hospital and dispensary which it organizes with that in view.

MISSISSIPPI

Population, 1,786,773. Number of physicians, 2054. Ratio, 1: 887.
Number of medical schools, 2.

MERIDIAN : *Population, 22,415.*

(1) MISSISSIPPI MEDICAL COLLEGE. Organized 1906. A stock company.

Entrance requirement: Nominal.

Attendance: 100, 94 per cent from Mississippi.

Teaching staff: 19, of whom 12 are professors, 7 of other grade.

Resources available for maintenance: Fees, amounting to $7500 (estimated).

Laboratory facilities: At the date of visit, there was no outfit at all. Subsequent reliable report credits the school with a vat containing four cadavers in a room without other contents, a simple outfit for elementary chemistry, and twenty brand-new microscopes, but no material to use with them.

Clinical facilities: Practically none. Some of the faculty have places on the staff of a small hospital over a mile distant.
There is no dispensary.

Date of visit: January, 1909.

OXFORD–VICKSBURG: (*Population:* Oxford, 2104; Vicksburg, 16,800).

(2) UNIVERSITY OF MISSISSIPPI, MEDICAL DEPARTMENT.[1] A divided school. First half organized 1903; second half organized 1909. An organic part of the university.

Entrance requirement: A four-year high school education or its equivalent. Over one-half of this year's entering class had had two or more years of college work.

Attendance: 39.

---

[1] As this report goes to press, it is announced that the clinical end of this school (at Vicksburg) is discontinued. The first two years will continue to be given at Oxford.

Teaching staff: At Oxford, 8 professors, 3 of whom give entire time to this department, and 3 assistants; at Vicksburg, 6 professors and 10 of other grade.

Resources available for maintenance: The department shares the general funds of the university. Its budget calls for $15,000. Fees amount to $3500.

Laboratory facilities: (Oxford.) Laboratories, adequate to the needs of the instruction offered, are provided for physiology, pharmacology, histology, and anatomy; pathology and bacteriology are less satisfactory. Chemistry is well cared for in the university laboratory. The teachers need a larger number of competent assistants and helpers; a beginning has been made towards a departmental library.

Clinical facilities: (Vicksburg.) The clinical end has been so recently started that no attempt will be made here to deal with it. It will probably be discontinued.

Date of visit: November, 1909.

General Considerations

OF the two schools, that at Meridian is without merit. At a time when the state has already more doctors than it needs, the starting of a didactic school, conducted by the local practitioners of a small town, is absolutely unjustifiable. The state laws ought to be promptly amended so as to make such ventures impossible.

The state is indeed not favorably situated for the entire training of its own doctors. The state university, the only institution to which the task could fall, is unfortunately located. Its present experiment with a divided school is even more problematical than similar ventures elsewhere; for to the inherent disadvantage of division is to be added the fact that Vicksburg itself is a small town. Moreover, the first half of the school, at Oxford, though distinctly creditable, is far from satisfying its faculty. It is a question whether the university would not do more wisely to concentrate its outlay on the Oxford branch.

Up to this time, the medical profession of Mississippi has been educated mainly in the proprietary schools of the southern states. It would be fortunate indeed if henceforth its members should get at least their first two years at Oxford. To make itself the main factor in the education of the physicians of the state, the university should keep its entrance requirement in touch with the secondary school system. Its present and prospective facilities do not really warrant a higher requirement. Besides, it can perform a more useful service by training a relatively large body of students at the high school level than by training a few on a higher standard. McGill and Toronto do not prove that a high school standard is as good as a college standard; but they do prove that where a high school standard, or even less, is enforced, well chosen teachers, well equipped and liberally sustained laboratories, are capable of producing a very useful type of physician. The present duty of the southern state universities is not to press prematurely to a standard that either cannot be enforced or that, if enforced, will relegate the main army of students to medical schools without either facilities or ideals, but to endeavor themselves to get hold of a sufficient body of students to meet the demand on an enforceable basis, to improve their facilities so that this number can be well trained, and to urge the legislature to make their standard the practice standard of their respective states. Under more favorable circumstances, a decade hence, the state can and should ask more. But just now it is more important to develop the medical department of the state university at the high school level than to push it higher, leaving the training of southern physicians to schools without ideals or resources.

MISSOURI

Population, 3,491,397. Number of physicians, 6323. Ratio 1: 552.

Number of medical schools, 12 (*plus* 1 postgraduate school).

COLUMBIA: *Population, 7302.*

(1) UNIVERSITY OF MISSOURI SCHOOL OF MEDICINE. A two-year school. Organized 1872. An organic department of the university.

Entrance requirement: One year of college work.

Attendance: 47, all from Missouri.

Teaching staff: 14, 8 being professors, 6 of other grade.

Resources available for maintenance: The department shares the general income of the university. Its budget calls for $31,000; fees amount to $2820.

Laboratory facilities: The medical department occupies a new and well equipped building, excellently adapted to its purposes. The teaching is in charge of full-time instructors of modern training and ideals. A university hospital of 45 beds gives the department the advantage of clinical material and connection, even though the actual instruction is limited to the work of the first two years, a feature of great importance. There is a library, supplied with important current periodicals, domestic and foreign.

Date of visit: April, 1909.

KANSAS CITY: *Population, 205,022 (plus Kansas City, Kan., 81,052).*

(2) UNIVERSITY MEDICAL COLLEGE. Organized 1881. An independent institution.

Entrance requirement: Less than a high school education.

Attendance: 174, 82 per cent from Missouri and Kansas.

Teaching staff: 65, 30 being professors, 35 of other grade. There is one full-time teacher.

Resources available for maintenance: Fees, amounting to $17,600 (estimated).

Laboratory facilities: A single large laboratory is set aside for chemistry of all kinds, and urinalysis: huge bottles are furnished instead of separate reagent sets; histology, pathology, and bacteriology occupy a second room, equipped for routine work in each of these branches. Physiology is similarly provided for. There is the usual dissecting-room, large, clean, and well lighted. There are no books. There is a small museum and a large supply of pathological material.

Clinical facilities: Adjoining the school is the University Hospital, most of the work of which is surgery; but as there are no free beds, it is of no real use to students. The main reliance for clinical instruction is the City Hospital, a beautiful modern structure, in which clinics are held, mainly in the amphitheater, one day weekly from 8 to 12. The school has no access to the clinical laboratory, to autopsies, obstetrics, or infectious diseases, but an out-patient department and a Rescue Home furnish obstetrical opportunity in abundance. Other institutions furnish additional material. The school dispensary — fairly clean — has a large attendance; but it is poorly equipped and loosely conducted. The clinical facilities are, therefore, unsatisfactory in both quality and extent.

Date of visit: November, 1909.

(3) KANSAS CITY HAHNEMANN MEDICAL COLLEGE. Homeopathic. Organized 1888, an independent institution.

Entrance requirement: Less than a high school education.

Attendance: 59.

Teaching staff: 41, of whom 33 are professors, 8 of other grade.

Resources available for maintenance: Fees only, amounting to $5900 (estimated).

Laboratory facilities: All laboratory work is conducted by one teacher, who serves in the same capacity in the local eclectic and osteopathic schools. The chemical laboratory is small and poor; that for pathology, histology, bacteriology, and embryology, urinalysis and blood work combined, is worse — meagerly equipped and in utter disorder. Anatomy had not as yet started (November). There are a few books.

Clinical facilities: Amphitheater instruction is given one morning a week at the City Hospital.

In the school building is a small dispensary, with an estimated attendance of 6 or 7 a day. A neatly kept card index is employed.

Date of visit: November, 1909.

(4) CENTRAL COLLEGE OF OSTEOPATHY. Established 1902. An independent institution.

Entrance requirement: Nominal.

Attendance: 40.

Teaching staff: 20. ·

Resources available for maintenance: Fees only, amounting to $4500 (estimated).

Laboratory facilities: Practically none at all: hopelessly meager appointments in two rooms are denominated respectively chemical and pathological laboratories. Dissection was not in progress at the time of the visit. It is held that "students ought to know anatomy before they dissect,—they get more out of it." A single cadaver. was dissected in September and October; another was expected in February.

Clinical facilities: A pay-dispensary is operated, senior students giving "treatments" to patients who pay three dollars a month. Students may on payment of fee attend public clinics at the City Hospital, but the school has no hospital facilities or connections of its own at all.

Date of visit: November, 1909.

KIRKSVILLE: *Population,* 8422.

(5) AMERICAN SCHOOL OF OSTEOPATHY. Established 1892 and owned by two individuals.

Entrance requirement: Less than a common school education.

Attendance: 560 (ranging in age from 18 to 54 years).

Teaching staff: 12, with 11 student assistants.

Resources available for maintenance: Fees, amounting to $89,600 (estimated).

Laboratory facilities: These are absurdly inadequate for the number of students, as is likewise the teaching staff. A single room, with a corresponding preparation room, is used as bacteriological and physiological laboratory, a six weeks' course being given by one teacher to successive squads of 32. In the same way separate additional laboratories are provided for chemistry, anatomy, and pathology. Material for pathological demonstration is bought; there is no museum, and no effort is made to save gross material. The dissecting-room is foul. The "professors" in charge of histology, pathology, and bacteriology are senior students.

Clinical facilities: A hospital of 54 beds adjoins, but its work is practically all "surgery;" the ward cases are "occasionally used for clinics. Students witness operations." Obstetrical work is comparatively scanty. There is no other hospital in the town.

A large dispensary is operated. An instructor is at hand the first time the student administers a "treatment;" after that, "only if summoned." A course of twenty lectures on the fallacies of medicine is given, so that the graduate will know why he does not use "drugs."

The school is a business in which a large margin of profit is secured by its owners. The teaching furnished is of the cheapest kind. Its huge income is therefore largely profit.

Date of visit: November, 1909.

ST. JOSEPH: *Population, 132,954.*

(6) ENSWORTH MEDICAL COLLEGE. Organized in 1876, it has twice merged with other schools. An independent institution.

Entrance requirement: Less than a four-year high school education.

Attendance: 72, 68 per cent from Missouri.

Teaching staff: Numbers 40, 32 being professors, 8 of other grade.

Resources available for maintenance: Fees only, amounting to $7060 (estimated).

Laboratory facilities: These are very weak. The chemical laboratory is of elementary character; there is a small outfit for physiological demonstration; a single room with little material is provided for pathology, bacteriology, and histology. There is the usual ill kept dissecting-room. There is no museum, books, or teaching accessories. The building is very dirty.

Clinical facilities: These are wholly inadequate. The adjoining hospital, containing six free beds, is of little use. Fifty beds, of which 14 were occupied at the time of visit, are accessible at a Catholic institution, but four-fifths of its work is surgical. Obstetrical work is entirely inadequate; post-mortems are very rare. The available material, scant as it is, is poorly used, as far as teaching is concerned.

There is a small dispensary, without records, organization, or equipment.

Date of visit: November, 1909.

ST. LOUIS: *Population, 698,706.*

(7) WASHINGTON UNIVERSITY MEDICAL DEPARTMENT. Organized 1842. United in 1891 with Washington University, of which it has been since 1907 an organic department. Completely reorganized on modern lines 1910.

Entrance requirement: Four-year high school education. Credentials are passed on and examinations conducted by the university.

Attendance: 178, 60 per cent from Missouri.

Teaching staff: 99, 48 being professors, 51 of other grade. There had been four full-time professors and a few full-time assistants, but as this report goes to press, the entire faculty is undergoing reconstitution. All the laboratory branches, as well as the departments of medicine, surgery, and pediatrics, have been already reorganized on a strict university basis.

Resources available for maintenance: The school shares the general funds of Washington University. Its fee income is $21,000; its budget (1909–10) $51,265, (not including $30,000 spent on the University Hospital). Productive endowments to the extent of $1,500,000 will become available in 1910–11.

Laboratory facilities: These have hitherto sufficed for only routine work in the fundamental branches, but the reorganization on productive modern lines, already under way, will shortly be completely effected. The museum, though small, is good; a start towards a modern medical library has been made.

Clinical facilities: The school has its own hospital of 98 beds, one-fourth of them free; and has access to other hospitals on the usual footing. The amount of material thus available was fair; but the close affiliation which has been made with the trustees of the Barnes and the Children's Hospitals revolutionizes the clinical situation of the school.

The school controls two dispensaries,—one connected with the University Hospital, the other situated in the medical school building. Their combined attendance is very large.

Date of visit: April, 1909.

(8) St. Louis University. The school, organized 1901 by merger, was in 1903 purchased for cash by the university, of which it is now an organic part.

Entrance requirement: Less than a high school education.

Attendance: 243, 42 per cent from Missouri.

Teaching staff: 121, 39 being professors, 82 of other grade. There are six full-time instructors with competent helpers; but the assistants are as a rule students.

Resources available for maintenance: Fees, amounting to $26,630 (estimated), supplemented by small allotment from the university treasury. During a period of seven years (1903–10), the university devoted $40,817 to its medical school. $20,000 have been recently subscribed towards an endowment fund for the department.

Laboratory facilities: Excellent teaching laboratories are provided for all the fundamental branches, in addition to which provision has been made for research in several directions.

Clinical facilities: The school has a small hospital of its own (12–16 free beds), and has access on the usual terms to several other institutions. The material, while fair in amount, is scattered and under imperfect control. The hospitals used are not organized, equipped, or conducted with a view to the requirements of modern medical teaching.

The dispensary is fair.

Date of visit: April, 1909.

(9) St. Louis College of Physicians and Surgeons. Organized 1869. An independent institution.

Entrance requirement: Nominal.

Attendance: 224.

Teaching staff: 49, of whom 25 are professors, 24 of other grade.

Resources available for maintenance: Fees only, amounting to $16,035 (estimated).

Laboratory facilities: The school occupies a badly kept building, the inner walls covered with huge advertisements. A single ordinary laboratory is provided for chemistry; there is a make-believe laboratory for experimental physiology; for the school owns the equipment stipulated by the state board, though the dust-covered tables do not indicate use. Rows of empty reagent bottles are also to be seen. The "museum" consists of some cheap photographs and drawings and a few badly preserved wet specimens,—all carefully arranged so as to occupy as much space as possible. Microscopes appear to indicate a laboratory of pathology or bacteriology; but the "individual lockers" were empty. It was explained that "students have to bring slides, holders, and cover-glasses with them, for they furnish their own and keep them at home." Anatomy was "over"—only empty tables were found in the dissecting-room, the sole access to which is by way of a fire-escape.

Clinical facilities: A small, poorly lighted, badly ventilated, and overcrowded hospital is part of the school building. Its operating amphitheater is good. Clinics of slight value are also held at the City Hospital. A few other opportunities of inferior importance are obtained in the usual way.

A dark and dingy suite of rooms serves for a dispensary. The room devoted to gynecology, for instance, is without a window, and contains no equipment except a deal table covered with a sheet.

The school is one of the worst in the country.

Date of visit: April, 1909.

(10) Barnes Medical College. Organized 1892. An independent institution.

Entrance requirement: Less than a high school education.

Attendance: 124.

Teaching staff: 64, of whom 39 are professors, 25 of other grade.

Resources available for maintenance: Fees only, amounting to $12,400 (estimated).

Laboratory facilities: A huge "chemical laboratory, the largest in the world devoted to medical education," is the most striking feature; its equipment suffices for elementary work only; another large room with ordinary equipment is devoted to bacteriology, histology, and pathology. A physiological laboratory is equipped in literal compliance with the state board stipulations. The dissecting-room is spacious and well lighted. There is no museum; few books and few teaching accessories.

Clinical facilities: These are wholly inadequate. The Centenary Hospital, adjoining the school, is without educational importance. Its work is mainly private and almost altogether surgical. The school has access to the City Hospital, too, but its clinics, held one afternoon a week, are of little value.

The college buildings contain a suite of rooms used as a dispensary. A considerable attendance is claimed, but the arrangements are shockingly bad. The rooms are in poor condition and almost devoid of proper equipment.

Date of visit: April, 1909.

(11) AMERICAN MEDICAL COLLEGE. Eclectic. Organized 1873. An independent school.

Entrance requirement: Nominal.

Attendance: 28.

Teaching staff: 28, of whom 25 are professors.

Resources available for maintenance: Fees, amounting to $3801 (estimated).

Laboratory facilities: Meager equipment is provided for anatomy, chemistry, pathology, and bacteriology. A small amount of apparatus for physiology demonstration, as required by the state board, is displayed in a case. There is no suggestion of use.

Clinical facilities are equally scanty. A weekly clinic can be held at the City Hospital; the rest depends on the professor's connections.

A dispensary room is also provided, and "almost every day some one comes."

Date of visit: April, 1909.

(12) HIPPOCRATEAN COLLEGE OF MEDICINE. A night school. An independent institution, in its third year.

Entrance requirement: Nominal.

Attendance: 31.

Teaching staff: 30 professors, 8 of other grade.

Resources available for maintenance: Fees, amounting to $3315 (estimated).

Laboratory facilities: A brand-new outfit is visible in the shape of a few microscopes, physiological apparatus, chemical reagents, etc. But though two classes were in session, none of the equipment was in use, nor did its appearance indicate previous use. One of the classes mentioned was receiving eloquent didactic instruction in osteology, the other in anesthesia.

Clinical facilities: Being not yet needed, these are not yet arranged for.

Date of visit: April, 1909.

KANSAS CITY:

(13) POSTGRADUATE HOSPITAL SCHOOL. This institution has a hospital of 25 ward beds, containing 15 patients,—2 medical, 13 surgical. There were no students in attendance at the date of the visit. The institution is really a private hospital, but incorporation as a school gives its faculty privileges at the City Hospital.

Date of visit: April, 1909.

General Considerations

MEDICAL education in Missouri is at a low ebb. The state board lacks authority to enforce even a high school preliminary,—the more regrettable as, under the stimulating influence of the state university, an excellent high school system has been developed. Missouri is therefore in the attitude of requiring every boy and girl who wishes to attend the state university to spend four years in good secondary schools supported by the people, but men and women who are charged to safeguard public health may attend medical schools chartered by the state without the assurance of any definite training whatever.[1] In consequence, the state is badly overcrowded with practitioners trained in poor schools, and still maintains some of the poorest schools in the country. Utterly wretched are (1) Kansas City Hahnemann Medical College, (2) Central College of Osteopathy, (3) American School of Osteopathy (Kirksville), (4) St. Louis College of Physicians and Surgeons, (5) American Medical College, (6) Hippocratean College of Medicine; feeble and without promise are (7) Barnes Medical College, (8) Ensworth Medical College, and (9) University Medical College, though the last named is distinctly superior to the other eight. There remain the two-year school conducted by the state university, the medical department of Washington University, and the St. Louis University School of Medicine.

There are in the state of Missouri fifty-odd academic institutions, of which only two have resources adequate to support medical schools, viz., the state university and Washington University. Of the several towns in the state capable of supplying clinical material, only one—St. Louis—contains a strong resident university. Washington University, St. Louis, is therefore at this writing marked out as the natural patron of medical education in Missouri.

Its importance is bound to be more than local. Aside from its obvious possibilities as a productive scientific center, Washington University must be the main factor in the training of physicians for the southwest country; the city of St. Louis has in this section an even clearer opportunity than has Chicago in the middle west, New York in the east, or Boston in New England. For there is no other large city

[1] That is what a certificate from a county school commissioner amounts to, no matter what it pretends to certify.

south of Minneapolis or as far west as the Pacific which as completely meets all the requirements of the case.

There is abundant evidence to indicate that those interested in Washington University appreciate its "manifest destiny;" it bids fair shortly to possess faculty, laboratories, and hospital conforming in every respect to ideal standards. It is, however, worth asking whether it may not supplement its own resources by some form of coöperation. The state university formerly conducted a four-year school at Columbia; realizing that its clinical instruction could not without immense expenditure be brought to the present level of the scientific years, it has had the wisdom and courage to confine its efforts to the first two years. The easy expedient of a clinical end at Kansas City or elsewhere, it has with equal wisdom and firmness rejected. Its resources and influence, however, may not impossibly be enlisted in behalf of the medical work of Washington University, for the latter institution is in position to use effectively whatever can be placed at its disposal. Should St. Louis University receive financial support enabling it to enforce the same entrance standard as the other two institutions mentioned, it also would be wise to forego clinical instruction, turning over its students in their last two years to Washington University. A second clinical establishment on the same scale is neither desirable nor likely. Nor will St. Louis University or its students be permanently satisfied with an old-fashioned clinical department superposed on its modern laboratory foundation.

NEBRASKA

Population, 1,069,579. Number of physicians, 1776. Ratio, 1: 602.

Number of medical schools, 3.

LINCOLN–OMAHA : (*Population:* Lincoln, 53,667; Omaha, including South Omaha, 164,519).

(1) COLLEGE OF MEDICINE, UNIVERSITY OF NEBRASKA. Organized 1881. Affiliated in 1902 with the state university, of which it is now an organic part. A divided school, the first two years being given at the university (Lincoln), the last two at Omaha.

Entrance requirement: Two years of college work.

Attendance: 122.

Teaching staff: 84, of whom 38 are professors, 46 of other grade. The laboratory branches are taught by full-time teachers, using in the main student or practitioner assistants.

Resources available for maintenance: The department is supported by state appropriations. Its income in fees for the year ending June, 1909, was $4905; its budget amounts to $20,612, reckoning only items due directly to the medical department.

Laboratory facilities: (Lincoln.) The department has the necessary laboratories, on the whole fairly equipped. The instructors are active men of modern training, eager to do research work. They are, however, in position to accomplish little in this direction for lack of space, proper assistance, and funds. The opportunities are nevertheless adequate for good routine undergraduate teaching. Animals are provided in abundance; there is a good library and a fair collection of necessary teaching adjuncts.

Clinical facilities: (Omaha.) The school has the privilege of the County Hospital for half the year, and staff privileges at the Methodist Hospital and several other institutions. These institutions are, of course, not equipped or conducted with regard to teaching. For example, the clinical pathologist of the school is not now a member of the staff of either institution; in consequence of which fact, the teaching of this important branch is isolated. Section visits are, however, arranged. There is little scientific intercourse or pedagogical interplay between the severed laboratory and clinical ends at Lincoln and Omaha respectively.

The dispensary has a fair attendance, but is not well organized.

Date of visit: April, 1909.

(2) LINCOLN MEDICAL COLLEGE. Eclectic. Organized 1890. Nominally the medical department of Cotner University.

Entrance requirement: Nominal.

Attendance: 42, 77 per-cent from Nebraska.

Teaching staff: 34, all of whom are professors.

Resources available for maintenance: Fees, amounting to $3794 (estimated).

Laboratory facilities: There are practically no laboratory facilities beyond a separate room set aside for dissecting and the meager chemical laboratory of Cotner University. Some little microscopical work may also be carried on at the latter institution.

Clinical facilities: There are no definite clinical opportunities, not even a dispensary.

Date of visit: April, 1909.

OMAHA

(3) JOHN A. CREIGHTON MEDICAL COLLEGE. Organized 1892. Integral part of Creighton University.

Entrance requirement: Less than a four-year high school education.

Attendance: 175.

Teaching staff: 49, 28 of whom are professors, 21 of other grade. One teacher devotes his entire time to medical instruction.

Resources available for maintenance: Mainly fees, amounting to $17,850 (estimated).

Laboratory facilities: Student laboratories, with individual equipment adequate to routine instruction, are provided for chemistry, pathology, histology, and bacteriology; the professors of the last three subjects have private laboratories besides. The provision for anatomy is poor; it comprises an ordinary dissecting-room and a lecture-room, equipped with a papier-mâché model, charts, a defective skeleton, and some odds and ends of bones. The outfit for experimental physiology and pharmacology is small. Animals are obtained as needed. There is a small museum and a small library. Quiz-compends are sold on the premises.

Clinical facilities: The school has access to several hospitals where clinical material is obtained. Its use is subject to the customary limitations. The main hospital is two miles from the school. Though 90–100 beds are there available for ward teaching, students cannot work in the clinical laboratory of the hospital. Opportunities at the other hospitals are not considerable.

Several large and well arranged rooms in the college building are used for dispensary work, one hour daily. The attendance is fair.

Date of visit: April, 1909.

General Considerations

In Nebraska, as in most of the western states, the hope of sound instruction in medicine lies with the state university. There is apparently no other institution in the state which can confidently count on spending much more on a medical department than fees bring in, though Creighton has succeeded in obtaining gifts for building purposes. The problem confronting the state university, however, is not simple. It has undertaken to require two years of college work for entrance, while the state law does not contemplate the enforcement of even a high school standard. The strengthening of the law, by way of backing the state university, ought not, however, to be difficult, for the eclectic school is surely without influence and Creighton has promised to come to the higher standard in 1910.

A more perplexing problem arises from the division of the state university department between Omaha and Lincoln. The edges of the two halves do not now touch. If our position in respect to divided schools is correct, the state must choose between wholly dropping clinical instruction and organizing a complete school on one of the two sites now partially occupied. An entire department at Omaha seems at this moment the more feasible.

NEW ENGLAND

The medical schools of Massachusetts, Maine, Vermont, New Hampshire, Connecticut (nine in all), may profitably be considered together, for the reputable ones among them are largely engaged in training local students, 85 per cent of their enrolment coming from this section. At present, the ratio of physicians to population in this section is 1: 592, not reckoning osteopaths. The section is thus badly overcrowded with physicians; and as population is increasing slowly, there is no possibility that its increase will within a generation bring about a satisfactory adjustment. In the matter of distribution, the usual conditions prevail: cities and small towns are alike oversupplied.[1]

It is clear, then, that New England will need no more physicians for years to come; it can of course begin none too soon the process of substituting a higher grade of physician for what it now has. To bring about a gradual reconstruction of the profession, it is important that certain legal changes be promptly made. Massachusetts, for example, remains one of three states which obstructs the improvement of medical education by permitting non-graduates to be examined for license. The law should not only require graduation from a reputable medical school, but should, in the interest of the public, fix with due warning a minimum basis for admission thereto, as Connecticut has wisely done, and should empower and require the state boards to refuse examination to graduates of schools whose facilities are inadequate. Of course, a thorough practical examination would still further increase the effectiveness of the boards in protecting the public against ill trained practitioners.

If, now, the law prescribed a thorough knowledge of physics, chemistry, and biology —surely feasible in New England if feasible in Minnesota and Indiana —as the minimum basis of medical education, attendance in medical schools would promptly shrink in number and improve in quality. A more critical attitude on the part of the state boards and the student body in reference to the educational advantages offered by the several schools would probably result in a reconstruction of the situation somewhat along these lines:

A thoroughly wretched institution, like the College of Physicians and Surgeons of Boston, would be at once wiped out. The clinical departments of Dartmouth, Bowdoin, and the University of Vermont would certainly be lopped off; there is no good reason why these institutions —colleges all of them—should be concerned with medicine at all. The mere fact that they are all old schools is a poor reason for continuing them if they fail to do justice to the student, and thereby fail to subserve

[1] By way of example, the following are cited at random:

		population	number of physicians
Massachusetts: *State ratio,* 1: 567	Onset Westport	621 900	4 3
Maine: *State ratio,* 1: 600	Saco Springfield Lisbon Falls	6270 582 200	14 2 3
New Hampshire: *State ratio,* 1: 651	Centerville Lisbon Orford	88 2100 794	2 6 3
Vermont: *State ratio,* 1: 584	Plainfield Newhaven Randolph	940 640 2000	3 3 8
Connecticut: *State ratio,* 1: 740	Stetney Depot Suffield	480 3400	2 7
Rhode Island: *State ratio,* 1: 784	Centerdale Thornton Wickford	970 415 1515	2 2 4

the public interest. They originated as didactic schools, and as such were quite as well off in small communities as anywhere else. They find themselves now compelled to teach clinical medicine by practical methods. They cannot command the necessary material nor the financial resources required to procure it. Why should either the students or the public make a sacrifice merely to enable them to continue, when it is easily possible for both to do better? The argument that these small schools train all-round doctors who go out into the country, prepared to do everything, is refuted by the obvious fact that schools, unable to command obstetrical cases, contagious diseases, and the ailments that throng dispensaries, are not really sending out the type of practitioner which, by their own admission, the rural districts need.

Whether even Boston will or should continue to support two regular schools— Harvard and Tufts—is decidedly doubtful. The enrolment of Tufts, even on the high school basis, is much swollen. The strict enforcement of that standard—and why should it not be enforced?—will greatly reduce the attendance. The inevitable elevation of requirements will still further cut it down. The school has no resources but fees; out of them it cannot possibly provide for the legitimate demands of the near future. It is difficult to see how the department in question can avoid being seriously crippled; for its remarkable prosperity has depended to no slight extent on the inducement held out by low entrance standards. Its only hope of escape is through endowment, first, so that it may develop its laboratories independently of fee income, next, that it may secure its own hospital. Why should such an expensive step be recommended? If New England is in future to be supplied with high-grade doctors, the quickest and cheapest road to that end is to complete Harvard and to develop Yale, rather than to maintain several more or less imperfect institutions. Whatever may once have been the case, local competition needs no longer be relied on to expose defects and to stimulate improvement. Keen scientific and educational emulation over a wide area provides a sharper incentive and involves no waste. It is, therefore, of supreme importance that higher standards be legalized in New England and that the clinical independence of the Harvard Medical School be established. The medical department of Yale is modestly working in the same spirit and to the same end. To these two institutions the future of medical education in New England may for many years to come be safely left.

New Hampshire

Population, 443,140. Number of physicians, 680. Ratio, 1 : 651.
Number of medical schools, 1.

HANOVER : *Population*, 1951.

DARTMOUTH MEDICAL SCHOOL. Organized 1798. The medical department of Dartmouth College.

Entrance requirement: A four-year high school education.

Attendance: 58, 91 per cent from New England.

Teaching staff: 24, of whom 17 are professors, 7 of other grade. There are two professors giving entire time to medical subjects, viz., pathology, bacteriology, and physiology. Chemistry, botany, embryology, and comparative anatomy are taught in the regular college laboratories. Ten clinical professors and one lecturer are nonresident.

Resources available for maintenance: The department is carried by the general resources of Dartmouth College. The income in fees is $5583 (estimated).

Laboratory facilities: Excellent working laboratories are provided for pathology, bacteriology, histology, physiology, and for the medical subjects cared for in the academic department. Every student serves four weeks during his second year as assistant in the pathological laboratory and thus gets an admirable practical experience. Anatomy, taught by a practitioner, has not as yet been developed on modern lines. There are good departmental libraries, supplied with books and current periodicals, foreign and domestic.

Clinical facilities: These are very limited. The college controls a hospital of 40 beds, of which 24 are in wards at reduced rates. These are available for teaching; to some extent private cases may also be demonstratively used. Still further to weaken the teaching value of the hospital, surgery predominates to the extent of 80 per cent of all cases. Students are employed to assist in surgical operations, but the backbone of clinical instruction — an adequate clinic in internal medicine—is lacking.

An isolation pavilion of fourteen beds for college use is employed for teaching as occasion presents. For obstetrical work, students sojourn for a period in Boston or New York. There are 12–14 post-mortems a year.

There is no dispensary.

Date of visit: March, 1910.

General Considerations

DARTMOUTH is already providing excellent modern instruction in most of the work of the first two years. The development of its clinical work presents a serious difficulty. The village is rather inaccessible; the surrounding country is thinly populated, —containing perhaps 50,000 people in a zone 100 miles north and south. Surgical cases are attracted easily enough. Can medical cases be attracted too? Certainly not without a very large outlay in the form of professional salaries and hospital expense. To what extent a compulsory fifth year spent as interne in a large hospital would answer in compensation of defective facilities is a question: much depends on the hospitals available for the purpose. That the school cannot much longer continue in its present stage is clear: for with the requirement of two years of college work for entrance in 1910, it asks a student to spend six years to get a degree in medicine, in attaining which he can enjoy only a very limited opportunity to learn internal medicine. It is safe to predict that on that basis the present facilities will not hold the student body together during the third and fourth years.

[*See "New England," p. 261.*]

NEW YORK

Population, 8,706,039. Number of physicians, 14,117. Ratio, 1: 617.

Number of medical schools, 11, *plus* 4 postgraduate schools.

ALBANY: *Population*, 101,461.

(1) ALBANY MEDICAL COLLEGE. Organized 1838. Nominally the medical department of Union University; actually an independent institution in all but form.

Entrance requirement: The Regents' Medical Student Certificate.

Attendance: 180, 91 per cent from New York state.

Teaching staff: 94, of whom 16 are professors, 78 of other grade. The professor of chemistry, the associate professor of physiology, and the director of the Bender Laboratory are non-practitioners.

Resources available for maintenance: Practically fees only, amounting to $20,276. $10,000 have been bequeathed to the school as the nucleus of a building fund.

Laboratory facilities: The Bender Laboratory, at a considerable distance from the school,—with endowment sufficient to keep up insurance and repairs,—provides instruction in pathology, bacteriology, histology (not including embryology), clinical microscopy, and a small amount of demonstrative work in physiology. There is no course in pharmacology. The head of the laboratory is pathologist to the Albany Hospital and other institutions; autopsies are thus procured. The laboratory has made itself practically self-supporting through board of health and similar work. The college, after equipping it, now contributes to its support no more than it absolutely must in order to keep it going. In consequence, there is now little active research in progress.

At the medical school building good laboratories are provided for chemistry and physiological chemistry, and the usual dissecting-room with a few charts, models, etc. Otherwise equipment is scant. The laboratory branches have been slighted in pursuance of the policy of paying annual dividends to the faculty.

Clinical facilities: The main clinical reliance is the Albany Hospital, in which perhaps 200 beds are available. But three-fourths of the work of the hospital is surgery. The service in medicine and surgery rotates every three months. On the medical side, students work up assigned cases. In general surgery, students can only "look on." They have no access to the obstetrical ward, though students serving as externes are allowed to observe free cases. Other institutions furnish supplementary material in obstetrics, pediatrics, mental diseases, etc.

The school uses two dispensaries: that at the hospital is unimportant; the South End Dispensary has a fair attendance and is conducted in an orderly manner.

Date of visit: January, 1910.

BROOKLYN: *Population,* 1,543,630.

(2) Long Island College Hospital. Organized 1858. An independent institution.

Entrance requirement: The Regents' Medical Student Certificate.

Attendance: 360, 89 per cent from New York state.

Teaching staff: 94, 9 being professors, 85 of other grade. There is no full-time instructor belonging to the school.

Resources available for maintenance: Fees, amounting to $61,398. Practically this amount is supplemented by advantageous arrangements to be described below in connection with laboratory and clinical facilities.

Laboratory facilities: The Hoagland Laboratory (endowment $131,000), independent of but affiliated with this school, sets aside a suite of rooms, in which pathology, bacteriology, and histology are taught to medical students. The college is thus partly relieved of the expense involved in the equipment and teaching of these branches. The opportunities provided are of routine character. The research work of the laboratory and its teaching are entirely distinct.

The college itself contains a good and well kept dissecting-room, in which drawing and modeling are employed, and two good, though ordinary, chemical laboratories.

There is no library, no museum, no physiological or pharmacological laboratory, though a demonstration course in physiology is offered. Freed from the necessity of providing certain laboratories, fees might have been used to provide others; instead of that, the surplus is annually divided among the faculty. What gifts have not provided, the college goes on lacking.

Clinical facilities: The school adjoins, and is legally one with, the Long Island College Hospital, with 200 beds usable in teaching. The hospital, though new, is not designed to serve modern ideas in medical teaching. It lacks adequate laboratories; specimens must be carried by students to the college building for examination.

For dispensary purposes, the college gets the use of the Polhemus Clinic, built at a cost of $500,000, having a productive endowment of $400,000.

The entire plant—school and clinic—is admirably kept.

Date of visit: March, 1909.

BUFFALO: *Population,* 401,441.

(3) UNIVERSITY OF BUFFALO MEDICAL DEPARTMENT. Organized 1846. Despite the university charter, the University of Buffalo is a fiction. Schools of medicine, law, dentistry, and pharmacy are aggregated under the designation; but they are to all intents and purposes independent schools, each living on its own fees.

Entrance requirement: Admission is on the basis of the Regents' Medical Student Certificate, being the equivalent of a high school education.

Attendance: 193.

Teaching staff: 97, of whom 38 are professors.

Resources available for maintenance: Fees amounting to $31,984.

Laboratory facilities: The school has a conventionally adequate equipment for anatomy, ordinary laboratories for chemistry, bacteriology, and pathology, a meager outfit in physiology,—it having been found that the students cannot profitably do much experimental work themselves,—nothing for pharmacology. The "whole-time" teachers have in the main other duties besides teaching in medicine: the professor of pathology and bacteriology is registrar, the chemist officiates in the pharmacy department, the anatomist in the dental department. There is a small museum, but a good library of 8000 volumes, current German and English periodicals, with a librarian in charge.

Clinical facilities: For clinical teaching, the school relies mainly on the Buffalo General Hospital close by. It has access to some 200 beds, used for demonstrative teaching in the wards. Records are made by internes. Students do no clinical laboratory work in connection with special patients, the teaching in clinical microscopy being separately given at the college. Infectious diseases are didactically taught. Clinical obstetrics is imperfectly organized. Besides the Buffalo General Hospital, a weekly clinic is held at the County Hospital, four miles distant, four clinics at the Sisters' Hospital, one and a half miles away, etc.

Despite the size of the city, the college dispensary is wretched. It has an attendance of perhaps 3000 during the college year, skin, eye, and ear cases mainly. A definite statement is impossible because there are no systematic records. The rooms are ill equipped. Records consist of brief pencil notes in separate books, usually without index. The work is hastily and superficially done, and its influence on the students, so far as it goes, must be thoroughly bad. The catalogue states, however, that as attendance in the dispensary is obligatory, each student "will secure an unusually thorough training in the taking and recording of histories."

Date of visit: October, 1909.

NEW YORK: *Population, 4,563,604.*

(4) COLLEGE OF PHYSICIANS AND SURGEONS. The Medical Department of Columbia University. Organized in 1807; affiliated with Columbia College 1860; an organic part of Columbia University since 1891.

Entrance requirement: The Regents' Medical Student Certificate, which must include physics and chemistry. Of the present first-year class of 86, 48 have the bachelor's degree, 11 more have had at least two years of college work: the department is therefore already close to the two-year college basis, which goes into effect 1910–11.

Attendance: 312, 56 per cent from New York state.

Teaching staff: 176, of whom 38 are professors, 138 of other grade.

Resources available for maintenance: The department has special endowments amounting to $832,351. Fees amount to $75,500. The budget calls for $239,072, including maintenance of Sloane Maternity Hospital and the Vanderbilt Clinic.

Laboratory facilities: The school laboratories are of modern equipment and organization, conducted by full-time instructors, amply assisted. Teaching and research are thus actively prosecuted in all departments. Anatomy deserves to be especially mentioned, as perhaps the most elaborate plant of its kind in the country. The school lacks a general library, though books and periodicals are available in several departments and in the students' study.

Clinical facilities: The school is admirably situated in respect to the Sloane Maternity Hospital (to which gynecology is now to be added) and the Vanderbilt Clinic (dispensary), which adjoin it and are under its control. Both philanthropically and pedagogically, they are effectively conducted on modern lines.

In other respects, the clinical department labors under the disadvantages common to the schools of New York. The situation will be more fully discussed below; suffice it here to say that various hospitals furnish an abundance of clinical material of all kinds under limitations that interfere with effective scientific or pedagogic use, and make exceedingly difficult anything like intimate interplay between laboratory and clinical teaching. Nowhere has the school rights; at Bellevue (municipal hospital), custom establishes a qualified security, liable, however, to be disregarded; elsewhere the basis is purely personal. Permission has recently been obtained to institute clinical clerking in a few places.

Date of visit: October, 1909.

(5) CORNELL UNIVERSITY MEDICAL COLLEGE. Organized 1898. An organic department of Cornell University.

Entrance requirement: Three years of college work.

Attendance: 207.

Teaching staff: 132, 32 being professors, 100 of other grade.

Resources available for maintenance: The department is liberally supported. Its budget (New York city) calls for $209,888; income from fees, $24,410; Ithaca: budget, $32,840; income from fees is negligible.

Laboratory facilities: The school laboratories in New York are, in general, of modern equipment and organization, anatomy and chemistry being, however, less elaborately developed than physiology and pathology. The professor of anatomy is a practising surgeon. Otherwise the laboratories are in charge of full-time teachers, properly assisted, devoting themselves unreservedly to teaching and research. Despite geographical separation from the university at Ithaca, the department is animated by university ideals: in part, this is ascribable to actual intercourse, in part, to the selection of teachers devoted to science, whom the university has so generously supported that they have reproduced the university spirit. At Ithaca—the seat of Cornell University—the first year's instruction is also offered: the departments of anatomy and physiology as there organized and conducted are thoroughly admirable, with their own additional teaching staff, supported by separate funds.

Clinical facilities: The major part of the clinical instruction is given at the Bellevue Hospital, directly opposite the college, in which the school enjoys the same privileges as Columbia and New York Universities. The service is good in point of extent; limitations which render it unsatisfactory will be discussed below. Supplementary hospitals increase the amount of available material, but always under serious pedagogic restrictions. Intimate correlation of laboratories and clinic is thus not feasible.

A thoroughly satisfactory dispensary, well conducted, occupies part of the school building.

Date of visit: February, 1910.

(6) UNIVERSITY AND BELLEVUE HOSPITAL MEDICAL COLLEGE. Formed in 1898 by merger of University Medical College (established 1841) and Bellevue Hospital Medical College (established 1861). An integral part of New York University.

Entrance requirement: The Regents' Medical Student Certificate, representing a four-year high school education.

Attendance: 408, 74 per cent from New York state.

Teaching staff: 164, 37 being professors, 127 of other grade.

Resources available for maintenance: The school is mainly dependent on fees, amounting to $76,115; these are supplemented by gifts and income from endowment amounting to about $11,000.

Laboratory facilities: The laboratories are developed unevenly, as the resources of the school are not equal to uniform promotion of all the medical sciences. Pathology is excellently organized and equipped both for teaching and research; in other branches good teaching facilities rather than any considerable opportunity for investigation have been aimed at. The departments of pathology, physiology, pharmacology, and chemistry are in charge of full-time teachers. Anatomy, including histology and embryology, has just been reorganized on the same basis. Available laboratory accommodations are being largely increased by an addition now in process of erection.

Clinical facilities: The major part of the clinical instruction is given at Bellevue Hospital, opposite the college, in which the school enjoys the same privileges as Cornell and Columbia. The service is good in point of extent. Limitations which make it unsatisfactory will be discussed below. Supplementary hospitals increase the amount of available material, but always under serious pedagogic restrictions. Intimate correlation of laboratories and clinic within the hospital is thus not feasible.

A thoroughly satisfactory dispensary, well conducted, occupies part of the school building.

Date of visit: November, 1909.

(7) FORDHAM UNIVERSITY SCHOOL OF MEDICINE. Organized 1905. An organic part of Fordham University.

Entrance requirement: Something over a four-year high school education.

Attendance: 42, 83 per cent from New York state.

Teaching staff: 72, of whom 32 are professors, 40 of other grade. Two instructors give their entire time to the medical school. Chemistry and physiology are taught in the university by full-time teachers.

Resources available for maintenance: Fees, amounting to $7330 (estimated 1908–9), supplemented by appropriations amounting to several thousand dollars annually from the general funds of the university.

Laboratory facilities: Chemistry and physiology are explained above. The equipment in pathology, bacteriology, and histology is adequate for the routine instruction of the small student body. Anatomy is limited to dissection. There is a library with current scientific journals.

Clinical facilities: Much of the clinical work of the school is carried on at Fordham Hospital, a municipal institution close by; the school has no voice in making its staff appointments. Supplementary opportunities are obtained at other institutions,—scattered, as is generally the case, with the medical schools of the city. The amount of material available is adequate, but it cannot be organized or controlled.

There is a good and growing dispensary service connected with Fordham Hospital.

Date of visit: October, 1909.

(8) NEW YORK MEDICAL COLLEGE AND HOSPITAL FOR WOMEN. Homeopathic. Organized 1863. An independent school.

Entrance requirement: Regents' Medical Student Certificate, equivalent to a four-year high school course.

Attendance: 24.

Teaching staff: 45, 23 being professors, 22 of other grade. No teacher devotes entire time to the school.

Resources available for maintenance: Fees, amounting to $2545.

Laboratory facilities: Attractive and well kept laboratories are provided for pathology, bacteriology, and histology together, chemistry and physiology and anatomy. The equipment is simple, but recent. There are a small library, a number of anatomical charts, and some normal and pathological preparations. Autopsy material is reported as scarce.

Clinical facilities: These consist of the hospital, occupying the same building and containing 35 available beds, most of the cases being surgical, and of the usual rotating services scattered among other hospitals, public and private. They do not include infectious diseases.

Most of the first floor of the school building is given over to a dispensary.

Date of visit: October, 1909.

(9) ECLECTIC MEDICAL COLLEGE. Organized 1865. An independent school.

Entrance requirement: Regents' Medical Student Certificate.

Attendance: 96, 84 per cent from New York state.

Teaching staff: 45, 16 being professors, 29 of other grade. No one devotes full time to teaching.

Resources available for maintenance: Mainly fees, amounting to $8311.

Laboratory facilities: The chemical laboratory, adequate for routine teaching, is active. Otherwise the facilities are weak: one room is used for bacteriology, histology, pathology, and clinical microscopy; this with the dissecting-room completes the laboratory outfit. There is no museum; but the school possesses a small collection of models, a materia medica cabinet, a stereopticon, and a fair-sized library, of which the books are mostly not recent.

Clinical facilities: There is no eclectic hospital. Twice weekly three students spend their entire afternoon at the Sydenham Hospital (80 free beds). There are some supplementary clinics of the usual kind. There is a small dispensary in the school building and an outside dispensary is also used. The clinical facilities are utterly inadequate in respect to both extent and control.

Date of visit: March, 1909.

(10) New York Homeopathic Medical College and Flower Hospital. Organized 1858. An independent institution.

Entrance requirement: Regents' Medical Student Certificate.

Attendance: 159, 88 per cent from New York.

Teaching staff: 65, of whom 31 are professors, 34 of other grade. The professors of chemistry, physiology, pathology, and bacteriology are full-time teachers.

Resources available for maintenance: The school and hospital budgets are combined. The institution has an endowment of $600,000, which carries a hospital of 125 free beds, dispensary with ambulance service, etc. Income from student fees amounts to $18,658.

Laboratory facilities: An attractive, well kept laboratory with models and bone-mounts is provided for anatomy; a single laboratory for chemistry; one, with a small museum, for pathology and histology; and others, with ordinary equipment, for bacteriology and physiology. There is a library of several thousand volumes.

Clinical facilities: Though the school possesses its own hospital, clinical teaching has not hitherto been so organized as to take the fullest advantage of it. The records are meager; the clinical laboratory inadequate. Improvements are, however, under way.

The dispensary enjoys a very large attendance.

Date of visit: December, 1909.

SYRACUSE: *Population, 127,281.*

(11) College of Medicine, Syracuse University. Organized 1872. An integral department of the university.

Entrance requirement: A year's work in science in addition to the Regents' Medical Student Certificate. Credentials are passed upon by the academic authorities. Of the present class of 40, the first on the new basis, 20 had had a year or more of college work; the rest presented high school or preparatory school certificates in the required sciences.

Attendance: 151, 90 per cent from New York state.

Teaching staff: 57, of whom 15 are professors and 42 of other grade. The sciences are taught by full-time teachers.

Resources available for maintenance: Income, almost wholly from fees, amounting to $28,861.

Laboratory facilities: Chemistry is well cared for in the university laboratories. The equipment in anatomy, physiology, pathology, including clinical microscopy and bacteriology, is adequate for instruction; the income of the school has been consistently and intelligently used to develop these departments. They are all in charge of full-time teachers, each provided with a competent helper. There is a good library, in charge of a librarian, but no museum.

Clinical facilities: Clinical facilities have not yet been put on the same modern basis as the laboratory branches. They are insufficient in respect to both extent and control. The school relies mainly on two local hospitals of about 150 beds, providing ward and bedside work in general medicine, surgery, and pediatrics, surgery predominating. The hospitals do not contain a working clinical laboratory for students. Supplementary opportunities are provided by several other institutions in the usual manner. The work in obstetrics is not sufficient.

Students attend the city dispensary, which is, from an educational point of view, of doubtful value. It has an attendance of 10,000; but the records, though systematic, are so brief that the experience would hardly conduce to thorough and careful habits. The head clinical professors have apparently been indifferent to it.

Date of visit: October, 1909.

POSTGRADUATE SCHOOLS

(1) BROOKLYN POSTGRADUATE MEDICAL SCHOOL. Established 1907.

Entrance requirement: The M.D. degree.

Attendance: Students are scarce; four or five may be in attendance at any one time.

Teaching staff: 52, of whom 19 are professors, 33 of other grade.

Resources available for maintenance: Fees.

Laboratory facilities: None.

Clinical facilities: The school offers graduate courses mainly in the Williamsburg Hospital, most of the cases in which are surgical. The hospital itself is wretched and has no teaching facilities worth mentioning. It is even without a clinical laboratory.

The existence of the school is a reproach to the state. It now operates on a limited charter from the state department of education, and is enabled to continue because it is aided by the city. It deserved no charter in the first place, and it deserves no recognition from the city now.

Date of visit: January, 1910.

(2) NEW YORK POSTGRADUATE SCHOOL. Established 1881.

Entrance requirement: The M.D. degree.

Attendance: There is an average attendance of 90 students in winter, 50 in summer. Short courses, usually six weeks in length and of a practical nature, are given. Formerly, the so-called "general" ticket was most popular; now, specialties are in demand and the medical courses are gaining on the surgical.

Teaching staff: 156, of whom 38 are professors, 118 of other grade.

Resources available for maintenance: The school, long without productive resources, has recently received a gift of $1,600,000, which, after paying debts and providing needed extensions, will leave a productive endowment of perhaps $400,000.

Laboratory facilities: These are very meager. A single room is devoted to laboratory work; little or no research or experimental work is carried on.

Clinical facilities: The Postgraduate Hospital is of modern construction and is excellently conducted. It contains 225 beds, 75 per cent of which are free. The new building will add 170 beds and space for clinical and laboratory teaching. Other hospitals are also used.

There is a good dispensary, very largely attended.

Date of visit: January, 1910.

(3) NEW YORK POLYCLINIC MEDICAL SCHOOL AND HOSPITAL. Organized 1881.

Entrance requirement: The M.D. degree.

Attendance: 25 to 50 students are in attendance usually.

Teaching staff: 149, of whom 24 are professors, 125 of other grade.

Resources available for maintenance: Fees.

Laboratory facilities: There is a pathological laboratory for practical work.

Clinical facilities: Postgraduate instruction is offered in the Polyclinic Hospital (100 beds), in the dispensary, which is largely attended, and in a considerable number of other hospitals, with which members of the faculty are connected as staff officers. The instruction is practical in character.

Date of visit: December, 1909.

(4) MANHATTAN EYE, EAR, AND THROAT HOSPITAL POSTGRADUATE SCHOOL. Established 1869. An independent institution.

Entrance requirement: The M.D. degree.

Attendance: There is an average attendance of 12 students. Courses range from one to six months or more in length. Students who attend at least three months are eligible to appointment as clinical assistants.

Teaching staff: 11.

Resources available for maintenance: Fees and income from endowment of $170,000, the latter yielding income sufficient to carry mortgage.

Laboratory facilities: These consist of two laboratories, one for pathological, the other for bacteriological, examinations.

Clinical facilities: There is an excellent modern hospital, with 125 ward beds. The teaching is demonstrative and practical in character, though assistants enjoy larger opportunities.

The dispensary has a very large daily attendance.

Date of visit: April, 1910.

General Considerations

NEW YORK has a double duty and a double opportunity in medical education. It must in the first place produce most of its own physicians and a considerable share of those who practise in neighboring states, which, like New Jersey, are without medical schools. Its eleven medical schools have so energetically done their part in this matter that New York itself and all the adjoining states are suffering from plethora.[1] There is, therefore, no section of the Union which is at this moment readier for an upward step: population is comparatively well distributed, communication is easy, roads are good, educational facilities abundant, and doctors superabundant. In the city of New York the two-year college requirement can be met at Columbia, New York University, and without expense at the College of the City of New York. Students outside the metropolis are, up to a certain number, similarly cared for by Cornell University.

But New York may be fairly asked to do more than produce doctors, however excellent the type. Its vast hospital and university resources should make it the Berlin or Vienna of the continent; a genuinely productive contributor to medical progress; the center to which, in the intervals of a busy life, physicians will repair to freshen their knowledge and to renew their professional youth; to which the young graduate from the interior — from the schools of Pittsburgh, Ann Arbor, Madison, Iowa City — will look for the extension of his scientific and clinical experience.

Little has as yet been done to realize this opportunity. The postgraduate schools are of very limited scope; the great New York schools have been in the main clinically unproductive. Why?

The reason is a matter of history. The schools that are now called university departments grew up as proprietary institutions. They have never been adequately financed. They obtained, and still obtain, their clinical facilities at each other's expense: that is to say, what one gets, the other loses. In the Bellevue Hospital a *modus vivendi* was found by division, with an arrangement that enables two schools to watch and obstruct the third and a lay board to oversee all three; in the great

[1] The ratios prove this: New York, 1 : 617; New Jersey, 1 : 950; Delaware, 1 : 906; Connecticut, 1 : 740; Rhode Island, 1 : 724; Vermont, 1 : 534.

private hospitals personal considerations nominate the staff, and the school subsequently negotiates with the appointees. Competition, professional and institutional, has molded the hospital situation, and in consequence clinical faculties are organized on a personal rather than a scientific or educational basis. Doubtless if Columbia, New York University, and Cornell had at this moment a free hand, they would retain some of their clinical teachers in their present positions. But at bottom this is a fortunate accident rather than a natural result: it just happens that some competent teachers find themselves in prominent hospital positions; but the system is not designed to pick them out. In the event of their withdrawal, their successors in the hospital would not be sought on the basis of scientific eminence, and if not in the hospital, then not in the school. Under these conditions, the schools can hardly be said to have ideals, policy, or genuinely organized departments, except by fortunate accident. For the nonce, there may be a continuous medical service here, clinical clerks there, post-mortems elsewhere. But the favoring conditions are perishable. The schools skate on thin ice. An accident may shatter the arrangement and convert a "department" into a congeries of courses lacking unity in conduct and aim. Indeed, most of the clinical departments now conform to just this description: there are a half-dozen professors of medicine and surgery in place of one; and no possibility of team-work on their part.

For many years nothing more than this was asked; but meanwhile the school point of view has changed. Doubtless there are professors who are satisfied to go on producing doctors and to let other institutions produce knowledge; but the productivity of the first and second years has suggested another ideal. The problems of clinical medicine have been the more sharply formulated as the pathologist and the bacteriologist have passed up to the clinician the results of their own scientific activity. The teachers of medicine must attack these problems. To attack them, they require quite another environment. The *modus vivendi* which enabled rival schools to lecture in the same hospitals does not provide the conditions in which a clinical scientist can work.

We have now suggested two results that medical schools in New York must attain: (1) they must make doctors in sufficient number; (2) they must actively participate in the advance of medical science. If the standpoint previously expounded is correct, the same institutions must do both. Of the eleven medical schools now existing in the state, only the bona-fide university departments can then expect to survive: outside of New York city, Syracuse University alone has just now a chance. The schools of Buffalo, Albany, and Brooklyn belong to the past. None of the three has even yet entirely emerged from the fee-dividing stage. Syracuse, with a smaller total fee income than any of them, devotes every dollar to the development of the fundamental branches and has fairly earned support from outside.

Of the New York city schools, Columbia and Cornell alone have at this moment any financial strength. Neither of them, indeed, is in actual possession of sufficient endowment; but there is little reason to doubt that what is additionally requisite will be forthcoming. New York University is much less secure. Its maintenance at its present level is conditioned on adherence to a lower admission standard than is scientifically justifiable or educationally necessary. It cannot much longer resist the upward trend; for its scientific faculty—and thence the initial stimulus comes—is apt to chafe under the limitations which the lower standard imposes. Whether on the higher basis the school will be a permanent factor in the situation is thus largely a question of adequate support from the outside in the next few years. None of the other local schools have at this date a substantial foundation of any sort.

The ground being thus cleared, the clinical difficulty still presses. Institutional competition is reduced; but personal and professional competition remain. Why should non-schoolmen freely retire for the sake of schoolmen? The situation is curiously deadlocked. The school faculties are not now made up on educational lines, —they cannot be. If the number of schools were reduced to two or three, it would still be true that their clinical faculties would in the main be constituted of men very much like the more important men omitted from them. Such being the case, the hospitals and the doctors naturally refuse to yield to the universities; and until they do yield, the universities cannot freely reconstruct their clinical branches. The faculty men would themselves doubtless make common cause with the outsiders as against a university which asks a free hand in order to bring in a body of clinical teachers from the outside. The usual hospital staff will not vacate for the present type of clinical faculty, because the faculty lacks commanding scientific and pedagogical preëminence; nor will the present faculties surrender to the universities for the purpose of enabling the latter to fill the places with men of another type.

Under these circumstances, palliation may perhaps come through some coöperative effort. Tension and friction will at least decrease as the number of schools diminishes. Clinical teaching in the municipal hospitals, perhaps, could then be controlled under some form of federation. The vast resources of these great institutions might under combined management form a great postgraduate and special clinic; and the municipal authorities might conceivably relax, for the common benefit of a single organization and for the glory of a great enterprise, restrictions which they have found necessary in dealing with several institutions engaged simultaneously in training boys. Unquestionably such action would bring the present postgraduate schools into the university, where they ought to be.

With this arrangement consummated, however, the schools still lack teaching hospitals in which the undergraduate student can be vigorously disciplined while his freely chosen teachers are themselves engaged in intensive clinical research. The teaching hospital must be in close geographical proximity to, and in the most intimate intercommunication with, the scientific laboratories. In the case of Columbia, every physical and educational condition is already satisfied by Roosevelt Hospital: the scientific laboratories, the dispensary, the maternity hospital, are on one side of the street; the general hospital on the other. Together they would form an ideally compact and complete plant. That they are not so operated cannot but be deplored as a tragic mischance. It is to the world at large of no consequence how they happened to drift apart. There are interests at stake that are entitled to outweigh all personal and historic considerations.

That an effective affiliation is feasible between a department of medicine and an endowed hospital, Western Reserve and Lakeside Hospital assuredly prove, just as Toronto proves the same as between a medical school and a municipal hospital. There are in New York city a dozen hospitals, each of them capable of becoming a teaching hospital in the best sense of the term. Their usefulness from every point of view would increase in precisely the measure in which they lend themselves to this function. They are already comfortable and indeed charming retreats for the sick and injured. Why should they be satisfied to be that, and nothing more? They are favorably known to the poor and to the philanthropic of New York city; and they are deservedly proud of their repute. Is it a defect of intelligence or of imagination that prevents them from reaching out for more substantial laurels? Perhaps neither, so much as a disinclination to depersonalize the hospital staff management; for depersonalization, in hospital management as in faculty appointments, each involving the other, is the condition precedent to reconstitution of medical education in New York. Without sacrificing a jot of their local distinction, without limiting in the slightest degree their usefulness to the sick poor, the New York hospitals may — any or all of them — win a place as scientific laboratories beside Guy's and St. Bartholomew's, the Royal Infirmary of Edinburgh, the Charité of Berlin, the Hôtel-Dieu of Paris. Mount Sinai, the Presbyterian, St. Luke's, and Roosevelt Hospitals might under such conditions be familiar names in medical science; as well known to the progressive clinicians of St. Petersburg, Vienna, Edinburgh, St. Louis, and San Francisco, as they are to the stricken widows of the East Side of New York city itself. What the Sloane Maternity Hospital wisely does for a single department, the general hospitals can do for general medicine and surgery. The great universities on the ground can be trusted with the opportunities and responsibilities which effective affiliation would give them. In the absence of such affiliation, separate endowment, procured for the purpose, must provide teaching hospitals in which the universities will be supreme. Would any contend that these hospitals are likely to be less admirably conducted than the unattached hospitals we have named? or that the university faculty of medicine, freely recruited, is likely to prove a less competent staff than present methods procure?

The issue is one that cannot be much longer fought off: Columbia and Cornell are already graduate schools in medicine. Their laboratories produce a high-grade student, to whom the university is bound to furnish a clinical opportunity of the same quality. Neither school can now do it. An effective affiliation, or endowment adequate to support a teaching hospital and a scientific medical faculty, is therefore their immediate need and desert.

North Carolina

Population, 2,142,084. Number of physicians { 1761 (Amer. Med. Direct.). Ratio, 1:1216; 1932 (Polk). " 1:1110.
Number of medical schools, 4.

CHAPEL HILL: *Population,* 1181.

(1) UNIVERSITY OF NORTH CAROLINA MEDICAL DEPARTMENT. A half-school. Established 1890. An organic part of the university.

Entrance requirement: A year of college work — not, however, strictly enforced during this, the first session in which it has been required.

Attendance: 74; 95 per cent from North Carolina.

Teaching staff: 15, of whom 10 are professors who take part in the work of the department. The instructors are trained, full-time teachers.

Resources available for maintenance: The department is provided for in the university budget. Its budget calls for $12,000. Its income in fees is $6500.

Laboratory facilities: The laboratories at Chapel Hill are in general adequate to good routine teaching of the small student body. The equipment covers pathology, bacteriology, histology, physiology, and pharmacology. Anatomy is inferior. Animals are provided for experimental work. The general scientific laboratories of the university are excellent; a small annual appropriation is available for books and periodicals. The work is intelligently planned and conducted on modern lines.

Date of visit: February, 1909.

CHARLOTTE: *Population,* 36,320.

(2) NORTH CAROLINA MEDICAL COLLEGE. Organized 1887, it has given degrees since 1893. A stock company; professorships are represented by stock and can be sold subject to the concurrence (never yet refused) of the faculty.

Entrance requirement: Nominal.

Attendance: 94, 87 per cent from North Carolina.

Teaching staff: 32, of whom 19 are professors, 13 of other grade.

Resources available for maintenance: Fees, amounting to $8345 (estimated), a large part being required to carry a building mortgage and to retire the debt.

Laboratory facilities: These comprise a poor chemical laboratory, containing one set of reagents, a wretched dissecting room, and a meager outfit for pathology, bacteriology, and histology. There is no museum, no library, and no teaching aids of any kind whatever. No post-mortems are even claimed.

Clinical facilities: The school, in virtue of a subscription, holds four weekly clinics at a colored hospital of 35 beds; other hospital connections are unimportant. Obstetrical cases are rare.

There is a poor dispensary, with a small attendance, in the school building. It occupies a fair suite of rooms.

Date of visit: February, 1909.

WAKE FOREST: *Population, 900.*

(3) WAKE FOREST COLLEGE SCHOOL OF MEDICINE. A half-school. Organized 1902. An integral part of Wake Forest College.

Entrance requirement: Two years of college work, actually enforced, but resting upon the irregular secondary school education characteristic of the section.

Attendance: 53.

Teaching staff: 6 whole-time instructors take part in the work of the department; two of them devote their entire time to medical instruction.

Resources available for maintenance: The budget is part of the college budget. Fees amount to $2225.

Laboratory facilities: The laboratories of this little school are, as far as they go, models in their way. Everything about them indicates intelligence and earnestness. The dissecting-room is clean and odorless, the bodies undergoing dissection being cared for in the most approved modern manner. Separate laboratories, properly equipped, are provided for ordinary undergraduate work in bacteriology, pathology, and histology, and the instructor has a private laboratory besides. Chemistry is taught in the well equipped college laboratory; physiology is slight; there is no pharmacology. There is a small museum; animals, charts, and books are provided.

Date of visit: February, 1909.

RALEIGH : *Population, 20,533.*

(4) LEONARD MEDICAL SCHOOL. Colored. Organized 1882. An integral part of Shaw University.

Entrance requirement: Less than four-year high school education.

Attendance: 125.

Teaching staff: 9, of whom 8 are professors, one of other grade.

Resources available for maintenance: Mainly fees and contributions, amounting to $4721, practically all of which is paid to the practitioner teachers.

Laboratory facilities: These comprise a clean and exceedingly well kept dissecting-room, a slight chemical laboratory, and a still slighter equipment for pathology.

There are no library, no museum, and no teaching accessories. It is evident that the policy of paying practitioners has absorbed the resources of a school that exists for purely philanthropic objects.

Clinical facilities: These are hardly more than nominal. The school has access to a sixteen-bed hospital, containing at the time of the visit three patients. There is no dispensary at all. About thirty thousand dollars are, however, now available for building a hospital and improving laboratories.

Date of visit: February, 1909.

General Considerations

THE state of North Carolina makes a comparatively satisfactory showing in the matter of ratio between population and physicians; but this may, perhaps, in some measure be due to the fact that practitioners, unlicensed and unregistered, exist undisturbed in the remote districts. It is futile to maintain a low standard in order to prepare doctors for those parts; for the graduates, instead of scattering to them, huddle together in the small towns already amply supplied. It is admitted that all eligible locations are overcrowded. There is not the slightest danger that the necessary supply of doctors would be threatened if, for instance, the practice of medicine in the state were pitched on the plane of entrance to the state university; higher than that it probably ought not to be at this time.

The standard suggested — any real standard whatsoever, indeed — would quickly dispose of the thoroughly wretched Charlotte establishment. No clinical school would remain in the state. The two half-schools — at Wake Forest and at the state university — are capable of doing acceptable work within the limits of their present resources. Both of these schools now require college work for entrance. Is this step to be generally recommended at this time to southern universities with medical departments? Without attempting to arrive at a decision, it may be pointed out that there are two sides to the question. On the one hand, the college requirement is essential to the symmetrical development of the medical curriculum; on the other, a good medical course can be given at an actual high school level, provided that facilities and teaching are developed to a high point of efficiency. How will the university best serve the state,— by training a small number at the higher level, or by getting actual control of the state situation on a high school basis before pushing ahead to a basis just generally feasible in more highly developed sections of the country? The University of Michigan is only now requiring college work for entrance; it became a strong school of immense influence in its own community on a lower basis. Undoubtedly it is right now to go to the higher standard; perhaps it should have done so earlier. But its present efficiency and influence show— as McGill and Toronto show — that if a lower standard is felt to be a reason for better teaching and not an excuse for poor teaching, an institution unfavorably located for the initiation of the higher standard can do good work on the lower basis. In the south now is it more important to destroy commercial schools by collecting in good university institutions a sufficient body of students, or to provide high-grade teaching for a few, leaving utterly wretched teaching for the vast majority? The dilemma is worthy of very careful consideration.

A word as to the colored school at Raleigh. This is a philanthropic enterprise that has been operating for well-nigh thirty years and has nothing in the way of plant to show for it. Its income ought to have been spent within; it has gone outside, to reimburse practitioners who supposed themselves assisting in a philanthropic work. Real philanthropy would have taken a very different course. As a matter of fact, Raleigh cannot, except at great expense, maintain clinical teaching. The way to help the negro is to help the two medical schools that have a chance to become efficient,— Howard at Washington, Meharry at Nashville.

NORTH DAKOTA

Population, 536,103. Number of physicians, 552. Ratio, 1:971.

Number of medical schools, 1.

GRAND FORKS: *Population, 12,602.*

STATE UNIVERSITY OF NORTH DAKOTA, COLLEGE OF MEDICINE. Organized 1905. A half-school. An organic part of the state university.

Entrance requirement: Two years of college work.

Attendance: 9.

Teaching staff: 9 professors and 7 instructors take part in the work of the department. The professor of bacteriology is State Bacteriologist.

Resources available for maintenance: The department shares in the general funds of the university. Its budget amounts to $6300; income from fees, $450.

Laboratory facilities: The laboratory of bacteriology, being at the same time the public health laboratory of the state, is well equipped and very active. Subjects given in the regular university laboratories are likewise well provided for. For the specifically medical subjects—physiology, pathology, anatomy—the provision is slighter. The students are, of course, few. A library and museum have been started.

Date of visit: May, 1909.

[*See South Dakota, "General Considerations," p. 301.*]

Ohio

Population, 4,594,240. Number of physicians, 7838. Ratio, 1: 586.
Number of medical schools, 8.

CINCINNATI: *Population, 353,108.*

(1) OHIO–MIAMI MEDICAL COLLEGE OF THE UNIVERSITY OF CINCINNATI. Organized by merger, 1909. An organic department of the university.

Entrance requirement: A four-year high school education or its equivalent.

Attendance: 197, 80 per cent from Ohio.

Teaching staff: 126, of whom 50 are professors, 76 of other grade. There are nine professors of medicine and nine professors of surgery (not including gynecology). There are three whole-time teachers.

Resources available for maintenance: Mainly fees, amounting to $26,345 (estimated).

Laboratory facilities: The university has so recently obtained complete control that it is not fair to make an inventory of the situation at this moment in a critical spirit. A modern outfit adequate to routine teaching has been already installed in pathology, bacteriology, and physiology. The subjects are taught by whole-time modern teachers. Chemistry, including physiological chemistry, is given at the university by whole-time instructors. Anatomy is as yet unorganized.

Clinical facilities: These are likewise in a state of transition, not only because of the recent formation of the department, but further, because the city has just begun the erection of a new hospital, whose exact relation to the university remains to be determined. There is an apparent disposition to make the relation close enough to be educationally effective. In that event, the university must on its side reorganize its clinical departments. The various schools may have disappeared, but their professorial titles remain. There must be a single professor of medicine, a single professor of surgery, etc., if the hospital facilities in prospect are·to be deserved and properly utilized.

The school dispensary awaits proper organization.

Date of visit: December, 1909.

(2) ECLECTIC MEDICAL INSTITUTE. Chartered 1845. An independent institution.

Entrance requirement: For Ohio students, a four-year high school education or its equivalent. Students from outside states are not held to the same standard.

Attendance: 86.

Teaching staff: 24, of whom one-half are professors. None of the instructors devotes his entire time to teaching.

Resources available for maintenance: Fees, amounting to $7500.

Laboratory facilities: A new building has just been provided; it contains an ordinary laboratory for elementary inorganic chemistry and a good dissecting-room. Separate laboratories, as yet meagerly equipped, are set aside for histology, pathology, and bacteriology. There is a small museum and a small collection of books, but practically no other teaching accessories. The course of instruction is not graded.

Clinical facilities: The school adjoins the Seton Hospital, with which it is affiliated. This institution has 60 beds, of which not over 24 are usable,—those mostly surgical. Little medical material is accessible. The teaching is carried on mainly in the amphitheater.

Sophomores are required to attend public clinics at the city hospital (never given by eclectic teachers), but the school does not know whether they attend or not.

A dispensary with a small attendance is connected with the hospital.

Dates of visits: December, 1909; April, 1910.

(3) PULTE MEDICAL COLLEGE. Homeopathic. Established 1872. An independent institution.

Entrance requirement: A four-year high school education or its equivalent.

Attendance: 16.

Teaching staff: 36, of whom 24 are professors, 12 of other grade.

Resources available for maintenance: Fees, amounting to $1325 (estimated).

Laboratory facilities: Anything more woe-begone than the laboratories of this institution would be difficult to imagine. The dissecting-room is a dark apartment in the basement, in which (December 14) the year's dissecting had not yet begun; but the teaching of anatomy was not therefore halted. A disorderly room with a small amount of morbid material and equipment is known as the pathological and bacteriological laboratory. The chemical laboratory contains a few desks, with reagent bottles, mostly empty. There are a few old books in the faculty-room. No charts, museum, models, or other teaching accessories are to be seen.

Clinical facilities: There was formerly a hospital in the same building, but it is now closed. The school claims to hold clinics at certain private institutions, in which, however, the work is mainly surgical and the cases not free. Except by attending amphitheater clinics at the city hospital, it is not clear that the Pulte students can regularly see any hospital medical cases at all.

There is an inexpressibly bad dispensary in the school building.

Date of visit: December, 1909.

CLEVELAND: *Population, 522,475.*

(4) CLEVELAND HOMEOPATHIC MEDICAL COLLEGE. Organized 1849. An independent institution.

Entrance requirement: A four-year high school education or its equivalent.

Attendance: 46.

Teaching staff: 61, of whom 30 are professors, 31 of other grade.

Resources available for maintenance: Fees, amounting to $5750.

Laboratory facilities: These comprise a good laboratory for physiology, in which vigorous teaching was in progress. In other subjects—chemistry, anatomy, pathology, and bacteriology—the provision is only fair. There are several cases of old medical books in the office.

Clinical facilities: These are limited to the City Hospital,—a large institution three miles distant, in which one-fifth of the material is assigned to this school. Adjoining the school building is a homeopathic hospital, with which the school was once intimately connected; they have now drifted apart.

Several rooms in the basement and on the first floor of the college building are used for a dispensary. Their equipment is poor; no complete or lasting records are kept.

Date of visit: December, 1909.

(5) WESTERN RESERVE UNIVERSITY MEDICAL DEPARTMENT. Organized 1843; in 1881 joined Western Reserve University, of which it is now an organic part.

Entrance requirement: Three years of college work.

Attendance: 98, of whom 70 per cent are from Ohio.

Teaching staff: 100, of whom 18 are professors, 82 of other grade. The laboratories are, with the exception of anatomy, manned with teachers giving their entire time to the school.

Resources available for maintenance: The department has endowments aggregating $784,865. Its income from fees is $11,000. Its budget calls for $63,000.

Laboratory facilities: Excellent laboratories, in which teaching and research are both vigorously prosecuted, are provided for all the fundamental scientific branches. A special endowment carries the department of experimental medicine. Books, museum, and other teaching accessories, all in abundance, are at hand.

Clinical facilities: From the faculty of the school is appointed the staff of Lakeside Hospital, an endowed institution of 215 available beds, thoroughly modern in construction and equipment. The school has erected a clinical laboratory on the premises, so that close correlation of bedside and laboratory work is easily attainable. The relation of the two institutions has progressively become more intimate, and in the same measure mutually more helpful. The situation is one that might be reproduced with infinite advantage in New York, Boston, Chicago, etc.

In addition, the school holds clinics at the City Hospital, Charity Hospital, St. Ann's Maternity Hospital, etc. It commands, therefore, all the material that is necessary. It requires now only additional endowment in order that it may completely command the time of clinical teachers.

The Lakeside Dispensary, admirably conducted, is used by the school on the same terms as the Lakeside Hospital. The attendance is large and varied. There is also an excellent dispensary connected with the Charity Hospital.

Date of visit: December, 1909.

(6) COLLEGE OF PHYSICIANS AND SURGEONS.[1] Organized 1863; since 1896 nominally the medical department of Ohio Wesleyan University.

Entrance requirement: Four-year high school education or equivalent.

Attendance: 89, 92 per cent from Ohio.

Teaching staff: Numbers 59, of whom 18 are professors, 41 of other grade. There are no teachers devoting their entire time to the school.

Resources available for maintenance: Fees only, amounting to $9520 (estimated).

Laboratory facilities: These cover only routine needs in chemistry, anatomy, bacteriology, and pathology. There is a meager supply of apparatus for experimental physiology, no museum, few books, and little else in the way of teaching accessories.

Clinical facilities: The school holds clinics at the City Hospital during four months, and at several private institutions, in which, however, the work is largely surgical. It has access to a fair amount of material, but under limitations that greatly impair its value. All the hospitals are at considerable distance from the school; none of them is provided with clinical laboratories for student use. In consequence, the teaching is of the discontinuous demonstrative type. Close contact of student with patient or systematic following of cases is impossible. Obstetrical work is limited to an out-patient service.

The dispensary is small and poorly organized. The attendance is slight.

Date of visit: December, 1909.

COLUMBUS: *Population,* 158,649.

(7) STARLING-OHIO MEDICAL COLLEGE. Formed by merger in 1907. An independent institution.

Entrance requirement: A four-year high school education or its equivalent.

---

[1] As this report goes to press, it is announced that this school has been consolidated with the Medical Department of Western Reserve University.

Attendance: 220.

Teaching staff: 60, of whom 32 are professors, 28 of other grade. There are no teachers giving their whole time to medical instructions. Some of the laboratory instruction is given by men who also teach in Ohio State University.

Resources available for maintenance: Fees only, amounting to $27,500.

Laboratory facilities: The school has a large plant. Laboratories adequately equipped for routine instruction are provided for anatomy, chemistry, physiological chemistry, bacteriology, pathology, and histology. There is no experimental pharmacology. Student assistants are employed. There is no evidence anywhere of original activity or interest. The school has a library, museum, and a supply of teaching accessories.

Clinical facilities: The school controls two hospitals, in one of which — containing, however, only 40 usable beds — it might introduce modern teaching methods. The other hospital, containing 150 beds, is a Catholic institution. Neither hospital is built, organized, or equipped with the necessities of teaching in view. No pavilion for contagious diseases is accessible. The city has thus far done nothing to provide proper hospital facilities for the sick poor. The state institutions are, however, available.

The school dispensaries enjoy an abundance of material, but lack equipment, organization, and oversight.

The conditions described are doubtless to some extent due to the difficulty of welding two schools into one. Vigorous measures might, however, produce here a good institution.

Date of visit: December, 1909.

TOLEDO: *Population,* 178,753.

(8) TOLEDO MEDICAL COLLEGE. Organized 1883. The medical department of Toledo University, a municipal institution of uncertain status and without substantial resources.

Entrance requirement: A four-year high school education or its equivalent.

Attendance: 82.

Teaching staff: 48, of whom 16 are professors, 32 of other grade. No one gives entire time to medical classes.

Resources available for maintenance: Fees only, amounting to $3240 (estimated).

Laboratory facilities: The school has nothing that can be fairly dignified by the name of laboratory. Separate rooms, badly kept and with meager equipment, are provided for chemistry, anatomy, pathology, and bacteriology. The class-rooms are bare: no charts, bones, skeleton, or museum are in evidence. There is a small library in the office.

Clinical facilities: These are entirely inadequate. The school formerly held clinics at the County Hospital, but the connection has been severed in consequence of a political overturning. It still has access to two hospitals: in one of them it holds a small number of clinics, both medical and surgical; in the other it conducts a surgical clinic twice a week. In neither of them can such material as exists be thoroughly used for teaching purposes.

There is a wretched little dispensary in the college building.

Date of visit: February, 1910.

General Considerations

Of the eight medical schools of Ohio one has already won a permanent place and two more have possibilities. The present administration of the state law is tightening about the other five, and there is every reason to suppose that they will all shortly have to submit to the inevitable. Just why the law should be tenderly applied is not clear. The state is rich, prosperous, and well supplied with secondary schools, though the competition of state-supported institutions has hitherto interfered with their systematic organization; and two or three doctors now contest every field capable of decently supporting one. It would appear feasible at once to enforce a genuine four-year high school preliminary and forthwith to move towards the higher standard just declared in Indiana.

The most prosperous universities of the state are, from the standpoint of medical education, fortunately situated: Western Reserve, at Cleveland, the Ohio State University, at Columbus, the University of Cincinnati, at Cincinnati. Of the future of Western Reserve there is no doubt. It is already one of the substantial schools of the country. Its clinical problem has been solved on lines that create a precedent worthy to be generally followed. Its financial resources are, however, decidedly inferior to its deserts and ideals. A keener appreciation of its worth must surely result in substantial improvement of its position in this respect.

The state of Ohio has a duty in reference to medical education and public health, the performance of which is made comparatively simple by the appropriate location at Columbus of the most important of its three state universities. As for the rest, it is a question of money and ideals. The plant of the Starling-Ohio school can probably be readily secured. Its educational value though not large may be readily increased; its laboratories could be easily consolidated, remodeled, and reorganized under trained teachers with paid assistants. On the clinical side, the difficulties are more serious, though not improbably the present Protestant Hospital could be developed into a good teaching hospital if the state supplied the necessary funds. The problem of procuring clinical teachers of modern type would still remain.

The city of Cincinnati seems definitely committed to the project of a municipal university. Coincidently, the building of the new municipal hospital furnishes an unusual opportunity to its medical department. A municipal university has two obvious sources of support: taxation may well be employed at least to maintain departments calculated to meet local needs,—industrial, social, or cultural; the pride of its citizens ought to supplement its tax income by way of supporting departments like medicine, whose main function can hardly be circumscribed by local considerations. The future of the medical department is thus likely to depend on the intelligence and munificence of the private benefactors of the university. The city can contribute its hospital and part of the current maintenance. Thus far the university has surely deserved well for its success in bringing together the rival schools which long divided and demoralized the field; the schools themselves made generous sacrifice of property rights in order to consummate the merger. It should, however, be added that this impersonal attitude has yet to be applied to the organization of the faculty. Property rights were yielded; professorial titles remain. Now, if the professors of the medical department of the University of Cincinnati really desire—as the coming together of the schools signifies—that there should be one strong medical school in the city, they must realize that a school in which there are nine professors of medicine and nine professors of surgery is as yet without organization. They ought therefore to surrender their titles to the university with the request that each clinical department be reconstructed by placing at its head the single individual marked out for the position, in the best judgment of the trustees of the university, by his scientific eminence and pedagogic skill.

OKLAHOMA

Population, 1,592,401. Number of physicians, 2703. Ratio, 1: 589.
Number of medical schools, 2.

NORMAN: *Population, 3389.*

(1) STATE UNIVERSITY OF OKLAHOMA, SCHOOL OF MEDICINE. Organized 1898. A half-school. An integral part of the university.

Entrance requirement: One year of college work in sciences.

Attendance: 22, all but 2 from Oklahoma.

Teaching staff: The instruction is given mainly by whole-time university teachers, two of whom devote their entire time to the department; the dean of the department is a practising physician.

Resources available for maintenance: The department is supported out of the general revenues of the university; fees amount to $600.

Laboratory facilities: Modest laboratories, adequate to routine work, are provided in anatomy, physiology, physiological chemistry, pharmacology, histology, pathology, and bacteriology. The laboratory of the state board of health is in the department. There are a small museum and a small departmental library.

Date of visit: November, 1909.

OKLAHOMA CITY: *Population,* 49,899.

(2) EPWORTH COLLEGE OF MEDICINE.[1] Organized 1904. A stock company, nominally the medical department of Epworth University.

Entrance requirement: Nominal.

Attendance: 51.

Teaching staff: 42, of whom 28 are professors, 14 of other grade.

Resources available for maintenance: Fees, amounting to $4285.

Laboratory facilities: These are hardly more than nominal: a little apparatus has been procured for each of the several subjects, but all is disorderly and neglected.

Clinical facilities: Clinics are held in a private hospital, where perhaps 30 beds, mostly surgical, are available.

There is no school dispensary.

Date of visit: November, 1909.

General Considerations

THE new commonwealth of Oklahoma may, if wise, avoid most of the evils which this report has described; for though they have already appeared, they have not taken deep root. Immigration—of physicians, among others—has been so rapid that the state has easily three times as many doctors as it needs. They pour in from the schools of St. Louis, Kansas City, and Chicago. If, however, the state wishes a high-grade supply only, it must speedily define a standard such as will (1) suppress commercial schools,—as, for example, that now nominally belonging to Epworth University,—and (2) by the same action exclude inferior doctors trained elsewhere. Having done this, only an institution with considerable resources, derived either from taxes or from endowment, will even attempt to conduct a medical school in the state : which is as it should be.

The state university is of course marked out for the work. Its present modest beginning must be developed. Perhaps it will have at once to occupy Oklahoma City with a clinical department so as to obtain control of the field ; though, if its sole right could be established without that, the project might well be delayed for a time. A good medical school is so costly that a new university does not want to anticipate the responsibility. Possible expenditures on such a department have in a way been crippled in advance by the absurd duplication of state institutions. There are

[1] As this report goes to press, it is stated that this school has been consolidated with the medical department of the state university, which thus becomes a complete school of the divided type.

26 state-supported educational institutions in Oklahoma. In other respects the people of the state have been quick to profit by the experience of other sections. Oklahoma City has not in its building recapitulated the phases of growth elsewhere. Its streets are of asphalt, its large buildings are fire-proof, their plumbing modern; they have begun with enamel, not with tin or zinc, bathtubs. Why do they not in the same way avoid the weary and costly errors in educational organization that the states about them have one after the other made? Ordinary intelligence, surveying the states of the middle west to-day after their educational experience of the last thirty years, could reduce its lessons to a few simple propositions which would be universally accepted. No two judges would differ as to the principle that state institutions of higher learning should be concentrated in a town of assured future; that proprietary medical schools should be forbidden, etc. The older states are painfully correcting or paying for their blunders: should Oklahoma, to soothe the local pride of this little town or that, run up a bill of the same sort?

OREGON

Population, 505,889. Number of physicians, 782. Ratio, 1: 646.
Number of medical schools, 2.

PORTLAND: *Population*, 131,508.

(1) UNIVERSITY OF OREGON MEDICAL DEPARTMENT. Organized 1887. Nominally the medical department of the state university.

Entrance requirement: Less than a high school education.

Attendance: 72, 65 per cent from Oregon.

Teaching staff: 41, of whom 14 are professors, 27 of other grade. No teachers devote full time to the school.

Resources available for maintenance: An annual appropriation of $1000 from the funds of the state university, and fees amounting to $8000 (estimated).

Laboratory facilities: The school occupies a frame building, wretchedly kept. It has one good laboratory, that of bacteriology, conducted by the city bacteriologist. Other branches, like chemistry, anatomy, pathology, and histology, are provided in the usual perfunctory manner. There is a scanty equipment in physiology; one thousand to fifteen hundred books, mostly old text-books, form the library. Other teaching accessories there are none.

Clinical facilities: The school has access by courtesy to two hospitals, in which students may look on. They cannot work in the clinical laboratories of the hospital, and there is no clinical laboratory at the school. Obstetrical cases are entirely insufficient.

The dispensary has an attendance varying from two to seven daily.

Date of visit: May, 1909.

SALEM: *Population,* 7287.[1]

(2) WILLAMETTE UNIVERSITY MEDICAL DEPARTMENT. Organized 1865. An independent institution in all but name.

Entrance requirement: Less than a high school education.

Attendance: 29, 86 per cent from Oregon.

Teaching staff: 16, of whom 15 are professors.

Resources available for maintenance: Fees, amounting to $3580 (estimated).

Laboratory facilities: The school has a fairly well equipped laboratory for bacteriology and histology; a small laboratory, with little material and no running water for chemistry; and a dissecting-room. There are no museum, no books, no other teaching accessories. Inquiry on the subject of physiology elicited the response that the "apparatus is in a physician's office downtown."

Clinical facilities: These are hardly more than nominal. Students have some access to a private hospital of 30 beds in Salem and to the State Asylum and Penitentiary a few miles distant. "Medical clinics depend on cases." Obstetrical cases "depend on private practice."

There is no dispensary at all.

Date of visit: May, 1909.

General Considerations

NEITHER of these schools has either resources or ideals; there is no justification for their existence. The entire coast is oversupplied with doctors by immigration; unless something better can be made than can be thus readily obtained, the state will do well to let the field lie fallow.

The Salem school is an utterly hopeless affair, for which no word can be said. Portland may conceivably some day maintain a distant department of the state university. Until, however, the financial strength of the state university permits it to develop there a school equal, for instance, to that which the University of Texas supports at Galveston, it has no right to allow a group of local doctors to exploit its name in the conduct of a low-grade proprietary institution. That out of its own slender revenues it should divert a thousand dollars annually into the coffers of this concern is well-nigh incredible.

[1] Not estimated by U. S. Census Bureau.

PENNSYLVANIA

Population, 7,032,915. Number of physicians, 11,056. Ratio, 1: 636.

Number of medical schools, 8, *plus* 1 postgraduate school.

PHILADELPHIA: *Population*, 1,540,430.

(1) UNIVERSITY OF PENNSYLVANIA DEPARTMENT OF MEDICINE. Organized 1765. An organic part of the university.

Entrance requirement: One year of college work, in which, however, conditions have been very freely allowed.

Attendance: 546, 63 per cent from Pennsylvania.

Teaching staff: 157, of whom 26 are professors, 131 of other grade. The laboratory instructors, with a few of their assistants, devote their entire time to teaching and research.

Resources available for maintenance: The department shares the general funds of the university. Its budget—exclusive of the hospital and dispensary—is $131,255; the income from fees is $104,612.

Laboratory facilities: Five separate well equipped buildings are provided for the laboratories of the department: the first for histology, embryology, etc.; the second—new and admirably adapted to its purposes—for pathology, physiology, and pharmacology; the third for chemistry and anatomy, with a deservedly famous anatomical museum; the fourth for hygiene; the fifth is the clinical laboratory, never as yet adequately supported. Near by is the Wistar Institute, open to graduate students for research in anatomy. The department possesses an admirable library. Its scientific faculty has been recently strengthened by the creation of chairs of physiological chemistry and experimental medicine, specially endowed. The department has, therefore, an admirable material equipment.

Clinical facilities: The University Hospital of 350 beds, of which 280 are available for instruction, is contiguous to the laboratories. There is a separate maternity pavilion of 50 beds. Considerable use is also made of several other hospitals, notably the Philadelphia General Hospital and the Pennsylvania Hospital, extramural instruction being given at the latter. The recently established Phipps Institute for tuberculosis is also now part of the clinical plant. The equipment of the department thus fully satisfies all essential conditions.

Two dispensaries are used, one at, the other at a distance from, the university. Abundant material is thus obtained.

Date of visit: March, 1909.

(2) JEFFERSON MEDICAL COLLEGE. Organized 1825. An independent institution.

Entrance requirement: A high school education or its equivalent. Of all independent schools outside New York state, this institution comes nearest to obtaining its published entrance requirements. It lacks, however, an organization adapted to the evaluation of secondary school credentials. A fair percentage of those admitted have had some college work.

Attendance: 591, of whom 57 per cent are from Pennsylvania.

Teaching staff: 122, of whom 22 are professors, 100 of other grade. Seven instructors devote their entire time to the school.

Resources available for maintenance: Fees only, amounting to $102,995. Part of the school income is, however, diverted in order to pay off building mortgages. The hospital has independent sources of support.

Laboratory facilities: An attractive building contains separate laboratories for anatomy, physiology, chemistry, pathology, histology, bacteriology, and pharmacy. The equipment is in general modern and adequate to the needs of undergraduate instruction ; in certain departments, *e. g.*, anatomy and bacteriology, additional activity is in progress. Lack of space and means restricts the school to undergraduate teaching. There are an attractive library, museum, and other teaching accessories.

Clinical facilities: The Jefferson Hospital—a modern structure, with 223 teaching beds, belonging to the institution—adjoins the laboratory building; it is connected with a dispensary which supplies an abundance of material. The maternity department, with 17 beds, occupies a separate building. Students are freely admitted to the hospital wards and its clinical laboratory.

The plant of the institution is therefore modern and compact.

Date of visit: March, 1909.

(3) MEDICO-CHIRURGICAL COLLEGE OF PHILADELPHIA. Organized 1881. An independent school.

Entrance requirement: Less than a four-year high school education.

Attendance: 480, 82 per cent from Pennsylvania.

Teaching staff: 109, of whom 23 are professors, 86 of other grade. No teachers devote their entire time to medical instruction; three teachers, however, devote themselves entirely to the school, if the dental and pharmacy departments are counted in.

Resources available for maintenance: Fees, amounting to $48,281.

Laboratory facilities: Well equipped for ordinary undergraduate teaching are the laboratories of physiology, chemistry, pathology, and bacteriology. Anatomy is practically limited to dissecting, with some drawing and modeling, the professor being a practitioner. There is no museum beyond necessary specimens for pathological work. There is a library at the College Club. Students in dentistry, pharmacy, and medicine mingle in a number of classes. Student assistants are freely used. Except in bacteriology, little or no effort is made to cultivate original scientific activity; great stress is laid on effective drill.

Clinical facilities: The school has entire control of its own hospital, of 180 available beds, which is in close proximity to the other buildings. The Maternity Hospital is near by. Ward and section methods are in use. Classes are also held in the usual manner at other hospitals.

The dispensary attendance is large.

Date of visit: March, 1909.

(4) TEMPLE UNIVERSITY, DEPARTMENT OF MEDICINE. Organized 1901.

Entrance requirement: Less than a four-year high school education.

Attendance: 186.

Teaching staff: 85, of whom 15 are professors, 70 of other grade. There are no full-time teachers.

Resources available for maintenance: Fees only, amounting to $17,000 (estimated).

Laboratory facilities: These are entirely inadequate and in some departments quite wretched. There is an ordinary elementary laboratory for chemistry; a single room with slight equipment for histology, pathology, and bacteriology, and only a demonstration outfit for physiology. The dissecting-room is in bad condition. There is a small museum and a library of several thousand volumes of miscellaneous character, but no other teaching accessories. Dental, pharmacy, and medical students mingle in the same classes.

Clinical facilities: The school has access to two small hospitals, whose work is almost four-fifths surgical. The dispensary has a large attendance.

Date of visit: March, 1909.

(5) HAHNEMANN MEDICAL COLLEGE AND HOSPITAL. Organized 1848. An independent institution.

Entrance requirement: Less than a four-year high school education,—probably much less, for most of the credentials were passed on by the secretary.

Attendance: 182, 61 per cent from Pennsylvania.

Teaching staff: 72, of whom 27 are professors, 45 of other grade. One teacher devotes his entire time to the school.

Resources available for maintenance: Fees, amounting to $18,500.

Laboratory facilities: The school possesses an ordinary laboratory for general chemistry; a second, with slight equipment, for histology and physiology; and another, fairly equipped, for pathology and bacteriology. The dissecting-room is clean and odorless. Both regular and homeopathic pharmacy are taught. There is a large and very well kept museum.

Clinical facilities: The school is connected with the Hahnemann Hospital, containing some 150 beds; but no ward clinics are held. Patients are wheeled into the amphitheater. Students have no access to the clinical laboratory.

The dispensary has a large attendance, and there only, for the most, the student comes into close contact with patients.

Date of visit: March, 1909.

(6) Woman's Medical College of Pennsylvania. Organized 1850. An independent institution.

Entrance requirement: A high school education or its equivalent.

Attendance: 125.

Teaching staff: 52, of whom 25 are professors, 27 of other grade. One teacher devotes entire time to the schools; several others teach laboratory subjects elsewhere as well.

Resources available for maintenance: Fees, amounting to $15,480, and income from endowments, amounting to $13,820.

Laboratory facilities: Simply, but intelligently, equipped and conscientiously used laboratories are provided for physiology, bacteriology and pathology, histology and embryology, chemistry, pharmacy, and anatomy. There is striking evidence of a genuine effort to do the best possible with limited resources. There are a useful library and a good museum.

Clinical facilities: The school is now building a new hospital, part of which is already in use. This, with a temporary building, accommodates 27 beds. There is, besides a maternity of 16 beds, and an out-patient obstetrical service. Ward work, with assignment of individual cases, is regularly carried on. Supplementary opportunities are obtained at several other institutions. There is a fair dispensary service.

Date of visit: March, 1909.

(7) Philadelphia College and Infirmary of Osteopathy. Established 1898. An independent institution.

Entrance requirement: Nominal.

Attendance: 126.

Teaching staff: 18, of whom 11 are professors, 7 of other grade.

Resources available for maintenance: Fees, amounting to $18,900 (estimated).

Laboratory facilities: These are utterly wretched. They comprise a laboratory for histology, in which a small centrifuge is the only visible object of interest; a small laboratory for elementary chemistry in a dark cellar; and an intolerably foul dissecting-room in a dark building, once a stable. If there is any provision for pathology, physiology, or bacteriology, any books, or museum, or other teaching accessories except a few crude drawings, a model, and a skeleton, all was successfully concealed. Three separate class-rooms are provided,—containing necessary furniture only.

Clinical facilities: The infirmary, the address of which is not given in the catalogue, is some blocks distant; it contains three beds and has, it is claimed, 200 patients who come twice or thrice weekly for treatment. The catalogue announces that its students have the "privilege of witnessing operations at the University Hospital, Jefferson Hospital, etc." This is not the case. These students are intruders, without rights or privileges of any description whatsoever.

Date of visit: January, 1910.

PITTSBURGH: *Population, 570,065.*

(8) UNIVERSITY OF PITTSBURGH, MEDICAL DEPARTMENT. Organized 1886; affiliated with the University of Pittsburgh in 1892, it became an organic department thereof in 1909.

Entrance requirement: Four-year high school education or its equivalent.

Attendance: 315.

Teaching staff: 103, of whom 43 are professors, 60 of other grade. Five instructors give their entire time to the school. There is one research assistant.

Resources available for maintenance: Fees, amounting to $48,500.

Laboratory facilities: The school has within a year undergone a complete transformation. A more thorough piece of house-cleaning within so short a period is hardly credible. A year ago, before the University of Pittsburgh obtained control, the so-called laboratories were dirty and disorderly beyond description. Since the present management took hold last fall, the admission of students has been much more carefully supervised; the building has been put in excellent condition; laboratories for chemistry, physiology, bacteriology, and pathology have been remodeled and equipped with modern apparatus for both teaching and research; foreign and domestic periodicals have been subscribed for; a study-room in good order has been instituted in place of the lounging-room where last year "four dozen wooden chairs were broken." Whole-time instructors of modern training and ideals have been secured. This is the more remarkable, as only fees have been available. Despite the necessary defects of schools relying wholly on fees, the experience of this institution confirms our contention that the conscientious and intelligent use of fees would alone greatly improve existing conditions in most schools.

A new building is in process of erection.

Clinical facilities: The school has access to several hospitals in which an abundance of material is available, subject, however, to the usual limitations. The clinical instruction is therefore here, as generally elsewhere, put together of disconnected parts. This does not, however, apply to obstetrics; for the school controls a maternity hospital of 34 beds, which, quite slovenly a year ago, has also been transformed in the last few months. It is neat, clean, well managed, and has been improved by the addition of a new delivery-room, sterilizing outfit, etc. It is in charge of a resident obstetrician of modern training.

The dispensary has been similarly reorganized. A permanent nurse has been installed. Records are now in order; the rooms and equipment are attractive and, in the main, adequate.

Date of visit: February, 1910.

(9) THE PHILADELPHIA POLYCLINIC. A postgraduate independent school.

Entrance requirement: The M.D. degree.

Attendance: Short courses, ranging from six weeks to six months in length, are given, the attendance varying from time to time. The annual attendance is perhaps 150.

Teaching staff: 129, of whom 29 are professors, 100 of other grade.

Resources available for maintenance: Fees and donations.

Laboratory facilities: The school has what no other postgraduate school in the country possesses, — a laboratory building in which its classes in clinical microscopy, operative surgery, etc., are conducted. The instruction is of a practical character, aiming to meet the needs of physicians whose training has been defective. No animals are used and no active research is in progress. There are few books and periodicals in reach.

Clinical facilities: The Polyclinic Hospital, an excellently conducted institution, contains 81 beds available for teaching purposes. Ward classes receive demonstrative instruction.

The present dispensary consists of a suite of rooms quite inadequate to the amount of material to be handled. A new building is in process of erection.

Date of visit: February, 1910.

General Considerations

MEDICAL education in the state of Pennsylvania presents no unusual problems from the standpoint of theory. It is easy enough to decide what ought to happen. From a practical point of view, however, the situation is exceedingly difficult. The medical schools are in some respects strong institutions; moreover, education, philanthropy, and politics have become so interwoven that they make a combination too intricate to be readily dissolved.

The state is without an educational system; and the legislature has recently refused to pass a bill aiming to organize the common, secondary, and normal schools of the state. Ordinary educational values are therefore still obscure and confused. Though the last legislature improved the law regulating medical education to the extent of making a four-year high school course or its equivalent the legal minimum, the educational disorganization of the state makes its enforcement problematical.

There is still another source of apprehension on this score. The real standard depends on who evaluates the "equivalent." The agents to whom this function has been officially delegated in the past have conceded much to the wishes—real or supposed —of the schools. The Pittsburgh representative has been extremely lax; his "equivalent" to the four-year high school education has not been equal to a two-year high school education. The present incumbent at Philadelphia is newly appointed; conditions described in the text refer to previous years. Finally, some of the schools have been using their own judgment in dealing with credentials, referring only such as they did not accept themselves. It is impossible to ascertain how those referred were distinguished from those accepted in the medical school office.

If, now, a genuine four-year high school standard is enforced, out of the eight undergraduate schools in the state only two will avoid very serious damage: the University of Pennsylvania and the Jefferson Medical College, the former already beyond the standard in question, the latter probably strong enough to stand the shrinkage which would result,—for a large part of its enrolment now meets the requirement. The University of Pittsburgh is fully alive to the necessity of procuring endowment in order to meet the inevitable deficit, and will stand or fall on that issue. The other five schools have no future; their enrolment is so largely the make-believe equivalent that enforcement of a real four-year high school standard will seriously threaten their existence even at their present level of efficiency; progress would be altogether impossible.

The situation so far simplified by an actual entrance standard, another topic presses for consideration. The state of Pennsylvania has for years been engaged in distributing large sums to private and semi-private charities. These largesses have enabled several of the Philadelphia schools to build and partly to maintain their own hospitals. That this policy is thoroughly objectionable and demoralizing is beyond dispute. The state has neither right nor business to make presents to private corporations that it can neither regulate nor control. And the level of civic life in Pennsylvania has been greatly lowered by the log-rolling and favoritism that the possibilities of "pull" have created. One would be perhaps not over-sanguine to expect that the bounty and subsidy system will one day be replaced by strict payment for services rendered,—so strict, that the hospitals will, as in New York, lose rather than gain by the operation. The unendowed medical schools of the state cannot survive such a wholesome treatment of the state's philanthropic obligations. The extension of their hospitals would be prohibited; even their maintenance would be imperiled.

It is thus clear that a reasonable—not a high—standard of admission and a righteous public policy in dealing with charities would soon reduce the schools of the state to two,—the University of Pittsburgh, provided it secures endowment, and the University of Pennsylvania, whose resources available for medical education would also require to be increased. Fortunate indeed would it be, if broad views might bring about this increase in part through consolidation of the three large schools of Philadelphia, one or two of the three being liquidated as a means of liberating a considerable sum, applicable thenceforth to the development of the single surviving school. Into such a scheme—inevitable, in any case, unless the independent schools accomplish the heretofore impossible task of procuring endowment—the Polyclinic would easily fall. The day of independent and elementary postgraduate instruction is rapidly passing; the postgraduate school of the future will crown a substantial undergraduate school of medicine. The outcome here suggested can be averted only if the independent schools secure endowment,—for which there is no precedent in America, —or if some university outside Philadelphia form an alliance there. There is just now no academic institution in the state whose resources would warrant this step. Whatever these medical schools now offer, they would, singly or combined, shortly prove a drain on any university endeavoring to apply to medicine the standards and ideals cultivated in its other departments. Moreover, as two schools—one at Pittsburgh, the other at Philadelphia—can supply the state with physicians, no other university is justified in entering the field unless its resources, free to be applied to medicine, are sufficient to insure as a consequence a real advance in medical knowledge and practice.

SOUTH CAROLINA

Population, 1,510,566. Number of physicians, 1141. Ratio 1: 1324.[1]
Number of medical schools, 1.

CHARLESTON: *Population, ·56,659.*

MEDICAL COLLEGE OF THE STATE OF SOUTH CAROLINA. Founded 1823. An independent institution.

Entrance requirement : Nominal.

Attendance : 213.

Teaching staff: 34, of whom 11 are professors, 23 of other grade. There are no whole-time teachers.

[1] Polk's statistics make the ratio 1: 1168.

Resources available for maintenance: Fees, amounting to $19,447 (estimated).

Laboratory facilities: Comprise very meager equipment for elementary chemistry, pharmacy, and anatomy — the dissecting-room in bad condition. The instructor in pathology and bacteriology has a fair private laboratory, to which students have no access; student work in those subjects is mostly confined to looking through the microscope at slides that he prepares. There is no museum, except old papier-mâché and wax models, no library, except some antiquated publications. It is without other teaching aids.

Clinical facilities: The school has access to the Roper Hospital, an unusually attractive institution of about 200 beds a mile distant. There were 80 patients at the time of the visit. Complaint is made that it is difficult to induce graduates to serve as internes. Obstetrical work is rare.

There is no school or other organized dispensary.

Date of visit: February, 1909.

SOUTH DAKOTA

Population, 498,077. Number of physicians, 607. Ratio, 1: 821.
Number of medical schools, 1.

VERMILION: *Population, 2183.*

UNIVERSITY OF SOUTH DAKOTA COLLEGE OF MEDICINE. Organized 1907. A half-school. An organic department of the state university.

Entrance requirement: 2 years of college work.

Attendance: 7.

Teaching staff: 5 professors and 5 instructors, who take part in the work of the department.

Resources available for maintenance: The department shares in the general funds of the university. No separate budget is prepared. Fees amount to $660.

Laboratory facilities: The necessary equipment is at hand for painstaking routine instruction in the laboratory branches. A library and museum have been started.

Date of visit: November, 1909.

General Considerations

THE two Dakotas have taken time by the forelock: before any vested proprietary interest could be created, they have fixed the state practice requirement at two years of college work, thus fortifying the medical department of the state university. The state, though thinly settled, is prosperous, and no anxiety is felt that the high standard will deplete the medical profession of the state. On the contrary, it has been adopted as a means of protecting a people already supporting twice as many doctors as it needs.

Though the students are few, the present provision for their teachers is on too unpretentious a scale. Unfortunately, like all the western states, South Dakota is already scattering its financial resources among half a dozen competing state institutions. Of its seven tax-supported institutions of higher grade, three give the A.B. degree and the others desire to do so. It will prove decidedly unfortunate if these institutions are not in their infancy coördinated, so as to form a genuine system rather than a number of separate, warring units. A population of half a million in a new country will do well to sustain one substantial state college with departments of law, medicine, etc. It can do that only by concentrating its outlay.

TENNESSEE

Population, 2,248,404. Number of physicians, 3303. Ratio, 1: 681.

Number of medical schools, 9.

CHATTANOOGA: *Population, 34,773.*

(1) CHATTANOOGA MEDICAL COLLEGE. Organized 1889. The medical department of the University of Chattanooga.

Entrance requirement: Nominal.

Attendance: 112.

Teaching staff: 25, of whom 11 are professors, 14 of other grade.

Resources available for maintenance: Fees, amounting to $4290.

Laboratory facilities: The school occupies a small building, externally attractive; the interior, dirty and disorderly, is almost bare, except for a fair chemical laboratory in good condition. The dissecting-room contains two tables; the single room assigned to histology, pathology, and bacteriology contains a few old specimens, mostly unlabeled, and one oil-immersion microscope. The instructor explained that they "study only non-pathogenic microbes; students do not handle the pathogenic." There is nothing further in the way of laboratory outfit; no museum, books, charts, models, etc.

Clinical facilities: Amphitheater clinics are held at the Erlanger Hospital, which averages about 50 free patients. Students may not enter the wards. Perhaps ten obstetrical cases annually are obtainable, students being "summoned,"—just how is not clear. The students see no post-mortems, no contagious diseases, do no blood or urine work, and do not always own their own text-books. They use quiz-compends instead.

There is no dispensary.

This is a typical example of the schools that claim to exist for the sake of the poor boy and the back country.

Date of visit: January, 1909.

KNOXVILLE: *Population, 38,328.*

(2) TENNESSEE MEDICAL COLLEGE. Organized 1889. A stock company; nominally the medical department of Lincoln Memorial University.

Entrance requirement: Nominal.

Attendance: 82, 70 per cent from Tennessee.

Teaching staff: 31, of whom 26 are professors, 5 of other grade.

Resources available for maintenance: Fees, amounting to $4994.

Laboratory facilities: The school building is externally attractive; within, dirty. In the basement is a small laboratory for inorganic chemistry. A few microscopes, a microtome, and some sterilizing apparatus—no cultures or pathological specimens were visible—constitute the laboratory for pathology, bacteriology, and histology. The dissecting-room is ordinary; there are no books, museum, charts, etc.

Clinical facilities: The school adjoins a neat hospital, recently constructed, which proves, however, to be simply the private hospital of the faculty for which student fees help to pay. It has an average of 40 patients, with no free wards. Five clinics weekly are scheduled, but it is admitted that "they are not always held." Practically, students "are called" when a case happens along which the doctor can arrange to have them see. Obstetrical instruction is limited "to a few deliveries before the class."

There is no dispensary.

Date of visit: January, 1909.

(3) KNOXVILLE MEDICAL COLLEGE. Colored. Established 1900. An independent institution.

Entrance requirement: Nominal.

Attendance: 23.

Teaching staff: 11, of whom 9 are professors.

Resources available for maintenance: Fees, amounting to $1020 (estimated).

Laboratory facilities: None. The school occupies a floor above an undertaker's establishment.

Clinical facilities: None. It was stated by a student that twice between October 1 and January 28 "a few students were taken to the Knoxville College Hospital."
There is no dispensary.

The catalogue of this school is a tissue of misrepresentations from cover to cover.

Date of visit: January, 1909.

MEMPHIS: *Population,* 140,145.

(4) COLLEGE OF PHYSICIANS AND SURGEONS. Organized 1906. A stock company, now calling itself the medical department of the University of Memphis, a fictitious affair.

Entrance requirement: None. "Accept students and try them out."

Attendance: 77.

Teaching staff: 47, of whom 22 are professors, 25 of other grade.

Resources available for maintenance: Fees, amounting to $7400 (estimated).

Laboratory facilities: The school occupies an excellent building, recently erected, fees being largely consumed in helping to pay for it. The dissecting-room is of modern design, consisting of small rooms with hot and cold water; but the work was conducted on antiquated lines, cadavers being in wretched condition. The chemical laboratory is good and quite adequate to instruction in elementary chemistry. Equipment for pathology and bacteriology is less than fair; for physiology, practically nothing. There are few books, no museum, charts, etc.

Clinical facilities: The schedule shows seven one-hour clinics (5 in surgery, 2 in medicine) per week at the City Hospital during one-half of the school year. At the date of the visit, perhaps 40 beds were thus accessible. Students "look on" at the obstetrical cases.
A suite of rooms in the college building is set aside for a dispensary.

Date of visit: November, 1909.

(5) MEMPHIS HOSPITAL MEDICAL COLLEGE. Organized 1880. A stock company.

Entrance requirement: Nominal.

Attendance: 442.

Teaching staff: 35, of whom 12 are professors, 23 of other grade.

Resources available for maintenance: Fees, amounting to $34,600 (estimated). The condition of the school laboratories shows what becomes of this sum.

Laboratory facilities: The school occupies an excellent building, heavily mortgaged. It is new and well kept. The chemical laboratory is good and adequate to elementary chemistry. An excellent room is assigned to dissecting, but the cadavers are putrid. One laboratory, with slight equipment and little material, answers for all microscopic work. It is obvious that large classes have paid in considerable sums that have been used to pay for an expensive building, not to provide even fair teaching facilities. The course of instruction is not graded.

Clinical facilities: The schedule shows nine one-hour clinics a week at the City Hospital, where the available material is divided between the two schools. At the date of the visit, perhaps 40 beds were thus accessible to each. Students "look on" at the obstetrical cases. The course of instruction is not graded; the amount of material is absurdly inadequate for the huge classes.

There is a dispensary in the school building. Its equipment is slight; there are no systematic records. The amount of material cannot possibly suffice for the student body; and there is nothing to indicate effective use, as far as it goes.

Date of visit: November, 1909.

(6) UNIVERSITY OF WEST TENNESSEE, MEDICAL DEPARTMENT. Colored. Organized 1900.

Entrance requirement: Nominal.

Attendance: 40.

Teaching staff: 14, all of whom are professors.

Resources available for maintenance: Fees, amounting to $2000 (estimated).

Laboratory facilities: There is meager equipment for chemistry, pharmacy, and microscopy. Otherwise the rooms are bare.

Clinical facilities: The students have access to eight or ten beds, twice weekly, in a small hospital close by.

There is a dispensary, without records, in the school building.

Date of visit: November, 1909.

NASHVILLE: *Population,* 107,076.

(7) VANDERBILT UNIVERSITY MEDICAL DEPARTMENT. Established 1874. An organic department of the university.

Entrance requirement: Less than high school graduation, though a fair proportion of the students have had some college work.

Attendance: 200.

Teaching staff: 40, of whom 17 are professors, 23 of other grade. The dean of the school is the professor of chemistry in the academic department—an undesirable arrangement at a time when medical education is so rapidly changing form. No instructor devotes entire time to the medical department.

Resources available for maintenance: Fees, amounting to $26,250. This sum, adequate to provide fair laboratory instruction, is not devoted to education alone. The medical department, although organically part of the university, is under contract to wipe out with its fees the cost of the building it occupies, and meanwhile it pays the university interest at six per cent on the unpaid balance.

Laboratory facilities: The school possesses satisfactory laboratories for pathology, bacteriology, and histology, and an energetic instructor has charge of them. A creditable beginning has been made in experimental physiology. Chemistry is well provided by the university. Anatomy is bad — the work being conducted on antiquated lines in a foul dissecting-room. There is a useful museum and a fair library.

Clinical facilities: The school has converted the basement of its own building into a ward of 35 beds; and has access to the City Hospital (65 beds) besides. The amount of material thus available is too restricted.

There is a dispensary with a fair attendance.

Date of visit: January, 1909.

(8) UNIVERSITIES OF NASHVILLE AND TENNESSEE MEDICAL DEPARTMENT. A combination under limited contract, formed in 1909, expiring 1912. One of the two institutions represented is the State University of Tennessee (Knoxville), the other the University of Nashville, — a university in name only.

Entrance requirement: Less than high school graduation.

Attendance: 207.

Teaching staff: 55, of whom 26 are professors, 29 of other grade. The distribution of chairs is significant: there are four professors of medicine, four professors of surgery (not including gynecology), and one whole-time teacher.

Resources available for maintenance: Fees, amounting to $26,000 (estimated), and subscriptions from the two universities, amounting to $8100 in cash. Of the two universities, the University of Tennessee is supported by legislative appropriation; the University of Nashville has an endowment of $60,000, yielding $3600 annually.

Laboratory facilities: These comprise a poor laboratory for elementary chemistry, an outfit, in part new, for bacteriology, pathology, histology, and physiology, and a poorly kept dissecting-room. There is a small museum.

Clinical facilities: The building formerly used by the medical department of the University of Tennessee has been converted into a hospital with a capacity of 70 beds. In view of the brief period that has elapsed since the merger, this improvement in clinical resources is most commendable, for the hospital is completely controlled by the school. The school has access to the City Hospital besides.

The first floor of the college hospital building is used as a dispensary. Though its equipment is still slight, it represents a great advance over the conditions that preceded.

Date of visit: January, 1909.

(9) MEHARRY MEDICAL COLLEGE. Colored. Organized 1876. The medical department of Walden University.

Entrance requirement: Less than a four-year high school education.

Attendance: 275.

Teaching staff: 26, of whom 12 are professors, 14 of other grade.

Resources available for maintenance: $23,946, representing income from endowment of $35,000, subscription from the Freedman's Aid Society, and fees, the last item being $20,310.

Laboratory facilities: The school possesses fair laboratories for chemistry and physiology and highly creditable laboratories for bacteriology, histology, and pathology, the outfit including animals, microscopes, microtome, and pathological material in excellent order. A separate frame building, well kept, is devoted to anatomy. The equipment and general conditions reflect great credit on the zeal and intelligence of those in charge of the school and its several departments.

Clinical facilities: These are restricted. The school has access to Mercy Hospital, 32 beds.

Date of visit: January, 1909.

General Considerations

THE state of Tennessee protects at this date more low-grade medical schools than any other southern state. It would be unfair and futile to criticize this situation without full recognition of local conditions. A standpoint that is entirely in order in dealing with Cincinnati, Chicago, or St. Louis is here irrelevant. The ideals held up must indeed be the same; but their attainment is much further in the future. The amount of money available for medical education is small; the preliminary requirement must be relatively low. Practically all that can be asked of Tennessee is that it should do the best possible under the circumstances.

This it does not do. The six white schools value their separate survival beyond all other considerations. A single school could furnish all the doctors the state needs and do something to supply the needs of adjoining states as well. Low as the entrance standard must be, it has been made lower in order to gather in students for six schools where one would suffice. The medical schools solicit and accept students who have not yet made the best of the limited educational opportunities their homes provide; and to this extent, not only injure the public health, but depress and demoralize the general educational situation.

The same is true in reference to laboratories and clinics. However small the sums applicable to building and equipping laboratories, conditions are needlessly aggravated when six plants are equipped instead of one. Fees that ought now to be used in providing better teaching are still paying for expensive buildings in Memphis and Nashville. The city hospitals of both places, small at best, are divided between two schools, though they do not furnish enough material for one.

Those who deal with medical education in Tennessee are therefore making the worst, not the best, of their limited possibilities. Their medical schools, treated on their merits, would speedily reduce to one: the utterly wretched establishments at Chattanooga and Knoxville would be wiped out; the more showy, but quite mercenary, concerns at Memphis would be liquidated. The University of Tennessee, with an annual income that does not as yet suffice for the legitimate needs of its own plant at Knoxville, should abandon for the present the effort to develop at Nashville a school that it can neither control nor support. The time may come when there will be a call for the state university to enter the field. But that time is not now. For the present it is dividing its own forces and hindering the most effective use of such resources as Nashville affords. The whole field is strangely confused: Lincoln Memorial University (which is an industrial school, not a university) at Cumberland Gap shelters a medical school at Knoxville; the University of Tennessee at Knoxville shelters an entirely superfluous school at Nashville.

If our analysis is correct, the institution to which the responsibility for medical education in Tennessee should just now be left is Vanderbilt University; for it is the only institution in position at this juncture to deal with the subject effectively. This does not mean that Vanderbilt has now any large sums of money available or that it should inaugurate impossible entrance standards. It can do neither, for the general situation countenances neither. The suggestion merely recognizes the facts that one school can do the work; that Vanderbilt occupies in Nashville the point of vantage; that, in the public interest, the field should be left to the institution best situated to handle it.

On the other hand, any such arrangement imposes upon Vanderbilt a very distinct responsibility. It would have to nurse its enrolment: having determined just how large a school local needs require, it must fix and enforce the strictest entrance requirement compatible therewith. At the present time this standard would be less than four-year high school graduation; but whatever it be, if only it is real and definite, it will operate to brace up general conditions. Improved teaching should compensate student defects. To this end, every effort should be made to secure endowment specifically applicable to the medical department; in the interval, fees must be employed not to wipe out old obligations, however incurred, but to improve the school. The contract between Vanderbilt University and its medical department should be canceled. The practitioner teachers must make good their ambition to advance medical education by being content with the indirect advantage accruing from school connections. If the entire fee income is used to equip the laboratories, to employ full-time teachers in the fundamental branches, to fit out and organize a good dispensary, there will still remain defects and makeshifts enough; but the school will wear a different aspect than is presented by any institution in the state to-day.

Let it be said ungrudgingly that these suggestions are offered in no spirit of unkindness. The State University and Vanderbilt have had their hands full. They have worked valiantly amidst conditions that might well appal the strongest hearts, They deserve no blame for the past, provided only they unselfishly and vigorously coöperate in forgetting it. In the last few years right courses of action in medical education have for the first time been defined. A decade hence it will be fair to look back and ask whether the universities of the state have followed them.

Of the three negro schools in the state, two are without merit. The third — Meharry — is a most creditable institution. The reader is referred to chapter xiv, "The Medical Education of the Negro," for a fuller discussion of its needs and deserts.

TEXAS

Population, 3,780,574. Number of physicians, 5789. Ratio, 1 : 653.
Number of medical schools, 4.

DALLAS: *Population*, 56,119.

(1) BAYLOR UNIVERSITY COLLEGE OF MEDICINE. Organized 1900. Since 1903 the medical department of Baylor University.

Entrance requirement: Nominally a three-year high school course or its equivalent.

Attendance: 53.

Teaching staff: 29, of whom 16 are professors, 13 of other grade. All the teachers are practitioners.

Resources available for maintenance: Fees, amounting to $7785 (estimated). The school has not thus far been assisted by the university.

Laboratory facilities: The school possesses a new laboratory adjoining the hospital to be noticed below; but at the date of the visit it was still quite bare. The dissecting-room was in good condition; a fair chemical laboratory and a meagerly equipped laboratory for pathology and bacteriology had been installed. There was nothing else, and no assurance of funds with which to provide additional laboratories or to maintain those already in part provided.

Clinical facilities: Adjoining the laboratory building is a new hospital of some 200 beds, in which the school has access to two free wards containing 32 beds, and to an additional negro ward of 22 beds in a pavilion close by. There is no clinical laboratory. Clinical opportunities are obtained at two other institutions, but no infectious diseases and little obstetrical work are obtainable. The clinical opportunities are thus decidedly inadequate.

A dispensary is just beginning.

Date of visit: November, 1909.

(2) SOUTHWESTERN UNIVERSITY MEDICAL COLLEGE. Organized 1903. Nominally the medical department of Southwestern University, which is protected by contract against liability for its debts.

Entrance requirement: Nominally a three-year high school course or its equivalent.

Attendance: 68.

Teaching staff: 32, of whom 17 are professors, 15 of other grade. All are practitioners.

Resources available for maintenance: Fees only, amounting to $7150 (estimated).

Laboratory facilities: The school possesses a new building, externally attractive but wretchedly kept. It contains a disorderly and incomplete chemical laboratory, a small amount of new physiological apparatus, a single laboratory fairly well equipped for pathology and bacteriology, and an ordinary dissecting-room. There is a "reading-room" with nothing to read. The lecture-rooms are bare, except for chairs; in a corner of one of them is an abused manikin.

Clinical facilities: Amphitheater clinics in surgery are held once weekly at an institution across the street, where perhaps 50 beds, mostly surgical, are accessible, and one afternoon a week at the City Hospital, one and a half miles distant. No infectious diseases are obtainable. Neither hospital contains a clinical laboratory. Clinical opportunities are therefore decidedly inadequate.

A dispensary is just starting.

Date of visit: November, 1909.

FORT WORTH: *Population, 27,096.*[1]

(3) FORT WORTH UNIVERSITY MEDICAL DEPARTMENT. Organized 1894. A nominal department of a local "university."

Entrance requirement: Nominally a three-year high school course or its equivalent.

Attendance: 100.

Teaching staff: 47, of whom 14 are professors, 33 of other grade. All are practitioners.

Resources available for maintenance: Fees only, amounting to $10,500 (estimated).

Laboratory facilities: These comprise a dissecting-room, ordinary laboratories for

[1] Not estimated by U. S. Census Bureau.

chemistry and bacteriology, and a single laboratory with routine outfit for pathology and histology; recent provision on a small scale has been made for physiology. The class-rooms are bare except for a reflectoscope and a defective skeleton. There are a small museum of unlabeled specimens and a small library.

Clinical facilities: The basement of the school building makes a wretched hospital of 50 beds, 20 of them free. There is no clinical laboratory. One surgical clinic weekly is held at a private hospital two miles distant.

For the dispensary a fair attendance is claimed, but no complete index is kept.

Date of visit : November, 1909.

GALVESTON: *Population, 37,834.*

(4) UNIVERSITY OF TEXAS, DEPARTMENT OF MEDICINE. Organized 1891. An organic department of the state university.

Entrance requirement: A four-year high school education, passed on by the state university.

Attendance: 206.

Teaching staff: 26, of whom 9 are professors, 17 of other grade. Three professors and seven instructors give entire time to the department. All instructors are on salary.

Resources available for maintenance: The department is carried by the general funds of the university. Its budget calls for $63,342, of which $6500 are derived from fees; the hospital budget requires $39,611 besides.

Laboratory facilities: The school has a complete series of admirable teaching laboratories, covering anatomy, physics, chemistry, physical chemistry, pathology, bacteriology, histology, and embryology. There is a large pathological museum, beautifully kept, every specimen classified, labeled, and indexed; and a notable anatomical museum in which special preparations are most advantageously arranged for teaching use. The library is good and is in regular receipt of foreign and domestic journals; animals in abundance are on hand. Competent helpers are provided for each floor. No effort, however, is made in the direction of research.

Clinical facilities: A university hospital of 155 beds adjoins the laboratories. Its organization is along sound lines—the service with a single chief being continuous, but students have not as yet been actively utilized in the wards. As elevated standards improve the student body, this innovation will become more feasible.

For lack of assistants, the dispensary is not so thoroughly organized. The attendance is fair.

Date of visit: November, 1909.

General Considerations

TEXAS is indubitably a state destined to a great development; its educational institutions must from time to time be readjusted to take account of its expanded needs. It is neither wise nor possible to provide now for requirements that will a generation hence become imperative. Sufficient for the people of Texas to-day to meet in the most effective way possible their own needs.

There is now only one educational institution in the state capable of maintaining a medical school whose graduates deserve the right to practise among its inhabitants; there is only one medical school in the state fit to continue in the work of training physicians. That institution is the state university; the medical school is its department at Galveston. The other three schools are without resources, without ideals, without facilities, though at Baylor the conjunction of hospital and laboratory might be made effective if large sums, specifically applicable to medical education, were at hand,—which is not, however, the case.

There is no indication on the face of things that any of the three inferior schools can live through the dry period to the opportunities of the future. Their enrolment is small; and the state is badly overcrowded with just the kind of doctor that they are engaged in producing. Should the loopholes in the present state standard be stopped up, all three would quickly disappear.

The course of the state university needs to be carefully considered. Whether a college requirement will soon be wise is a question to be pondered. The institution has not yet exhausted the possibilities of the high school standard; its laboratories— admirable for undergraduate teaching —need further development on the productive side; its hospital must be enlarged; more effective teaching methods can be introduced into it; the dispensary is not yet effective. It is worth asking whether from the four-year high school basis the university will not be wise to get complete control of the field, driving out the low-grade schools, educating the people of the state to regard it as their main source of supplies in the matter of doctors and the active conservator of public health, before endeavoring to push ahead to a higher standard, which may not be so well adapted to local conditions in a relatively new country.

Meanwhile, to the outsider it seems a regrettable mischance that located the medical department away from the university. Were it placed at Austin, it would apparently gain in every way: the town is as large, and various state institutions there would strengthen its clinical opportunities; it would be easier to attract and to hold outsiders in teaching positions; the stimulus of the university would assist the growth of a productive spirit. Whether at Galveston the school will ever be creative is a question; should it become so, isolation increases the liability to slip back into an unproductive groove. Perhaps it is not yet too late for the people of the state to concentrate their state institutions of higher learning in a single plant.

UTAH

Population, 336,122. Number of physicians, 359. Ratio, 1: 936.
Number of medical schools, 1.

SALT LAKE CITY : *Population, 65,464.*

UNIVERSITY OF UTAH, DEPARTMENT OF MEDICINE. Organized 1906. A half-school. An organic part of the state university.

Entrance requirement: One year of college work.

Attendance : 18.

Teaching staff : 6 professors and 10 of other grade, who take part in the instruction. The professors are all university teachers, of whom 3 give their entire time to medical subjects.

Resources available for maintenance : The department is supported out of the general funds of the university. It costs approximately $10,000; its income in fees is $1405.

Laboratory facilities: Laboratories are adequately equipped for the routine instruction of small classes in anatomy, physiology, physiological chemistry, chemistry, histology, pathology, and bacteriology. The spirit is excellent. A few books, scientific journals, charts, etc., are at hand ; a museum has been begun. More liberal support, however, is necessary if the department is to justify its high entrance standard.

It is to be hoped that whenever clinical instruction is started in Salt Lake City, it may be only for the purpose of completing the half-course now offered ; in that event Utah need never know the proprietary medical school.

Date of visit : April, 1909.

VERMONT

Population, 353,739. Number of physicians, 663. Ratio, 1 : 534.
Number of medical schools, 1.

BURLINGTON : *Population, 22,690.*

UNIVERSITY OF VERMONT COLLEGE OF MEDICINE. Organized 1822. Now an organic part of the university.

Entrance requirement : Less than a four-year high school education.

Attendance: 156, 42 per cent from Vermont.

Teaching staff : 33, of whom 18 are professors, 15 of other grade. Thirteen teachers are non-resident, among them the professors of medicine, obstetrics, pediatrics, physiology, and pathology. Some of the non-resident teachers go to Burlington weekly ; others give a concentrated course covering several weeks. The entire teaching staff never meets. There is one full-time teacher,—in the department of anatomy.

Resources available for maintenance : Fees, amounting to $21,388. The state has lately appropriated $10,000.

Laboratory facilities : The school has an attractive new laboratory building adequate to routine teaching of anatomy, pathology, histology, bacteriology, physiology, and chemistry. No research is in progress. There is no library, no museum, few teaching accessories, and no animals on the premises.

Clinical facilities : Two hospitals with 200 ward beds are in a limited way available, but the material is predominantly surgical: medical and obstetrical cases are relatively few. Infectious diseases are in the main didactically taught. There is little bedside work, patients being examined by assigned students in a small room and subsequently demonstrated in the amphitheater. The combined Senior and Junior classes attend a majority of the clinics in internal medicine and general surgery.

The dispensary has a small attendance.

Date of visit : May, 1909.

[For general considerations see " New England," p. 224.]

VIRGINIA

Population, 2,032,567. Number of physicians, 2215. Ratio, 1: 918.
Number of medical schools, 3.

CHARLOTTESVILLE: *Population, 7307.*

(1) UNIVERSITY OF VIRGINIA, DEPARTMENT OF MEDICINE. Organized 1827. An organic department of the university.

Entrance requirement: One year of college work in sciences.

Attendance: 89, 53 per cent from Virginia.

Teaching staff: 31 teachers, of whom 12 are professors, 19 of other grade, take part in the work of the department. The laboratory branches are taught by 8 instructors who give their entire time to them.

Resources available for maintenance: The budget of the department calls for $52,195, including hospital deficit; it is met out of the funds of the university. The income in fees amounts to $10,060.

Laboratory facilities: Up to three years ago the department was a didactic school.

Since then it has been revolutionized: good teaching laboratories in all necessary branches, with increased provision for research, have been equipped and put in charge of enthusiastic teachers of modern training and ideals. The main present lack is a suitable building and an adequate medical library.

Clinical facilities: The University Hospital of 100 beds (80 of them ward beds) is the laboratory of the clinical teachers.[1] Its relation to the medical school and its organization for teaching purposes leave nothing to be desired. Though the material has not yet reached proper proportions, it is increasing and is skilfully and effectively used to train the student body in the technique and methods of scientific medicine. The surgical side is in this respect more highly organized than the medical.

There is a small dispensary.

Date of visit: February, 1909.

RICHMOND: *Population,* 111,078.

(2) MEDICAL COLLEGE OF VIRGINIA. Organized 1838.

Entrance requirement: Less than a four-year high school education. The registration office is most systematically conducted.

Attendance: 206.

Teaching staff: 61, of whom 16 are professors, 45 of other grade. There are no teachers giving their entire time to medical instruction.

Resources available for maintenance: Fees, amounting to $22,490, and an annual state appropriation of $5000.

Laboratory facilities: The school occupies an imposing building with ordinary laboratories for pathology, histology, bacteriology, physiology, and chemistry. The dissecting-room is in poor condition. There is a fair museum and an attractive library with some recent books, in charge of a librarian.

Clinical facilities: These are inadequate. Close by is the Memorial Hospital, with about 40 beds available for teaching. Supplementary facilities are enjoyed in the City Hospital and elsewhere.

The dispensary occupies an excellent suite of rooms and has a fair attendance.

Date of visit: February, 1909.

(3) UNIVERSITY COLLEGE OF MEDICINE. Organized 1893. An independent institution.

Entrance requirement: Less than a four-year high school education.

Attendance: 121, 63 per cent from Virginia.

[1] A recent gift of $50,000 is now available for the extension of the hospital.

Teaching staff: 74, of whom 22 are professors, 52 of other grade.

Resources available for maintenance: Fees, amounting to $14,975.

Laboratory facilities: The school was recently destroyed by fire and now occupies temporary laboratory quarters.

Clinical facilities: These are inadequate. The school adjoins its own hospital, with less than 50 beds available for teaching. Supplementary facilities are enjoyed elsewhere. An out-patient obstetrical service is well organized.

The dispensary has a fair attendance.

Date of visit: February, 1909.

General Considerations

THE destruction by fire of the University College of Medicine at Richmond should precipitate the consolidation of the two independent schools. Separately neither of them can hope greatly to improve its present facilities, which, weak in respect to laboratories and laboratory teaching, are entirely inadequate on the clinical side. Their present hospitals utilized together, though still unsatisfactory, would at any rate be much more nearly adequate than is either hospital taken by itself; and the combined fees would furnish much better laboratory training than either school now gives. A single independent school of the better type might still have in Virginia a brief term of prosperity,—the more so as the medical department of the University of Virginia is on a considerably higher basis.

The rapid improvement of the medical department of the University of Virginia in the last three years is one of the striking phenomena of recent medical school history. The limitations of Charlottesville have been acutely felt; the university is pursuing the course calculated to surmount them. It faces indeed a much greater outlay than it has yet made, for larger clinics in internal medicine and obstetrics must be developed. The alternative of a remote department diminishes difficulty of one kind only to create difficulty of another. A remote department at Norfolk or Richmond would of course command abundant clinical material; but could it preserve university ideals? The present resources of the university are not large enough to stand the strain of such liberal support as a remote department needs if it is to be genuinely productive. The experience of a few years warrants the belief that a clinic in most lines, for a school of 200 students, can be developed at Charlottesville if the university can afford it. Graduating classes of 50 easily suffice for Virginia's demand. At any rate, so much is evident: in Virginia, as elsewhere, the teaching of medicine will fall to the universities; and at this writing, the only institution available is the University of Virginia.

West Virginia

Population, 1,135,206. Number of physicians, 1608. Ratio, 1 : 706.
Number of medical schools, 1.

MORGANTOWN, *Population, 2779.*

West Virginia University College of Medicine. Organized 1902. A half-school.
An organic department of the university.

Entrance requirement: A four-year high school education, though applicants not thus
qualified are admitted as special students.

Attendance: 18.

Teaching staff: 7 professors, who take part in the instruction offered, two of them
giving their entire time to this department.

Resources available for maintenance: The department is carried by the university. Its
income in fees is $1000 (estimated).

Laboratory facilities: The school is fairly equipped to do elementary work in anatomy,
chemistry, histology, pathology, and bacteriology; less well in physiology. There
is no library, no museum, no charts, no models, or other teaching accessories. The
work and interest are limited to routine.

    The school has an "affiliation" with the College of Physicians and Surgeons of
Baltimore, — an independent institution over which West Virginia University has
neither control nor influence. [*See* Maryland (2).]

Date of visit: March, 1909.

Wisconsin

Population, 2,356,874. Number of physicians, 2518. Ratio, 1 : 936.
Number of medical schools, 3.

MADISON : *Population, 28,438.*

(1) University of Wisconsin College of Medicine. Organized 1907. A half-school.
An organic part of the university.

Entrance requirement: Two years of college work, including sciences, rigidly enforced.

Attendance: 49.

Teaching staff: 23 instructors, who take part in the work of the department, of whom
17 give their entire time to it.

Resources available for maintenance: The department is maintained out of the general funds of the university. Its budget calls for $40,625.

Laboratory facilities: Though temporarily housed, the laboratories, complete in number, are admirably equipped with respect to both teaching and research. A successful effort has been made to provide facilities worthy of students on a two-year college basis and of teachers deserving opportunities for progressive work. The department lacks only a building which shall bring its parts together.

Date of visit: May, 1909.

MILWAUKEE: *Population, 337,117.*

(2) MILWAUKEE MEDICAL COLLEGE. A stock company, organized 1894, and now nominally the medical department of Marquette University.

Entrance requirement: A four-year high school education or its equivalent.

Attendance: 168, 91 per cent from Wisconsin.

Teaching staff: 67, of whom 30 are professors, 37 of other rank.

Resources available for maintenance: Fees only, amounting to $22,680.

Laboratory facilities: Meager facilities are provided for the teaching of pathology and bacteriology; there is the usual chemical laboratory; anatomy is better than ordinary. Experimental physiology and toxicology are taught at Marquette College near by; the equipment is slight.

Clinical facilities: These are extremely weak. The school adjoins Trinity Hospital, which is practically part of the same corporation. It has 75 beds, largely occupied by pay patients and given up almost wholly to surgery; teaching is limited to amphitheater clinics; weekly clinics are also held at the County Hospital, five miles distant.

An ill equipped dispensary in the college building has an attendance varying from ten to twenty a day. A card index is now kept.

Date of visit: February, 1910.

(3) WISCONSIN COLLEGE OF PHYSICIANS AND SURGEONS. Organized 1893. An independent institution, nominally the medical department of Carroll College.

Entrance requirement: A four-year high school education or its equivalent.

Attendance: 60, 85 per cent from Wisconsin.

Teaching staff: 66, of whom 26 are professors, 40 of other grade. No teacher devotes his entire time to the school.

Resources available for maintenance: Fees only, amounting to $8675 (estimated).

Laboratory facilities: The school occupies an attractive building which contains an ordinary laboratory for elementary chemistry, another—poor and very disorderly, without animals—for bacteriology; the room given to histology and pathology is clean, contains a small amount of well kept material, and is adequate to routine elementary work. Anatomy is very poor; there is not even a complete skeleton. No other teaching adjuncts are at hand. No provision is made for even demonstrative work in experimental physiology.

Clinical facilities: These are utterly wretched. The school gives amphitheater clinics only, at a Catholic hospital across the street, practically all of whose work is in surgery. Acute medical cases are seen, if at all, twice a week at the County Hospital, five miles off. A neat dispensary, with poor records and with no laboratory or other equipment, adjoins the school building.

Date of visit: February, 1910.

General Considerations

WISCONSIN presents a simple problem : the two Milwaukee schools are without a redeeming feature. It is claimed that the examiner representing the state board enforces a four-year high school standard; but it has been impossible to procure any information at all from this official, though repeated efforts have been made to do so. Neither of the schools meets the most lenient standards in respect to laboratory outfit or teaching; and as for clinical facilities they are hardly more than nominal.

A western state so admirably organized on the educational side, furnishing excellent college opportunities without cost to the student, is surely in position to meet Minnesota and Indiana in the matter of practice standards. The requirement of a year or two of college work as preliminary to practice would quickly leave the medical department of the state university in sole control.

This department has wisely resisted efforts to make of it a divided instead of a half school; nothing worse could ever happen to it than that it should be rounded off with a clinical end at Milwaukee,—made up, perhaps, in part out of the two schools now there. When the time comes for the completion of the department, it must be completed at Madison. The difficulties due to the size and residential character of the town are not insuperable. There is not the least doubt that wise administration can develop on the site of the university a medical school large enough to train the doctors of the state. But its scope will run far beyond this primary duty; for it will inevitably be a producing department. Assuredly, Wisconsin, fortunate beyond almost all other states in the concentration of its higher institutions of learning, will not be guilty of the folly of detaching in whole or part the medical department from the university whose ideals it can share and help to create.

CANADA

Population, 6,945,228. Number of physicians, 6786. Ratio, 1 : 1030. Number of medical schools, 8.

Manitoba

WINNIPEG: *Population*, 150,000.

(1) Manitoba Medical College. Organized 1883. The medical department of the University of Manitoba, the connection being in process of becoming organic.

Entrance requirement: The University Matriculation Examination or its actual equivalent. The medical course covers five years.

Attendance: 115.

Teaching staff: 41, of whom 22 are professors, 19 of other grade.

Resources available for maintenance: Fees, amounting to $14,000.

Laboratory facilities: Instruction in chemistry, bacteriology, histology, and pathology is competently given by the University of Manitoba. Other branches are carried on by the medical faculty. The equipment is adequate to routine instruction, new, and steadily increasing. There is a beautifully kept collection of several hundred wet specimens. Appearances indicate a conscientious and intelligent employment of such resources as the school has had.

Clinical facilities: The excellent Winnipeg General Hospital of 400 beds adjoins the school. The school faculty is practically the staff of the free wards. The relation between school and hospital is admirable. Students work freely in wards, clinical laboratory, operating-rooms, obstetrical ward, etc.

There is a good dispensary.

Date of visit: May, 1909.

Nova Scotia

HALIFAX (Nova Scotia): *Population*, 45,000 (estimated).

(2) Halifax Medical College. Organized in 1867. An independent school with a peculiar relationship to Dalhousie University, which provides satisfactorily instruction in chemistry, physics, and biology, during part of the first two years of the five-year course. In respect to all else the medical school is an independent institution, though its students are practically all examined for their degree by Dalhousie University. The university thus furnishes part of the first two years' teaching and is the final examining body ; with the intervening years it has nothing to do.

Entrance requirement : On a par with that of Dalhousie University.

Attendance : 63, 90 per cent from Nova Scotia.

Teaching staff : 33, of whom 16 are professors. There are no full-time instructors. (This does not include the instructors in the scientific branches furnished by Dalhousie University.)

Resources available for maintenance : An annual appropriation of $1200 from the provincial government and fees amounting to about $5000. Three-fourths of the fees are distributed among the professors; one-fourth provides, with the government grant, for all other expense. A bequest yielding $200 per annum supports the college library.

Laboratory facilities : This disposition of funds is reflected in the condition of the medical college : it possesses an ordinary, ill smelling dissecting-room and a single utterly wretched laboratory for pathology, bacteriology, and histology. A microscope is provided for each student. Though this same " laboratory " serves for the provincial board of health, no animals are used. There is no museum worthy the name, and no laboratory work in physiology or pharmacology. The laboratory sciences have been starved that small dividends might be paid to generally prosperous practitioners.

Clinical facilities : Clinical instruction is provided at the Victoria General Hospital,— a government institution of some 200 beds, open to the medical school. About 70 per cent of the cases are surgical. The staff appointments are made by the government for its own reasons ; the medical college is forced to confer professorships on these appointees. Ward classes are conducted ; individual cases are assigned, and the student's notes become part of the hospital records. Instruction in clinical microscopy is very limited.

Obstetrical opportunities barely suffice. Autopsies are performed in the presence of students, who report on them. The college has no dispensary, but students are required to attend the city dispensary,—an institution within which the medical school has no authority. The attendance is fair.

It has been stated above that except during part of the first two years Dalhousie University has no teaching responsibility for or connection with Halifax Medical College. On the other hand, students of Halifax Medical College are examined by the medical faculty of Dalhousie University and obtain the Dalhousie medical degree. The question may fairly be asked: What is the value of the Dalhousie degree in medicine, won by students whose opportunities have been provided by Halifax Medical College ? The connection is, from the standpoint of Dalhousie University, highly objectionable.

Date of visit : October, 1909.

ONTARIO

KINGSTON: *Population, 20,000.*

(3) MEDICAL DEPARTMENT OF QUEEN'S UNIVERSITY. Organized 1854. The relation of the medical department to the university is anomalous, marking a period of transition that is likely soon to result in complete integration.

Entrance requirement : Heretofore somewhat below that of the arts department of the university, though students must comply with the requirements of the province in which they expect to practise. The medical course covers five years.

Attendance : 208, 71 per cent from Ontario.

Teaching staff : 38, 16 being professors.

Resources available for maintenance : Income in fees, $19,978. A fixed percentage of fees is annually expended on buildings, equipment, and maintenance. The remainder belongs to and is disbursed by the medical faculty.

Laboratory facilities : The laboratory building is new and the equipment is adequate to intelligent routine work. At present, physics, chemistry, and physiology are taught in the university, in return for which the university receives a part of the fees of the students instructed. Full-time professors in anatomy and pathology are provided by the medical school. A museum is in process of formation. There is a small collection of books and periodicals in the faculty room, open to students.

Clinical facilities : The clinical facilities are limited. The school relies mainly on the adjoining Kingston General Hospital, in which its faculty practically constitutes the staff. The average number of beds available is 80, but they are well used. In addition to ward work, students are required to work up individual cases in correct form, including the clinical laboratory aspects. There is a ward for infectious diseases. Obstetrical cases are too few. Post-mortems are secured mainly at the Rockwood Insane Asylum. Two supplementary hospitals provide additional illustrative clinical material. The opportunities for out-patient work are slight.

Date of visit : October, 1909.

LONDON: *Population, 41,500.*

(4) WESTERN UNIVERSITY MEDICAL DEPARTMENT. Established 1881. Practically an independent school.

Entrance requirement: Nominal. The student, for his own protection, is expected to fulfil the requirements of the place in which he intends to practise. The medical course covers four years.

Attendance: 104.

Teaching staff: 20, of whom 8 are professors, 12 of other grade.

Resources available for maintenance: Fees, amounting to $11,590 (estimated).

Laboratory facilities: These consist of a single room called the laboratory of pathology, bacteriology, and histology, whose equipment consists of microscopes and some unlabeled specimens,—no microtome, cut sections, incubator, or sterilizer being visible,—a wretched chemical laboratory, and an ordinary dissecting-room. There is no outfit for physiology, pharmacology, or clinical microscopy, and no museum deserving the name. There are a few hundred books, locked in cases to which the janitor carries the key.

Clinical facilities: These are entirely inadequate. They are confined almost wholly to a small number of beds in the municipal hospital.

The school has no dispensary.

Date of visit: October, 1909.

TORONTO: *Population, 328,911.*

(5) UNIVERSITY OF TORONTO FACULTY OF MEDICINE. Established 1887. An organic department of the university.

Entrance requirement: The Junior Matriculation Examination, strictly enforced. The course covers five years.

Attendance: 592.

Teaching staff: 68, of whom 27 are professors, 41 of other grade. Ten professors with fifteen assistants give their entire time to teaching and research.

Resources available for maintenance: The department is supported out of the general funds of the university, its cost being considerably in excess of fees received. The latter amount to $64,500.

Laboratory facilities: The laboratories are in point of construction and equipment among the best on the continent. Increasing attention has recently been devoted to the cultivation of research. There are both general and departmental libraries, an excellent museum, and all necessary teaching accessories.

Clinical facilities: The school has recently perfected a very intimate relationship with the new Toronto General Hospital, by which its faculty obtains complete control of the clinical advantages of some 500 beds. Students have free access to all wards, clinical laboratory, dispensary, etc. Other large local hospitals—general and special —are also available.

Date of visit: March, 1909.

QUEBEC

MONTREAL: *Population, 267,730.*

(6) McGILL UNIVERSITY MEDICAL FACULTY. Established 1824. An organic department of the university.

Entrance requirement: The University School Leaving Examination, strictly enforced. The medical course covers five years.

Attendance: 328.

Teaching staff: 99, of whom 19 are professors, 80 of other grade. Ten instructors devote their entire time to teaching.

Resources available for maintenance: The department has separate endowments aggregating $350,000 and is assisted out of the general university funds. Its fees amount to $43,750; its budget, $77,000.

Laboratory facilities: The laboratories having been recently injured by fire, the school is now waiting the completion of its new buildings, for which ample funds have been secured. Meanwhile its temporary quarters, well equipped for both teaching and research in all departments, show what energy and intelligence can accomplish in the face of disaster. The anatomical and pathological museums are among the most famous on the continent. The school possesses an excellent library and all necessary teaching accessories.

Clinical facilities: These are excellent. The school enjoys a most favorable relation to two large hospitals, of about 500 beds, besides several other institutions. Students work freely in all the wards and clinical laboratory.

    The dispensary service is large and admirable.

Date of visit: March, 1909.

(7) LAVAL UNIVERSITY MEDICAL DEPARTMENT. Organized 1878. The university connection is not intimate.

Entrance requirement: Indefinite, depending on the prospective location of the student. The medical course covers five years.

Attendance: 217.

Teaching staff: 8.

Resources available for maintenance: Fees, most of which are distributed among the teachers.

Laboratory facilities: Chemistry is given by the university. Anatomy is limited to dissecting. A single laboratory with meager equipment is assigned to pathology, bacteriology, and histology. There is a library and a small collection of specimens, not all labeled.

Clinical facilities: The school has access to two hospitals, containing together 250 beds. The dispensary has a fair attendance.

Date of visit: March, 1909.

QUEBEC: *Population,* 70,000.

(8) LAVAL UNIVERSITY MEDICAL DEPARTMENT. Organized 1848. An organic part of Laval University.

Entrance requirement: Indefinite, depending on the student's prospective location. As most graduates locate in the province—French being the language of instruction—they must comply with the provincial requirement. The medical course covers five years.

Attendance: 92.

Teaching staff: 22.

Resources available for maintenance: Fees and an appropriation by the university.

Laboratory facilities: Instruction in chemistry and physics is provided by the university; in the medical building, recent, though not extensive, laboratory provision is made for anatomy, histology, bacteriology, and pathology. There is no experimental physiology or pharmacology. A library for students and a museum have been started lately. The buildings are admirably kept.

Clinical facilities: Clinical instruction in medicine, surgery, and pediatrics is given at the Charity Hospital (Hôtel Dieu), to the free wards of which the faculty serves as staff. The amount of material is limited in quantity; the staff rotates monthly. The hospital contains a clinical laboratory, in which instruction is given in connection with ward work. The fifth year, now required, and a proposed reorganization of staff and teaching arrangements promise to improve the instruction. Obstetrical opportunity is abundant.

The dispensary has a sufficient attendance.

Date of visit: October, 1909.

General Considerations

IN the matter of medical schools, Canada reproduces the United States on a greatly reduced scale. Western University (London) is as bad as anything to be found on this side the line; Laval and Halifax Medical College are feeble; Winnipeg and Kingston represent a distinct effort toward higher ideals; McGill and Toronto are excellent. The eight schools of the Dominion thus belong to three different types, the best adding a fifth year to their advantages of superior equipment and instruction.

At this moment the needs of the Dominion could be met by the four better English schools and the Laval department at Quebec. Toronto has practically reached the limits of efficiency in point of size; McGill and Manitoba are capable of considerable expansion. The future of Kingston is at least doubtful. It could certainly maintain a two-year school; for the Kingston General Hospital would afford pathological and clinical material amply sufficient up to that point. But the clinical years require much more than the town now supplies. Its location—halfway between Montreal and Toronto, on an inconvenient branch-line—greatly aggravates the difficulties due to the smallness of the community. The rapid development of the Northwest Territory will undoubtedly hasten the growth of the Winnipeg school; other institutions will in time be established nearer the Pacific coast as the country grows in population.

The legal standard in the Dominion has not thus far been high; but it has practically been elevated a year by the general movement to prolong the course to five years. Meanwhile, the high quality of instruction offered by McGill and Toronto to students who enter on less than a four-year high school education proves that our trouble in the United States has been at bottom not less one of low ideals than of low standards. Indeed, where ideals are low, there are no standards; and where ideals are high, the standard, even though low, is at any rate so definite that it furnishes a sure starting-point towards a clearly apprehended goal. The low standard school in the United States has had no such starting-point and no such goal.

APPENDIX

TABLE SHOWING NUMBER IN FACULTY, ENROLMENT,
. FEE INCOME, BUDGET OF SCHOOLS BY STATES

INSTITUTION (Half-schools marked *)	Number of Professors	Number of Other Instructors	Number of Students	Total Annual Income from Fees	Annual Budget [2]
ALABAMA					
1. Birmingham Medical College	18	12	185	$ 14,550 [1]	
2. University of Alabama, Medical Department	8	17	204	17,300 [6]	
ARKANSAS					
3. University of Arkansas, Medical Department	18	17	179	14,100 [1]	
4. College of Physicians and Surgeons (Little Rock)	25	9	81	6,450 [1]	
CALIFORNIA					
5. College of Physicians and Surgeons (Los Angeles)	28	13	32	4,075 [1]	
6. California Eclectic Medical College	26	1	9	1,060 [1]	
7. Los Angeles College of Osteopathy	19		"More than 250"	37,500 [1]	
8. Pacific College of Osteopathy	19	19	85	12,750 [1]	
9. Oakland College of Medicine and Surgery	18	19	17	2,760 [1]	
10. Hahnemann Medical College of the Pacific	13	22	23	2,685 [1]	
11. College of Physicians and Surgeons (San Francisco)	23	30	70	7,715 [1]	
12. Leland Stanford Junior University, College of Medicine	16	5	16 [3]		
13. University of California, Medical Department	12	48	36	7,004	$83,396
COLORADO					
14. University of Colorado, School of Medicine	25	20	85	4,043	28,000
15. Denver and Gross College of Medicine (University of Denver)	44	35	109	12,624 [1]	
CONNECTICUT					
16. Yale Medical School	14	50	138	15,325	43,311
DISTRICT OF COLUMBIA					
17. George Washington University, Department of Medicine	25	44	117	21,833	23,779
18. Georgetown University, Department of Medicine	20	54	89	11,000	
19. Howard University, Medical Department	22	30	205	26,000	40,000 [4]
GEORGIA					
20. Atlanta College of Physicians and Surgeons	20	31	286	28,000	
21. Atlanta School of Medicine	17	27	230	20,000 [1]	
22. Georgia College of Eclectic Medicine and Surgery	14	6	66	5,655 [1]	
23. Hospital Medical College	16		43	3,950 [1]	
24. Medical College of Georgia (University of Georgia)	18	15	99	6,835	
ILLINOIS					
25. Rush Medical College (University of Chicago)	89	141	488	60,485 [5]	82,452
Forwarded	562	665	3,142	$343,699	

[1] *Estimated.* [2] *First year in operation.*
[3] *Absence of information under this heading may mean one of several things: in proprietary schools there is no budget, because no plans are made, — necessary expenses are met and the balance is divided or is used to reduce debts; in many university departments the expense incurred, while much greater than fee income, is so involved with expense incurred for other laboratory purposes that it cannot be separated. In such instances, it cannot be definitely stated what the cost of the department is.*
[4] *Includes state appropriation of $5000 which pays for scholarships.*
[5] *First two years, University of Chicago: $55,000. Third and fourth years, Rush Medical College: $27,455.*

INSTITUTION (Half-schools marked *)	Number of Professors	Number of Other Instructors	Number of Students	Total Annual Income from Fees	Annual Budget
Carried forward	562	665	3,142	$343,699	
ILLINOIS (Continued)					
26. Northwestern University Medical School	54	89	522	89,076	$88,861
27. College of Physicians and Surgeons (University of Illinois)...................	42	156	517	80,155[1]	....
American Medical Missionary College................................	....	*See Michigan*	....	....	....
28. Hahnemann Medical College and Hospital of Chicago.................	38	46	130	14,300[1]	....
29. Chicago College of Medicine and Surgery	37	34	366	43,430[1]	....
30. Hering Medical College................................	30	14	32	3,360[1]	....
31. Illinois Medical College................................	38	35	69	9,175[1]	....
32. Bennett Medical College	21	21	181	19,380[1]	....
33. College of Medicine and Surgery—Physio-medical................	33	9	33	2,935[1]	....
34. Jenner Medical College	28	9	112	12,680[1]	....
35. National Medical University................................	36	....	150	22,500[1]	....
36. Reliance Medical College................................	23	21	88	9,945[1]	....
37. Littlejohn College of Osteopathy	43	....	75	11,250[1]	....
INDIANA					
38. Indiana University, School of Medicine	99	76	266	31,240[1]	....
39. *Valparaiso University, Medical Department................	....	....	25	....	....
IOWA					
40. Drake University College of Medicine................	16	29	106	9,505	12,417
41. Still College of Osteopathy................................	13	2	115	17,250[1]	....
42. State University of Iowa, College of Medicine................	12	20	267	13,707	35,316[2]
43. State University of Iowa, College of Homeopathic Medicine................	10	15	42	1,864	5,453[1]
KANSAS					
44. University of Kansas, School of Medicine................	24	39	89	5,030	40,000
45. Western Eclectic College of Medicine and Surgery................	30	2	21	1,600[1]	....
46. Kansas Medical College (Washburn College)................	31	16	65	4,876	....
KENTUCKY					
47. University of Louisville, Medical Department................	40	50	600	75,125	....
48. Southwestern Homeopathic Medical College................	12	15	18	1,100[1]	....
49. Louisville National Medical College................	17	6	40	2,560[1]	....
Forwarded................	1,289	1,269	7,061	$325,942	

[1] *Estimated.*   [2] *The university hospital budget is $33,745.*   [3] *Hospital budget, $7847.*

INSTITUTION (Half-schools marked *)	Number of Professors	Number of Other Instructors	Number of Students	Total Annual Income from Fees	Annual Budget
Carried forward	1,289	1,269	7,061	$825,942	
LOUISIANA					
50. Tulane University of Louisiana, Medical Department.........................	17	58	439	67,500	$101,781
51. Flint Medical College..........................	6	9	24	1,300	....
MAINE					
52. Medical School of Maine (Bowdoin College)........................	14	21	81	8,100	15,700
MARYLAND					
53. Johns Hopkins University, Medical Department...............................	23	89	297	60,542	102,429
54. College of Physicians and Surgeons (Baltimore)........................	21	38	252	39,000[1]	....
55. University of Maryland, School of Medicine........................	24	37	316	44,530	....
56. Baltimore Medical College........................	20	43	392	33,424	....
57. Woman's Medical College of Baltimore........................	18	13	22	2,000[1]	....
58. Maryland Medical College........................	21	18	95	7,460[1]	....
59. Atlantic Medical College........................	12	35	43	3,905[1]	....
MASSACHUSETTS					
60. Harvard University Medical School........................	23	150	285	72,037	251,389
61. Boston University School of Medicine........................	29	35	90	12,762[1]	....
62. Tufts College Medical School........................	33	70	384	59,093	....
63. College of Physicians and Surgeons (Boston)........................	30	15	172	10,000[1]	....
64. Massachusetts College of Osteopathy........................	19	15	90	11,400[1]	....
MICHIGAN					
65. University of Michigan, Department of Medicine and Surgery.........	22	41	389	34,093	83,000[2]
66. University of Michigan Homeopathic College........................	15	11	80	4,515	16,400[3]
67. American Medical Missionary College........................	22	10	75	4,778[1]	....
68. Detroit College of Medicine........................	25	79	161	22,000[1]	....
69. Detroit Homeopathic College........................	17	18	34	3,010[1]	....
MINNESOTA					
70. University of Minnesota, College of Medicine and Surgery........................	49	71	174	16,546	71,336
MISSISSIPPI					
71. Mississippi Medical College........................	12	7	100	7,500[1]	....
72. University of Mississippi, Medical Department........................	14	13	39	3,500	15,000
MISSOURI					
73. *University of Missouri, School of Medicine........................	8	6	47	2,820	31,000
Forwarded................	1,783	2,171	11,142	$1,857,757	

Estimated.   [1] *Not including university hospital budget of $70,000.*   [2] *Hospital budget, $31,000.*

INSTITUTION (Half-schools marked *)	Number of Professors	Number of Other Instructors	Number of Students	Total Annual Income from Fees	Annual Budget
Carried forward	1,783	2,171	11,142	$1,357,757	
MISSOURI (CONTINUED)					
74. University Medical College................	30	35	174	17,600 [1]	....
75. Kansas City Hahnemann Medical College.......	33	8	59	5,900 [1]	....
76. Central College of Osteopathy.............	20	....	40	4,500 [1]	....
77. American School of Osteopathy...........	12	11	560	39,600 [1]	....
78. Ensworth Medical College..............	32	8	72	7,060 [1]	....
79. Washington University, Medical Department.........	48	51	178	21,000	$51,265 [1]
80. St. Louis University School of Medicine........	39	82	243	26,630 [1]	37,000 [1]
81. St. Louis College of Physicians and Surgeons..........	25	24	224	16,035 [1]	
82. Barnes Medical College...............	39	25	124	12,400 [1]	
83. American Medical College...............	25	3	28	3,801 [1]	....
84. Hippocratean School of Medicine............	30	8	31	3,315 [1]	....
NEBRASKA					
85. University of Nebraska, College of Medicine	38	46	122	4,905	20,612
86. Lincoln Medical College (Cotner University)..........	34	....	42	3,794 [1]	....
87. John A. Creighton Medical College (Creighton University)............	28	21	175	17,850 [1]	....
NEW HAMPSHIRE					
88. Dartmouth Medical School (Dartmouth College)............	17	7	58	5,583 [1]	....
NEW YORK					
89. Albany Medical College (Union University)............	16	78	180	20,276	
90. University of Buffalo Medical Department	38	59	193	31,984	
91. College of Physicians and Surgeons, New York City (Columbia University)	38	138	312	75,500	239,072 [3]
92. Cornell University Medical College	32	100	207	24,410	309,888 (New York) 32,840 (Ithaca)
93. Eclectic Medical College of the City of New York	16	29	96	8,311	....
94. Fordham University School of Medicine............	32	40	42	7,330 [1]	....
95. Long Island College Hospital	9	85	360	61,398	....
96. New York Homeopathic Medical College...........	31	34	159	18,658	....
97. New York Medical College for Women	23	22	24	2,545	....
98. University and Bellevue Hospital Medical College (New York University)	37	127	408	76,115	87,115
99. Syracuse University, College of Medicine............	15	42	151	28,861	....
Forwarded................	2,520	3,254	15,404	$1,953,118	

[1] Estimated.   [2] Hospital budget, $30,000.   [3] Including Sloane Maternity Hospital and Vanderbilt Clinic.

INSTITUTION (Half-schools marked *)	Number of Professors	Number of Other Instructors	Number of Students	Total Annual Income from Fees	Annual Budget
Carried forward	2,520	3,254	15,404	$1,953,118	
NORTH CAROLINA					
100. *University of North Carolina, Medical Department...............	10	5	74	6,500	$ 12,000
101. North Carolina Medical College...	. 19	13	94	8,345 [1]	....
102. Leonard Medical School (Shaw University)...........................	8	1	125	2,846	
103. *Wake Forest College, School of Medicine............................	6	....	53	2,225	
NORTH DAKOTA					
104. *State University of North Dakota, College of Medicine...........	9	7	9	450	6,300
OHIO					
105. Ohio-Miami Medical School (University of Cincinnati)...............	50	76	197	26,345	....
106. Eclectic Medical Institute...	12	12	86	7,500 [1]	
107. Pulte Medical College...	24	12	16	1,325 [1]	....
108. Cleveland College of Physicians and Surgeons.......................	18	41	89	9,520 [1]	
109. Cleveland Homeopathic Medical College................................	30	31	46	5,750 [1]	
110. Western Reserve University, Medical Department....................	18	82	98	11,000	68,000
111. Starling-Ohio Medical College..	32	28	220	27,500 [1]	....
112. Toledo Medical College...	16	82	32	3,240 [1]	....
OKLAHOMA					
113. *State University of Oklahoma, School of Medicine.................	9	....	22	600	....
114. Epworth University College of Medicine	28	14	51	4,285 [1]	
OREGON					
115. University of Oregon, Medical Department............................	14	27	72	8,000 [1]	....
116. Willamette University, Medical Department...........................	15	1	29	3,580 [1]	
PENNSYLVANIA					
117. University of Pennsylvania, Department of Medicine...............	26	131	546	104,612	131,255 [2]
118. Jefferson Medical College	22	100	591	102,995	
119. Medico-Chirurgical College of Philadelphia	23	86	480	48,281 [1]	....
120. Woman's Medical College of Philadelphia	25	27	125	15,480	
121. Hahnemann Medical College, Philadelphia.............................	27	45	182	18,500	
122. Temple University, Department of Medicine	15	70	136	17,000 [1]	....
123. Philadelphia College of Osteopathy....................................	11	7	126	18,900 [1]	....
124. University of Pittsburgh, Medical Department........................	43	60	315	48,500	....
Forwarded................	3,030	4,162	19,218	$2,456,397	

[1] *Estimated.*   [2] *Exclusive of hospital and dispensary.*

INSTITUTION (Half-schools marked *)	Number of Professors	Number of Other Instructors	Number of Students	Total Annual Income from Fees	Annual Budget
Carried forward..........................	3,030	4,162	19,218	$2,456,397	
SOUTH CAROLINA					
125. Medical College of the State of South Carolina	11	23	213	19,447	....
SOUTH DAKOTA					
126. *University of South Dakota, College of Medicine	5	5	7	660	
TENNESSEE					
127. Chattanooga Medical College (University of Chattanooga)....................	11	14	112	4,290[1]	....
128. Tennessee Medical College (Lincoln Memorial University)......................	26	5	82	4,994	....
129. Knoxville Medical College......................	9	2	23	1,020[1]	....
130. College of Physicians and Surgeons (Memphis)..............	22	25	77	7,400[1]	....
131. Memphis Hospital Medical College...............	12	23	442	34,600[1]	....
132. University of West Tennessee, Medical Department...............	14	....	40	2,000[1]	....
133. Universities of Nashville and Tennessee, Medical Department....................	26	29	207	26,000[1]	....
134. Vanderbilt University, Medical Department...............	17	23	200	26,250	....
135. Meharry Medical College (Walden University)	12	14	275	20,310	$23,946
TEXAS					
136. Baylor University, College of Medicine	16	13	58	7,735[1]	....
137. Southwestern University, Medical College	17	15	68	7,150[1]	....
138. Fort Worth University, Medical Department...............	14	33	100	10,500[1]	....
139. University of Texas, Medical Department................	9	17	206	6,500	63,343[1]
UTAH					
140. *University of Utah, Department of Medicine	6	10	18	1,405	10,000
VERMONT					
141. University of Vermont, College of Medicine	18	15	156	21,388	
VIRGINIA					
142. University of Virginia, Department of Medicine...............	12	19	89	10,060	53,195[1]
143. Medical College of Virginia.................	16	45	206	22,490[1]	....
144. University College of Medicine	22	52	121	14,975	....
WEST VIRGINIA					
145. *West Virginia University, College of Medicine...............	7	....	18	1,000[1]	....
WISCONSIN					
146. *University of Wisconsin, College of Medicine...............	7	16	49	....	40,635
147. Milwaukee Medical College (Marquette University)...........................	30	37	168	22,680[1]	....
Forwarded.....................	3,369	4,597	22,148	$2,729,251	

[1] *Estimated.* [2] *Hospital budget, $59,611.* [3] *Including hospital deficit.*

INSTITUTION (Half-schools marked *)	Number of Professors	Number of Other Instructors	Number of Students	Total Annual Income from Fees	Annual Budget
Carried forward..	3,369	4,597	22,148	$2,729,251	
SCONSIN (Continued)					
Wisconsin College of Physicians and Surgeons	26	40	60	8,675	....
NITOBA					
Manitoba Medical College (University of Manitoba)[1]............................	22	19	115	14,000	....
VA SCOTIA					
Halifax Medical College (Dalhousie University).......................................	16	17	63	5,000	$6,200
TARIO					
University of Toronto, Faculty of Medicine[1]...	27	41	592	64,500	....
Queen's University, Medical Faculty[1]...	16	22	208	19,978	....
Western University, Medical Department[2]...	8	12	104	11,590	....
EBEC					
McGill University, Medical Faculty[1]...	19	80	328	43,750	77,000
Laval University, Medical Department[1] { Montreal	8	....	217 }		
Quebec	22	....	92 }	....	....
Total....................	3,533	4,828	23,927	$2,896,744	

u-year course.   [2] Four-year course.

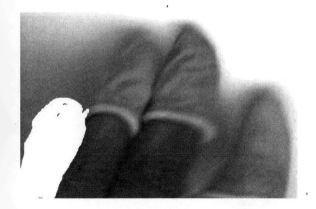

INDEX

—

CPSIA information can be obtained
at www.ICGtesting.com
Printed in the USA
BVHW041350100920
588458BV00004B/121